Essential Lists

f MRCP

Second Edition

Stuart McPherson BSc MBChB MRCP
Specialist Registrar in Gastroenterology/General Medicine
Northern Deanery

Duncan Fullerton MBChB DTM&H MRCP
Specialist Registrar in Respiratory/General Medicine
North Western Deanery

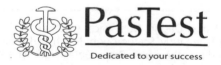

PasTest

Dedicated to your success

© 2006 PASTEST LTD
Egerton Court
Parkgate Estate
Knutsford
Cheshire
WA16 8DX

Telephone: 01565 752000

First published 2002
Second Edition 2006

ISBN: 1904627544

A catalogue record for this book is available from the British Library.

The information contained within this book was obtained by the authors from reliable sources. However, while every effort has been made to ensure its accuracy, no responsibility for loss, damage or injury occasioned to any person acting or refraining from action as a result of information contained herein can be accepted by the publishers or authors.

PasTest Revision Books and Intensive Courses

PasTest has been established in the field of postgraduate medical education since 1972, providing revision books and intensive study courses for doctors preparing for their professional examinations.

Books and courses are available for the following specialties:

MRCGP, MRCP Parts 1 and 2, MRCPCH Parts 1 and 2, MRCPsych, MRCS, MRCOG Parts 1 and 2, DRCOG, DCH, FRCA, PLAB Parts 1 and 2.

For further details contact:

PasTest, Freepost, Knutsford, Cheshire WA16 7BR
Tel: 01565 752000   Fax: 01565 650264
www.pastest.co.uk   enquiries@pastest.co.uk

Cover design by Parker Design, Northwich, Cheshire.
Text prepared by Type Study, Scarborough, North Yorkshire, UK.
Printed and bound by Athenauem Press, Gateshead, Tyne & Wear.

Contents

Tables

Introduction

This book is a compilation of clinical, diagnostic and prognostic features of the symptoms and diseases that cover the whole spectrum of general medicine. It is aimed at the MRCP candidate and provides comprehensive lists in subject areas that commonly appear in both part 1 and part 2 of the examination. It will be particularly useful for last-minute revision and will also be a useful reference for doctors on the ward when they come across a clinical problem for which there are a number of causes. Even though MRCP exams do change, lists will remain a vital resource in the candidates' preparation.

The lists are compiled systematically in a subject-based manner and are as 'user friendly' as possible with a comprehensive index to provide a quick reference.

In this second edition the lists have been expanded and updated in line with recent advances in clinical practice. In addition, there is a new chapter that comprises 100 best of five multiple-choice questions to give readers a taste of the exam and put the lists into clinical context.

Finally, I would like to thank Dr James Greenwood and Dr Tom Ledson for their contribution to the first edition, and Dr Kirstin Scott and Dr Rasha Omar for reviewing the manuscript.

Abbreviations

Ab	antibody
ABG	arterial blood gas
ABPA	allergic bronchopulmonary aspergillosis
ACC	American college of cardiology
ACE(I)	angiotensin converting enzyme (inhibitor)
ACTH	adrenocorticotrophic hormone
AD	autosomal dominant
ADH	anti-diuretic hormone
ADP	adenosine diphosphate
AF	atrial fibrillation
AFP	alpha-fetoprotein
Ag	antigen
AIDP	acute inflammatory demyelinating polyneuropathy
ALL	acute lymphoblastic leukaemia
ALP	alkaline phosphatase
ALT	alanine aminotransferase
AML	acute myeloid leukaemia
ANA	antinuclear antibody
ANCA	anti-neutrophil cytoplasmic antibody
ANP	atrial natriuretic peptide
APC	antigen presenting cell
APKD	adult polycystic kidney disease
APTT	activated partial thromboplastin time
AR	aortic regurgitation (Cardiology)
AR	autosomal recessive (elsewhere)
ARB	angiotensin receptor blocker
ARDS	acute respiratory distress syndrome
ARF	acute renal failure
AS	aortic stenosis (Cardiology)
AS	ankylosing spondylitis (Rheumatology)
ASA	amino-salicylic acid
ASD	atrial septal defect
ASO	antistreptolysin O
ASOT	antistreptolysin O titre
AST	aspartate aminotransferase
AT2	angiotensin 2
ATN	acute tubular necrosis
AVNRT	atrio-ventricular nodal reentry tachycardia

AVR	aortic valve replacement
AVRT	atrio-ventricular reentry tachycardia
AXR	abdominal X-ray
BAL	bronchoalveolar lavage
BCC	basal cell carcinoma
BCG	bacillus Calmette-Guérin
BE	base excess
BHL	bilateral hilar lymphadenopathy
BHS	British Hypertension Society
BNP	brain natriuretic peptide
BT	bleeding time
BTS	British Thoracic Society
CABG	coronary artery bypass graft
CAH	congenital adrenal hyperplasia
cAMP	cyclic adenosine monophosphate
Cca	corrected calcium
CCF	congestive cardiac failure
CCK	cholecystokinin
CD	cluster designation
CDC	Center for Disease Control
CEA	carcinoembryonic antigen
CF	cystic fibrosis
CFA	cryptogenic fibrosing alveolitis
CHB	complete heart block
CIDP	chronic inflammatory demyelinating polyneuropathy
CK, CK-MB	creatine kinase (MB isoenzyme)
CLL	chronic lymphoid leukaemia
CML	chronic myeloid leukaemia
CMV	cytomegalovirus
CNS	central nervous system
COPD	chronic obstructive pulmonary disease
COX	cyclo-oxygenase
CPAP	continuous positive airways pressure (ventilation)
CPR	cardiopulmonary resuscitation
CRC	colorectal cancer
CREST	calcinosis, Raynaud's, oesophageal dysfunction, scleroderma, telangiectasia
CRF	chronic renal failure
CRH	corticotrophin-releasing hormone
CRP	C reactive protein
CSF	cerebrospinal fluid
CT	computerised tomography
CTD	connective tissue disease
CVA	cerebro-vascular accident
CWP	coal workers' pneumoconiosis
CXR	chest X-ray

DAF	decay accelerating factor
DDAVP	arginine vasopressin (desmoprsssin)
DI	diabetes insipidus
DIC	disseminated intravascular coagulation
DIDMOAD	diabetes insipidus, diabetes mellitus, optic atrophy and deafness
DKA	diabetic ketoacidosis
DM	diabetes mellitus
DMARDs	disease modifying anti-rheumatoid drugs
DMD	Duchenne muscular dystrophy
DMSA	dimercaptosuccinic acid
DTPA	diethylenetriamine penta-acetic acid
DU	duodenal ulcer
EAA	extrinsic allergic alveolitis
EBV	Ebstein–Barr virus
ECT	electroconvulsive therapy
EDM	early-diastolic murmur
EDTA	ethylenediaminetetraacetic acid
EEG	electroencephalogram
ELISA	enzyme linked immunosorbent assay
EMD	electromechanical dissociation
EMG	electromyography
EPO	erythropoietin
ERCP	endoscopic retrograde cholangio-pancreatography
ESC	European society of cardiology
ESM	ejection systolic murmur
ESR	erythrocyte sedimentation rate
ESRF	end-stage renal failure
EUS	endoscopic ultrasound
FAP	familial adenomatous polyposis
FEV_1	Forced expiratory volume in one second
FFP	fresh frozen plasma
FH	family history
FNA	fine needle aspiration
F-O	faecal–oral
FSGN	focal segmental glomerulonephritis
FSGS	focal segmental glomerulosclerosis
FSH	follicle stimulating hormone
FVC	forced vital capacity
GABA	gamma aminobutyric acid
GAD	glutamic acid decarboxylase
GBM	glomerular basement membrane
GBS	Guillain–Barré syndrome
GCSF	granulocyte colony stimulating factor
GFR	glomerular filtration rate
GH	growth hormone

GHRH	growth hormone releasing hormone
GIP	gastric inhibitory peptide
GMCSF	granulocyte macrophage colony stimulating factor
GN	glomerulonephritis
GnRH	gonadotrophin releasing hormone
GORD	gastro-oesophageal reflux disease
G6PD	glucose-6-phosphate dehydrogenase
GP11b	receptor on platelets
GTN	glyceryl trinitrate
GU	gastric ulcer
GVHD	graft versus host disease
HACEK	Haemophilus species Actinobacillus actinomycetemcomitans, Cardiobacterium hominis, Eikenella corvodens and kingella species
HAV	hepatitis A virus
Hb	haemoglobin
HbA_{1c}	glycosylated haemoglobin
HBV	hepatitis B virus
HCC	hepatocellular carcinoma
HCG	human chorionic gonadotrophin
HCM	hypertrophic cardiomyopathy
HCV	hepatitis C virus
HDL	high density lipoprotein
HELLP	haemolysis, elevated liver enzymes and low platelets
HIAA	5-hydroxyindoleacetic acid
HHV	human herpes virus
HLA	human leucocyte antigen
HMG CoA	hydroymethylglutaryl coenzyme A
HONK	hyperosmolar non-ketotic state
HPV	human papilloma virus
HSMN	hereditary sensorimotor neuropathy
HSP	Henoch–Schönlein purpura
HSV	herpes simplex virus
HTLV	human T lymphocyte virus
HUS	haemolytic uraemic syndrome
IBD	inflammatory bowel disease
ICAM	intracellular adhesion molecule
ICP	intracranial pressure
IDA	iron deficiency anaemia
IDDM	insulin dependent diabetes mellitus
IFN	interferon
Ig	immunoglobulin
IGF	insulin-like growth factor
IHD	ischaemic heart disease
IL	interleukin
INR	international normalised ratio

ITP	immune thrombocytopenic purpura
ITU	intensive therapy unit
IUGR	intrauterine growth retardation
IVDU	intravenous drug user
IVU	intravenous urogram
JC	Jamestown Canyon (virus)
JVP	jugular venous pulse
KUB	kidneys ureters and bladder (X-ray)
LA	left atrium
LAD	left axis deviation
LBBB	left bundle branch block
LDH	lactate dehydrogenase
LDL	low density lipoprotein
LE	lupus erythematosus
LFT	liver function test
LH	luteinizing hormone
LICS	left intercostal space
LMN	lower motor neurone
LMWH	low molecular weight heparin
LOS	lower oesophageal sphincter
LRTI	lower respiratory tract infection
LSE	left sternal edge
LT	leukotriene
LTOT	long term oxygen therapy
LV	left ventricle
LVEDP	left ventricular end diastolic pressure
LVF	left ventricular failure
LVH	left ventricular hypertrophy
MAC	*Mycobacterium avium intracellulare*
MAHA	microangiopathic haemolytic anaemia
MALT	mucosa-associated lymphoid tissue
MAOI	monoamine oxidase inhibitor
MCGN	mesangiocapillary glomerular nephritis
MCP	metacarpophalangeal (joint)
MCT	medullary carcinoma of the thyroid
MCTD	mixed connective tissue disorder
MCV	mean corpuscular volume
MDM	mid-diastolic murmur
MDS	myelodysplastic syndrome
MEN	multiple endocrine neoplasia
MG	myasthenia gravis
MGUS	monoclonal gammopathy of undetermined significance
MHC	major histocompatibility complex
MI	myocardial infarction
MIBG	metaiodobenzylguanidiene
MMSE	mini mental-state examination

MND	motor neurone disease
MPO	myeloperoxidase
MPTP	1-methyl-4-phenyl 1,2,3,6-tetrahydropyridine
MR	mitral regurgitation
MRCP	magnetic resonance cholangio-pancreatography
MRI	magnetic resonance imaging
MRSA	methicillin-resistant *Staphylococcus aureus*
MS	mitral stenosis (Cardiology)
MS	multiple sclerosis (elsewhere)
MSH	melanocyte stimulating hormone
MTP	metatarsophalangeal (joint)
MUGA	multiple gated acquisition (scan)
MV	mitral valve
MVP	mitral valve prolapse
MVR	mitral valve replacement
NA	noradrenaline
NADPH	nicotinamide-adenine dinucleotide phosphate
NAFL	non-alcoholic fatty liver
NAPQI	N-acetylbenzoquinoneimine
NASH	non-alcoholic steatohepatitis
NBM	nil by mouth
NF	neurofibromatosis
NHL	non-Hodgkin's lymphoma
NIDDM	non-insulin dependent diabetes mellitus
NK	natural killer
NNRTI	non-nucleoside reverse transcriptases inhibitor
NRTI	nucleoside reverse transcriptase inhibitor
NSAIDs	non steroidal anti-inflammatory drugs
NSTEMI	non-ST elevation myocardial infarction
NSU	non-specific urethritis
N+V	nausea and vomiting
NYHA	New York Heart Association
OA	osteoarthritis
OCP	oral contraceptive pill
PA	pulmonary artery (Cardiology)
PA	pernicious anaemia (elsewhere)
PABA	para-aminobenzoic acid
PAN	polyarteritis nodosa
PAS	periodic acid Schiff
PBC	primary biliary cirrhosis
PCOS	polycystic ovarian syndrome
PCP	*Pneumocystis carinii* pneumonia
PCR	polymerase chain reaction
PDA	patent ductus arteriosus
PE	pulmonary embolism
PEA	pulseless electrical activity

PEEP	positive end expiratory pressure
PEFR	peak expiratory flow rate
PFO	patent foramen ovale
PG	prostaglandin
PHX	pulmonary histiocytosis X
PI	protease inhibitor
PID	pelvic inflammatory disease
PIP	proximal interphalangeal (joint)
PML	progressive multi-focal leukoencephalopathy
PMR	polymyalgia rheumatica
PND	paroxysmal nocturnal dyspnoea
PP	pancreatic polypeptide
PPAR	peroxisome proliferator activated receptor
PPI	proton pump inhibitor
PPM	permanent pacemaker
PR3	proteinase-3
PRV	polycythaemia rubra vera
PS	pulmonary stenosis
PSC	primary sclerosing cholangitis
PSM	pansystolic murmur
PSP	progressive supranuclear palsy
PT	prothrombin time
PTCA	percutaneous angioplasty
PTH	parathyroid hormone
PU	passed urine
PUO	pyrexia of unknown origin
PUVA	psoralens and ultraviolet A
PVD	peripheral vascular disease
RA	rheumatoid arthritis
RAAS	renin–angiotensin–aldosterone system
RAD	right axis deviation
RBBB	right bundle branch block
RBC	red blood cell
RF	rheumatoid factor
RHF	right heart failure
RICS	right intercostal space
RNP	ribonucleic protein
RSV	respiratory syncytial virus
RTA	renal tubular acidosis
RUQ	right upper quadrant
RV	right ventricle
RVEDP	right ventricular end diastolic pressure
RVH	right ventricular hypertrophy
RVSP	right ventricular systolic pressure
SAH	subarachnoid haemorrhage
SAP	serum amyloid protein

SBE	subacute bacterial endocarditis
SeHCAT 23	selinium 75 homocholinic acid taurine
SIADH	syndrome of inappropriate anti-diuretic hormone secretion
SLA	soluble liver antigen
SLE	systemic lupus erythematosus
SMA	smooth muscle antibody
SOB	shortness of breath
SSRI	selective serotonin reuptake inhibitor
SVT	supraventricular tachycardia
SVC	superior vena cava
TCA	tricyclic antidepressant
TCC	transitional cell carcinoma
TG	triglycerides
TIA	transient ischaemic attack
TIBC	total iron binding capacity
TIPS	transjugular intrahepatic portocaval shunt
TLC	total lung capacity
TNF	tumour necrosis factor
TOE	trans-oesophageal echocardiogram
tPA	tissue plasminogen activator
TPMT	thiopurine-methyl-transferase
TPN	total parenteral nutrition
TR	tricuspid regurgitation
TRH	thyrotrophin releasing hormone
TSH	thyroid stimulating hormone
TT	thrombin time
TTP	thrombotic thrombocytopenic purpura
TURBT	transurethral resection of bladder tumour
UC	ulcerative colitis
UFH	unfractionated heparin
UIP	usual interstitial pneumonitis
UMN	upper motor neurone
URTI	upper respiratory tract infection
USS	ultrasound scan
VC	vital capacity
VDRL	Venereal Disease Reference Laboratory (test for syphillis)
VF	ventricular fibrillation
VIP	vasoactive intestinal peptide
VLDL	very low density lipoprotein
VSD	ventricular septal defect
VT	ventricular tachycardia
vWF	von-Willebrand factor
VZV	varicella zoster virus
WCC	white cell count
WHO	World Health Organisation
WPW	Wolff–Parkinson–White

Normal Values

Haematology

Haemoglobin	
Males	13.5–17.5 g/dl
Females	11.5–15.5 g/dl
MCV	76–98 fl
PCV	33–55%
WCC	$4\text{–}11 \times 10^9/l$
Neutrophils	$2.5\text{–}7.58 \times 10^9/l$
Lymphocytes	$1.5\text{–}3.5 \times 10^9/l$
Platelets	$150\text{–}400 \times 10^9/l$
Reticulocytes	0.5–2%
ESR	0–10 mm in the first hour
PT	10.6–14.9 s
APTT	23.0–35.0 s
TT	10.5–15.5 s
Fib	125–300 mg/dl
Vitamin B_{12}	160–900 pmol/l
Folate	1.5–10.0 µg/l
Ferritin	
Males	20–250 µg/l
Females	10–120 µg/l

Biochemistry

Na^+	135–145 mmol/l
K^+	3.5–5.0 mmol/l
U	2.5–6.5 mmol/l
Cr	50–120 µmol/l
ALT	5–30 IU/l
AST	10–40 IU/l
Bilirubin	2–17 µmol/l
Alk P	30–130 IU/l
Alb.	35–55 g/l

| γGT | 5–30 IU/l |
| αFP | < 10 kU/l |

| CCa | 2.20–2.60 mmol/l |
| PO_4^{2-} | 0.70–1.40 mmol/l |

| CK | 23–175 IU/l |
| LDH | 100–190 IU/l |

Caeruloplasmin	1.0–2.7 mmol/l
Antitrypsin	1.1–2.2 g/l
Serum osmolality	285–295 mmol/kg

| CRP | 0–10 mg/l |

Diabetes

Glucose
     Random   3.5–5.5 mmol/l*
     Fasting   < 7 mol/l
HbA_{1c} < 7.0%

Endocrinology

TSH	0.17–302 mU/l
T_4	11–22 pmol/l
Cholesterol	< 5.2 mmol/l
Triglycerides	0–1.5 mmol/l
LDL	< 3.5 mmol/l
HDL	> 1.0 mmol/l
Total/HDL	< 5.0

Blood gases

pH	7.35–7.45
PCO_2	4.6–6.0 kPa
PO_2	10.5–13.5 kPa
HCO_3	24–30 mmol/l
BE	–2–2.0 mmol/l

CSF

Protein	0.2–0.4 g/l
Glucose	2.5–3.9 mmol/l (two-thirds plasma)
Cells	< 5/mm^3 (WCC)
Opening pressure	6–20 cmH$_2$O

* If > 5.5 then OGTT 2 hrs: 7–11.1 = IGT
                               > 11.1 = DM

AIDS/HIV Medicine

MODES OF TRANSMISSION

1 Sexual intercourse
   (a) Including oral sex
   (b) Uncircumcised men are at higher risk of becoming infected than circumcised
2 IV drug abuse with shared needles
3 Blood and blood products
4 Maternal–fetal transmisson – avoid breastfeeding, delivery by caesarean reduces risk

VIRUS BIOLOGY

1 Human retrovirus
2 Member of the lentivirus family
3 RNA virus, therefore contains enzyme reverse transcriptase
4 Two known types
   (a) HIV-1 – prevalent worldwide
   (b) HIV-2 – common in West Africa
5 HIV has tropism for the following CD4 cells
   (a) T-helper lymphocytes
   (c) B lymphocytes
   (d) Macrophages
   (e) CNS cells
6 Causes progressive immune dysfunction, characterised by CD4 cell depletion

SEROCONVERSION ILLNESS

1 Will occur in 90% within 3 months of infection
2 Features
  (a) Fever
  (b) Malaise
  (c) Diarrhoea
  (d) Meningoencephalitis
  (e) Rash
  (f) Sore throat
  (g) Lymphadenopathy
  (h) Arthralgia

CDC CLASSIFICATION OF HIV/AIDS

Usually progression from stage 1 to 4
1 Stage 1 – primary seroconversion illness
2 Stage 2 – asymptomatic
3 Stage 3 – persistent generalised lymphadenopathy
4 Stage 4a – AIDS-related complex (ie advanced HIV disease, but no features of 4b–d)
5 Stage 4b–d AIDS – patient has opportunistic infection or tumours; AIDS indicator illnesses

DIAGNOSIS

1 Anti-HIV antibodies in the blood
2 May not be present for 3-month 'window period'
3 HIV RNA or p24Ag may be present in blood earlier

INDICATOR DISEASES FOR AIDS

1 Bacterial chest infections (recurrent in 12-month period)
2 Candidiasis (trachea, bronchi, lungs)
3 Invasive carcinoma of the cervix
4 Coccoidomycosis, disseminated or extrapulmonary

5 *Cryptococcus* – extrapulmonary
6 Cryptosporidiosis with diarrhoea for more than 1 month
7 CMV disease (not in liver, spleen or nodes)
8 Encephalopathy (dementia due to HIV)
9 HSV ulcers for more than 1 month or bronchitis, pneumonitis, or oesophagitis
10 Histoplasmosis – disseminated or extrapulmonary
11 Isosporidiosis with diarrhoea for > 1 month
12 Kaposi's sarcoma
13 Lymphoid interstitial pneumonitis and/or pulmonary lymphoid hyperplasia in a child < 13 years
14 Mycobacteriosis, pulmonary TB
15 PCP
16 Progressive multifocal leukoencephalopathy
17 *Salmonella* (non-typhoid) septicaemia, recurrent
18 Toxoplasmosis of brain after 1 month of age
19 Wasting syndrome – > 10% loss with no other cause identified

DRUG THERAPIES IN HIV

Aims of treatment

1 Complete suppression of viral replication
2 Obtaining a synergistic effect from combination therapy
3 Reducing the risk of viral resistance emerging
4 Strict adherence to therapy is essential

Nucleoside reverse transcriptase inhibitors (NRTIs)

1 Zidovudine (AZT)
2 Lamivudine (ZTC)
3 Didanosine (DDI)
4 Stavudine
   (a) Inhibit HIV replication
   (b) Multiple side effects, including
      (i)   Pancreatitis
      (ii)   Lactic acidosis
      (iii) Lipodystrophy

Non-nucleoside reverse transcriptase inhibitors (NNRTIs)

1 Nevirapine
2 Efavirenz
   (a) Inhibit viral replication
   (b) Many drug interactions

Protease inhibitors (PIs)

1 Indinavir
2 Ritonivir
3 Saquinavir
4 Nelfinavir
   (a) Inhibit virus assembly
   (b) Multiple side effects, including
       (i) Pancreatitis
       (ii) Lipodystrophy

Fusion inhibitors

1 Eufuvitide
   (a) Inhibits HIV from fusing to the host cell
   (b) Hypersensitivity reactions common

When to initiate treatment?

1 Dependent on
   (a) CD4 count (< 350)
   (b) Plasma viral load (high viral load)
   (c) Clinical symptoms
2 Three drugs, including two NRTIs and *either* one PI *or* one NNRTI
3 Balance of preventing irreversible damage to the immune system
   against drug toxicity and viral drug resistance
4 This is an area of rapid change – consult an expert

REPIRATORY DISEASE IN HIV

HIV patients are at increased risk of all respiratory infections
1 *Pneumocystis carinii* pneumonia
   (a) Most common respiratory presentation
   (b) Dry cough, SOB, fever, malaise, chest pains

(c) Symptoms usually gradually worsen over 2–3 weeks
(d) Chest examination often normal
(e) Abnormal CXR in 90% (classically perihilar interstitial shadowing)
(f) Hypoxic (desaturation on exercise)
(g) Treatment is with high dose co-trimoxazole or pentamidine
(h) Severe cases should be given steroids
(i) Patients should be on prophylaxis if CD4 < 200
(j) Diagnosis
    (i) Induced sputum or BAL
    (ii) Immunofluorescence or PCR on sputum

2 Pulmonary TB (See also page 420)
  (a) Very common in sub-Saharan Africa at presentation
  (b) Can occur with any CD4 count
  (c) TB in early HIV usually presents with typical symptoms and signs
  (d) In more advanced HIV TB presents atypically, often with extrapulmonary disease
  (e) Multidrug resistance is more common
  (f) Treat with three- or four-drug regimen

3 *Mycobacterium avium intracellulare* (MAC)
  (a) Disseminated infection
  (b) Presents with fever, night sweats, weight loss and diarrhoea
  (c) CD4 usually > 50
  (d) Treat with azithromycin, ethambutol and rifabutin

4 Viral
  (a) CMV
  (b) HSV
  (c) EBV
  (d) Adenovirus
  (e) Influenza

5 Bacterial
  (a) *Streptococcus pneumoniae*
  (b) *Staphylococcus aureus*
  (c) Gram-negatives

6 Fungal
  (a) *Candida*
  (b) Histoplasmosis
  (c) *Cryptococcus*
  (d) *Nocardia*

7 Tumour
   (a) Kaposi's sarcoma
   (b) NHL

GASTROINTESTINAL DISEASE IN HIV

Oropharyngeal/oesophageal disease

99% of patients will develop an oral/oesophageal problem
1 Candidiasis
2 Oral hairy leukoplakia (EBV)
3 Aphthous ulcer
4 Periodontal disease
5 HSV
6 Lymphoma
7 Kaposi's sarcoma
8 CMV

Diarrhoeal disease

1 Bacteria
   (a) *Salmonella*
   (b) *Campylobacter*
   (c) *Shigella*
2 Protozoa
   (a) *Giardia lamblia*
3 Virus
   (a) CMV
4 Opportunistic organisms
   (a) Bacteria – atypical mycobacterium
   (b) Protozoal – *Isospora belli*, cryptosporidia

Gastrointestinal neoplasms

1 Kaposi's sarcoma
2 Intra-abdominal lymphoma

Biliary and pancreatic disease

1 Cholangiopathy – due to drugs or *Cryptosporidium*, CMV or *Microsporidium*
2 Pancreatitis

Anorectal conditions

Symptoms include
1 Anal discharge
2 Tenesmus
3 Pruritus ani
4 Rectal bleeding
5 Diarrhoea

Causative agents

1 HSV
2 Wart virus
3 Syphilis
4 Gonorrhoea
5 Chlamydia

NEUROLOGICAL DISEASE IN HIV

1 Can be first presentation of disease in up to 10%
2 Lymphocytic meningitis can be initial presentation
3 Can present with focal signs or generalised features. Often asymptomatic

Direct neurotropic effects

1 HIV encephalopathy
   (a) Direct neuronal loss
   (b) Leads to a dementia
   (c) Less common with antiretroviral therapy
2 Vacuolar myelopathy
3 Neuropathy
   (a) Mononeuritis multiplex
   (b) Peripheral neuropathy
   (c) AIDP
   (d) Drug induced

Neurological infections

Focal disease

1 *Mycobacteruim tuberculosis* (meningitis, abscess)
2 *Toxoplasma gondii*
   (a) Usually reactivation of toxoplasma cysts
   (b) CD4 < 200
   (c) Presents with headaches, seizures and fever
   (d) CT shows ring enhancing lesions (differential diagnosis is CNS lymphoma)
   (e) Treat with sulfadiazine and pyrimethamine

Generalised disease

1 *Cryptococcus neoformans* (meningitis)
   (a) Headache, vomiting, fever, with few neurological signs
   (b) CSF cryptococcal antigen or cryptococci seen on India ink stain
   (c) Treat with fluconazole or amphotericin
2 CMV (retinitis, peripheral neuropathy)
3 Progressive multifocal leukoencephalopathy (PML)
   (a) Demyelinating disorder that presents with personality change, ataxia and neurological signs
   (b) Caused by JC virus
   (c) Diagnosed by CSF PCR

Neurosyphilis – can cause aggressive and atypical neurosyphilis, leading to

1 Myelopathy
2 Retinitis
3 Meningitis
4 Meningovascular

Ophthalmic complications

1 Molluscum contagiosum of the lids
2 Episcleritis and keratitis
3 Uveitis
4 Kaposi's sarcoma – lids or conjunctiva
5 Retinal changes – haemorrhages/cotton wool spots/oedema/ vascular sheathing
6 Choroidal granulomas

7 CMV retinitis
8 Toxoplasmosis
9 *Candida* endophthalmitis
10 Neuro-ophthalmic manifestations

CUTANEOUS MANIFESTATIONS OF HIV

Affect up to 75% of all patients with HIV. During seroconversion may develop a marked seborrhoeic dermatitis. As disease progresses tumours and atypical infections are seen.

* Common

1 Infections
   (a) Tinea and onychomycosis*
   (b) Candidiasis*
   (c) Hairy leukoplakia*
   (d) Syphilis
   (e) Bacterial folliculitis
   (f) Condylomata acuminata (viral warts)
   (g) Molluscum contagiosum*
   (h) Cutaneous mycobacterial infection
   (i) HSV*
   (j) HPV*
   (k) VZV
2 Inflammatory dermatoses
   (a) Seroconversion toxic erythema
   (b) Psoriasis
   (c) Seborrhoeic dermatitis*
   (d) Severe drug reactions
   (e) Eosinophilic pustular folliculitis
   (f) Generalised granuloma annulare
   (g) Papular eruption of HIV
3 Neoplasia
   (a) Kaposi's sarcoma
      (i) Multiple purple nodular lesions on mucosal surfaces
      (ii) Can be in organs such as lungs or GI tract
      (iii) Caused by HHV8 virus
   (b) Cutaneous lymphoma
   (c) Melanoma and non-melanoma skin cancer

Cardiology

EXAMINATION

Pulses

1 Normal
2 Slow rising pulse
   (a) Aortic stenosis
3 Collapsing pulse (large amplitude; rapid rise and fall)
   (a) Aortic regurgitation
   (b) Patent ductus arteriosus
   (c) AV shunt
4 Pulsus paradoxus (exaggeration of the normal fall in pulse volume with respiration)
   (a) Cardiac tamponade
   (b) Constrictive pericarditis
   (c) Severe asthma
5 Pulsus bisferiens (double peak)
   (a) Combined aortic stenosis and regurgitation
   (b) Hypertrophic cardiomyopathy
6 Pulsus alternans (alternating large and small volume beats)
   (a) Left ventricular failure

JVP waves

1 a wave = atrial systole
2 c wave = closure of the tricuspid valve
3 v wave = atrial filling

Abnormalities of the JVP

1 Raised JVP
   (a) Right heart failure
   (b) Fluid overload
   (c) Pericardial tamponade ($\uparrow$ on inspiration – Kussmaul's sign)

11

(d) Constrictive pericarditis
(e) Superior vena cava obstruction (loss of waves in JVP)
2 Large a waves
   (a) Pulmonary hypertension
   (b) Pulmonary stenosis
   (c) Tricuspid stenosis
3 Absent a waves
   (a) AF
4 Large v waves
   (a) Tricuspid regurgitation
5 Cannon waves
   (a) Complete heart block
   (b) Extrasystoles
   (c) Atrial flutter

Causes of absent radial pulse

1 Arterial embolus
2 Congenital
3 Aortic dissection with subclavian involvement
4 Takayasau's arteritis
5 Iatrogenic (surgery, catheterisation)

Apex beat (most inferior and lateral cardiac pulsation)

1 Normal
   (a) Midclavicular line, fifth intercostal space
2 Displaced laterally
   (a) Dilatation of left ventricle (MR, AR, aneurysm) – thrusting apex
   (b) Mediastinal shift (pneumothorax etc.)
3 Hypertrophic (heaving, not markedly displaced)
   (a) Hypertension
   (b) AS
   (c) Coarctation of aorta
4 Tapping (palpable first heart sound)
   (a) MS

HEART SOUNDS

First heart sound

Closure of mitral and tricuspid valves
1 Loud
  (a) Mobile MS
  (b) Short PR interval, eg WPW
  (c) Left to right shunts
  (d) Hyperdynamic states
2 Soft
  (a) Immobile MS
  (b) MR
  (c) Prolonged PR interval

Second heart sound

Closure of aortic then pulmonary valves
1 Loud
  (a) Systemic hypertension (loud A2)
  (b) Pulmonary hypertension (loud P2)
  (c) ASD (loud P2)
2 Soft
  (a) Severe AS
  (b) Aortic root dilatation
3 Splitting
  (a) Inspiration (physiological)
  (b) RBBB
  (c) ASD (fixed splitting; does not vary with respiration)
  (d) LBBB (reverse splitting)
  (e) Prolonged LV systole (HCM, IHD, AS, PDA) – reverse splitting

Third heart sound

Best heard at left sternal edge or apex
1 Physiological
  (a) Due to passive ventricular filling on opening of the AV valves
    (i) Young people (< 40 yrs)
    (ii) Hyperdynamic states (eg thyrotoxicosis, pregnancy)
2 Pathological
  (a) Due to rapid ventricular filling

    (i)   LVF
    (ii) Cardiomyopathy
    (iii) MR
    (iv) VSD
    (v) Constrictive pericarditis

Fourth heart sound

Always pathological
Due to the increased atrial contraction that has to fill a stiff left ventricle
Does not occur in atrial fibrillation
1 LVH
2 Following MI
3 Amyloid heart disease
4 HCM

MURMURS

Systolic murmurs

1 Midsystolic murmurs
   (a) Innocent flow murmur
      (i)   Soft, short murmur at LSE
   (b) Aortic stenosis or sclerosis
      (i)   Aortic area (second RICS), radiating to neck
   (c) Pulmonary stenosis
      (i)   Second LICS, ↑ on inspiration, present in Fallot's tetralogy
   (d) Coarctation of the aorta
      (i)   Coarse murmur maximal over apex of left lung (anterior and posterior)
   (e) Hypertrophic cardiomyopathy
      (i)   Increased by Valsalva manoeuvre
2 Pansystolic murmurs
   (a) Mitral regurgitation
      (i)   Apex, radiating to axilla
   (b) Tricuspid regurgitation (LSE)
   (c) Ventricular septal defect
      (i)   Harsh at LSE

3 Late-systolic murmurs
   (a) Mitral valve prolapse (apex) associated with midsystolic click
   (b) Hypertrophic cardiomyopathy

Diastolic murmurs

1 Early-diastolic murmurs
   (a) Aortic regurgitation
       (i) Maximal third LICS in expiration
   (b) Pulmonary regurgitation
   (c) Graham Steell murmur
       (i) Pulmonary regurgitation secondary to pulmonary hypertension and mitral stenosis
2 Mid-diastolic murmurs
   (a) Mitral stenosis
       (i) Rumbling, mid–late diastole at apex
   (b) Austin Flint murmur (LSE)
       (i) Aortic regurgitant jet impairing diastolic flow through mitral valve
   (c) Tricuspid stenosis
   (d) Atrial tumours

Continuous murmurs

Maximal in systole but persistent into diastole
1 Patent ductus arteriosus
   (a) Machinery-like quality at second LICS, midclavicular line
2 Venous hum
   (b) Positional
3 AV shunts/fistulae (in lungs or coronary arteries)
4 Mixed aortic valve disease

ECG ABNORMALITIES

Left bundle branch block

1 Almost always pathological
2 Wide QRS
3 M pattern in V5
4 Causes

(a) Ischaemic heart disease
(b) LVH (hypertension)
(c) Aortic valve disease
(d) Cardiomyopathy
(e) Myocarditis

Right bundle branch block

1 RSR in V1
2 Causes
   (a) Normal variant
   (b) RVH/RV strain (eg pulmonary embolus)
   (c) IHD
   (d) Congenital heart disease (eg ASD)
   (e) Myocarditis

Causes of RVH

1 Cor pulmonale
2 Pulmonary embolism
3 Mitral valve disease
4 Pulmonary hypertension
5 Pulmonary stenosis
6 Fallot's tetralogy

Causes of a low-voltage ECG

1 Obesity
2 COPD
3 Pericardial effusion
4 Hypothyroidism
5 Dextrocardia
6 Cardiomyopathy

Causes of dominant R wave in V1

1 RBBB
2 PE
3 RVH
4 Posterior MI
5 Myocarditis
6 WPW (type A)
7 HCM

Short PR interval

1 Wolff–Parkinson–White syndrome
2 Lown–Ganong–Levine syndrome
3 P wave followed by ventricular ectopic
4 AV junctional rhythm (p wave usually negative)
5 Concealed accessory pathway

Wolff–Parkinson–White syndrome

1 Accessory pathway between atria and ventricles
2 Delta wave on ECG
3 Short PR interval
4 Type A positive R wave in V1
5 Associated with Ebstein's anomaly (apical displacement of the tricuspid valve leaflets leading to atrialisation of the RV)
6 Can cause AF, AVRT, VF
7 Prophylaxis of arrhythmias
   (a) Flecainide
   (b) Sotalol
8 Radiofrequency ablation of pathway will 'cure' patient
9 Digoxin or verapamil are contraindicated for pre-excited AF as they paradoxically accelerate ventricular rate

Prolonged QT interval

1 Associated with syncope and sudden death (from VT, especially polymorphic VT)
2 Causes
   (a) Familial (90%)
       (i)   Romano Ward syndrome (AD) – deafness
       (ii) Jervell–Lang–Neilsen syndrome (AR)
   (b) IHD
   (c) Myocarditis
   (d) Metabolic
       (i)   Hypocalcaemia
       (ii) Hypokalaemia
       (iii) Hypomagnesaemia
       (iv) Hypothermia
       (v)   Hypothyroidism

(e) Drugs
   (i) Erythromycin
   (ii) Amiodarone
   (iii) Sotalol
   (iv) Quinine/quinidine
   (v) Terfenadine
   (vi) TCAs
   (vii) Phenothiazines

ST depression

1 Myocardial ischaemia (including posterior MI)
2 Digoxin therapy (downsloping)
3 Hypertension
4 LVH with strain

ST elevation

1 Myocardial infarction
2 Pericarditis
3 Hyperkalaemia
4 Coronary artery spasm (variant/Prinzmetal angina)
5 Left ventricular aneurysm

T-wave inversion

1 Ischaemia
2 Digoxin therapy
3 LVH
4 Cardiomyopathy
5 PE

ECG variants in athletes

1 Sinus arrhythmia
2 First-degree AV block
3 Wenckebach phenomenon
4 Junctional rhythm
5 Slight ST elevation (high take-off)
6 Tall R waves
7 Prominent U waves

Pulseless electrical activity (PEA; previously electromechanical dissociation or EMD)

Cardiac arrest situation; cardiac rhythm compatible with an output but without any palpable pulse (4 Hs and 4 Ts)
1 Hypo- or hyperkalaemia (or other electrolyte disturbances)
2 Hypothermia
3 Hypovolaemia
4 Hypoxia
5 Cardiac tamponade
6 Tension pneumothorax
7 Pulmonary thromboembolus
8 Toxin/drug overdose
9 Aortic dissection
10 Myocardial infarction

ARRHYTHMIAS

Tachyarrhythmias

Sinus tachycardia

1 Anxiety
2 Fever
3 MI
4 Hypovolaemia/shock
5 Anaemia
6 Pregnancy
7 PE
8 Thyrotoxicosis
9 Phaeochromocytoma
10 Drugs, eg β-agonists, atropine, sympathomimetics

Atrial fibrillation

1 Causes
  (a) Cardiac
    (i) MI and IHD
    (ii) Valvular heart disease (especially mitral stenosis)
    (iii) Congenital heart disease
    (iv) Cardiomyopathy (especially dilated)

(v) WPW
(vi) Myocarditis
(vii) Pericarditis (constrictive or infiltrating carcinoma)
(b) Respiratory
(i) PE
(ii) Pneumonia
(c) Others
(i) Hypertension
(ii) Hyperthyroidism
(iii) Alcohol (and other drugs)
(iv) Idiopathic ('lone' AF)
2 Treatment
(a) Rate control is appropriate for most patients
(b) Patients with structurally normal hearts may be candidates for rhythm control
(c) Cardioversion (rhythm control)
(i) < 48 hrs after onset or after 6 weeks' anticoagulation
(ii) DC cardioversion
(iii) Flecainide
(iv) Sotalol
(v) Amiodarone
(d) Rate control
(i) Digoxin – does not control rate effectively alone in active patients
(ii) Verapamil
(iii) Beta blockers
(e) Prophylaxis for paroxysmal AF
(i) Sotalol
(ii) Flecainide
(iii) Amiodarone
(f) Anticoagulation (↓ risk of stroke threefold)

Broad complex tachycardia

Rate >140 bpm
QRS > 0.12 s
1 Ventricular tachycardia
2 SVT with bundle branch block
3 *Torsades de pointes* tachycardia

Junctional tachycardia (SVT)

1 AV nodal re-entry tachycardia (usually structurally normal hearts)
2 AV re-entry tachycardia (eg Wolff–Parkinson–White syndrome)

Ventricular tachycardia

1 Causes
   (a) Myocardial infarction or chronic IHD
   (b) Myocarditis
   (c) Cardiomyopathy
   (d) Hyper- or hypokalaemia
   (e) Left ventricular aneurysm
   (f) Prolonged QT interval
2 Treatment (medical emergency)
   (a) DC cardioversion/defibrillation
   (b) Overdrive pacing
   (c) Amiodarone
   (d) Lignocaine

Torsades de pointes tachycardia

1 Polymorphic VT with varying axis
2 May degenerate into VF
3 Patients at high risk of sudden death
4 Triggered in those with prolonged QT
5 Treatment
   (a) Correct underlying cause of long QT
   (b) Defibrillation
   (c) Intravenous magnesium
   (d) Beta blockers (only for those with congenital long QT)
   (e) Implantable cardioverter defibrillators

Features of tachyarrhythmias

[See Table 1, overleaf]

Features suggesting VT in broad complex tachycardia

1 VT should be suspected in all broad complex tachycardias
2 History of IHD
3 AV dissociation

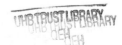

Table 1

Type	Rate	P wave	P:R	QRS complex
Sinus	> 100	Normal	1:1	Normal
Atrial	120–200	Abnormal shape	1:1	Normal and regular Can have broad complex if aberrant conduction
Atrial flutter	150	Flutter waves (300/min) Sawtooth pattern	1:1–4:1	Regular
AF	> 120	Absent	–	Irregular and normal Can have broad complex if aberrant conduction
AVNRT	140–220	None seen	–	Normal, regular
AVRT	140–220	Inverted p waves after QRS	–	Normal, regular
VT	120–250	Dissociated	–	Broad complex, regular

4 Very regular
5 Very wide QRS (> 140 ms)
6 Extreme axis deviation
7 Concordance in all leads (all up or down)
8 Fusion or capture beats

Bradyarrhythmias

Sinus bradycardia

Rate 40–50 bpm
1 Athleticism
2 Myocardial infarction (especially inferior)
3 Hypothyroidism
4 Hypothermia
5 Sinus node disease
6 Raised ICP
7 Increased vagal tone, eg vomiting
8 Drugs, eg. beta blockers, digoxin, verapamil

Heart block

1 First-degree heart block
  (a) Prolonged PR interval (> 0.20 s)
  (b) Usually benign
2 Second-degree heart block
  (a) Wenckebach (Mobitz 1)
     (i) Successively increasing PR interval until a p wave is not conducted
     (ii) Usually benign
  (b) Mobitz 2
     (i) Unpredictable failure to conduct p waves
     (ii) Often progresses to complete block
     (iii) Usually requires a PPM
3 Complete heart block (third-degree AV block)
  (a) 25–50 bpm (ventricular escape rhythm)
  (b) Narrow (more stable) or wide QRS complexes
  (c) Associated with large volume pulse and systolic flow murmurs
  (d) Requires PPM

(e) Causes
  (i) Congenital
  (ii) Acquired
    (1) Idiopathic fibrosis
    (2) MI/IHD
    (3) Acute inflammation (eg myocarditis)
    (4) Chronic inflammation (eg sarcoid)
    (5) Drugs (eg rate-limiting agents)

Indications for permanent pacemakers

1 Complete heart block
2 Mobitz 2 heart block
3 Sinus node dysfunction
4 Symptomatic sinus bradycardia
5 Bifascicular and trifascicular block accompanied by syncope
6 Hypertrophic cardiomyopathy
7 Post AV nodal ablation for arrhythmias

ISCHAEMIC HEART DISEASE

Criteria for diagnosis of an acute or recent MI (ESC/ACC 2000)

1 Typical rise and gradual fall, or more rapid rise and fall of biochemical markers of myocardial necrosis with one of the following:
  (a) Ischaemic symptoms
  (b) Development of pathological Q waves on the ECG
  (c) ECG changes indicative of MI (ST ↑ or ↓)
  (d) Coronary artery intervention (angioplasty)

Risk factors

1 Hypertension
2 Diabetes
3 Smoking
4 Hypercholesterolaemia (↑ LDL, ↑ TG, ↓ HDL)
5 Alcohol excess (moderate intake is protective)
6 Sedentary lifestyle

7 Obesity
8 Drugs (contraceptive pill)
9 Family history of premature heart disease
10 Chronic renal failure
11 Male gender
12 Increasing age
13 Ethnicity (Afro-Caribbean low, Indo-Asians high)
14 LVH
15 ↑ CRP
16 ↑ Homocysteine
17 ↑ Lipoprotein (a)
18 ↑ Plasminogen activator inhibitor
19 ↑ Fibrinogen
20 Poor oral hygiene
21 Metabolic syndrome
   (a) Hyperinsulinaemia
   (b) Abdominal obesity
   (c) Hypertension
   (d) ↑ Triglycerides
   (e) ↓ HDL
22 Type A personality

Causes of MI

1 Atherosclerotic plaque rupture (90%)
2 Coronary emboli
3 Coronary spasm
4 Cocaine
5 Severe hypotension, eg GI bleed

Management of MI

Acute

1 Oxygen
2 Aspirin
3 GTN
4 Diamorphine
5 Thrombolysis (PTCA if contraindication to thrombolysis)
   (a) Indications – chest pain with:
      (i) ST ↑ > 2 mm in two or more chest leads

      (ii) ST ↑ > 1 mm in two or more limb leads
      (iii) Posterior infarction
      (iv) New-onset LBBB
  (b) Contraindications
      (i) Bleeding/trauma
         (1) Internal bleeding
         (2) Heavy vaginal bleeding
         (3) Prolonged or traumatic CPR
         (4) Recent trauma or surgery
      (ii) GI
         (1) GI bleeding
         (2) Acute pancreatitis
         (3) Severe liver disease
         (4) Oesophageal varices
      (iii) Neurological
         (1) Head injury
         (2) Cerebral neoplasm
         (3) Recent haemorrhagic stroke
      (iv) Others
         (1) Active lung disease with cavitation
         (2) Severe hypertension (> 200/120)
         (3) Suspected aortic dissection
         (4) Previous allergic reaction
         (5) Pregnancy or < 18 weeks postnatal
  6 Beta blocker (not if heart failure)
  7 Insulin sliding scale if glucose > 11
  8 Diuretics and nitrates if heart failure
  9 ACEI (not if hypotensive)
10 LMWH (prophylaxis of thromboembolism)
11 If ongoing pain GP11b/111a inhibitors and angioplasty/stenting

Long term

1 Risk factor modification
  (a) Stop smoking
  (b) Weight loss
  (c) Exercise (cardiac rehabilitation)
  (d) Good diet and reduce alcohol
  (e) Good diabetic control
  (f) Treat hypertension

2 Post-infarct prophylaxis
   (a) Aspirin (↓ vascular events by 29% post MI)
   (b) Clopidogrel (NSTEMI with aspirin, or if intolerant of aspirin)
   (c) Beta blockers (reduces mortality by 25% post MI)
   (d) Statins (benefit post MI if cholesterol elevated or normal)
   (e) ACEI (full-thickness MI or LVF, ↓ 2 yr mortality by 25–30%)

Complications of MI

1 Arrhythmias (AF, VT/VF, CHB or other AV block)
2 Heart failure/cardiogenic shock
3 Hypertension
4 Thromboembolic disease (DVT/PE, mural thrombus)
5 Pericarditis or Dressler's syndrome
6 LV aneurysm
7 VSD
8 Mitral regurgitation
9 Papillary muscle rupture
10 Cardiac rupture

Cardiac enzymes

1 CK (including CK-MB)
   (a) Rises 3–12 hrs
   (b) Falls to baseline 48–72 hrs
2 Troponins (I, T)
   (a) Rises 3–12 hrs
   (b) Peak 24–48 hrs
   (c) Falls to baseline 5–14 days

Conditions that may be associated with a troponin rise

1 Coronary artery occlusion
2 Pericarditis
3 Myocarditis
4 Direct myocardial damage
   (a) Chest wall trauma
   (b) Surgical manipulation
   (c) Radiofrequency ablation
   (d) Drug toxicity (adriamycin)
5 Tachyarrhythmia

6 CCF
7 Severe PE
8 Severe exacerbation of COPD
9 Sepsis
10 Renal failure
11 GI haemorrhage
12 Ischaemic stroke or SAH

HEART FAILURE

Causes of heart failure

1 Cardiac
  (a) IHD
  (b) Arrhythmia
  (c) Valvular or congenital heart disease
  (d) Myocarditis or pericarditis
  (e) Cardiomyopathy (See page 43)
2 Drugs
  (a) Negative inotropes, eg beta blockers
  (b) Fluid-retaining properties, eg steroids, NSAIDs
3 Increased metabolic demand
  (a) Pregnancy
  (b) Hyperthyroidism
  (c) Anaemia
  (d) Obesity
4 Others
  (a) PE
  (b) Intercurrent illness
  (c) Inappropriate reduction of therapy

Pathophysiological abnormalities in heart failure

1 Remodelling of the LV
  (a) Hypertrophy
  (b) Loss of myocytes
  (c) Fibrosis
  (d) Beta adrenergic desensitisation
  (e) Leads to enlarged ventricular cavity (except diastolic dysfunction) with more spherical shape – less effective pump

2 ↑ peripheral vascular tone
  (a) ↑ sympathetic activity
  (b) Activation of renin–angiotensin–aldosterone system (RAAS)
  (c) ↑ vasopressin
  (d) ↑ endothelin-1
3 Fluid and sodium retention
  (a) RAAS
  (b) Vasopressin (water retention)
4 Secretion of BNP/ANP (opposing AT2 and vasopressin)
  (a) Vasodilatation
  (b) Natriuresis
5 Mitral regurgitation (due to dilatation of valve ring)
6 ↓ Cardiac output
7 ↑ Pulmonary venous pressure
8 ↑ TNF
9 ↑ Interleukins

NYHA classification of heart failure

Grade 1 No breathlessness, no effect on daily life
Grade 2 Breathless on severe exertion
Grade 3 Breathless on mild exertion
Grade 4 Breathless at rest, unable to do minimal exertion

Clinical features of heart failure

1 Symptoms
  (a) LVF
    (i)   SOB
    (ii) Cough (dry or pink frothy sputum)
    (iii) Cardiac wheeze
    (iv) Orthopnoea and PND
  (b) RVF
    (i)   Peripheral oedema
    (ii) Ascites
2 Signs
  (a) Left and right
    (i)   Hypotension
    (ii) Tachycardia
    (iii) Gallop rhythm
    (iv) Displaced apex (dilated heart)

(b) LVF
  (i) Bilateral crepitations
  (ii) Pleural effusions
(c) RVF
  (i) Peripheral oedema
  (ii) Raised JVP (may have giant V waves if TR)
  (iii) Hepatomegaly
  (iv) Ascites

Diagnosis

1 Chest X-ray
  (a) Upper lobe diversion
  (b) Cardiomegaly
  (c) Alveolar oedema
  (d) Kerley B lines
  (e) Pleural effusions
2 Echo
3 MUGA (very reliable measure of LV ejection fraction)
4 BNP (↑ in heart failure)
  (a) Women > men
  (b) ↑ with age
  (c) Correlates with NYHA grade
  (d) Reliable at differentiating between heart failure and pulmonary disease

Treatments for chronic heart failure

1 Low-salt diet
2 Fluid restriction
3 Loop/thiazide diuretics
4 ACE inhibitors (↓ mortality by 25%)
5 ARBs (↓ mortality, use in those intolerant of ACEI)
6 Beta blockers, eg bisoprolol, carvedilol (↓ mortality by 30%)
7 Spironolactone (↓ mortality)
8 Digoxin (↓ admissions but no ↓ mortality)
9 Vasodilators (nitrates, hydralazine)
10 Anticoagulation (AF)
11 Cardiac transplantation
12 Treat BP, lipids and diabetes

HYPERTENSION

Causes of systemic hypertension

1 Essential hypertension (90%)
2 Renal disease (4%)
   (a) Renal artery stenosis
   (b) Polycystic kidney disease
   (c) Renal parenchymal disease (eg glomerulonephritis etc.)
   (d) Chronic renal failure
3 Endocrine disease
   (a) Diabetes mellitus
   (b) Metabolic syndrome
   (c) Phaeochromocytoma
   (d) Conn's syndrome (primary hyperaldosteronism)
   (e) Cushing's syndrome
   (f) Acromegaly
   (g) Congenital adrenal hyperplasia
4 Drugs
   (a) Steroids (including OCP)
   (b) NSAIDs
   (c) Sympathomimetics
5 Pregnancy (pre-eclampsia)
6 Neurogenic (post head injury)
7 Coarctation of the aorta

Complications of systemic hypertension

1 Cardiac
   (a) Left ventricular hypertrophy/failure
   (b) IHD
2 Neurological
   (a) CVA (haemorrhage or infarct)/TIA
   (b) Retinopathy
   (c) Hypertensive encephalopathy (rare)
   (d) Increased frequency of subarachnoid haemorrhage
3 Others
   (a) Peripheral vascular disease
   (b) Aortic aneurysm
   (c) Renal impairment and proteinuria

CARDIOLOGY

Treatment guidelines (BHS guidelines 2004)

1 Treatment for all with sustained systolic >160 or diastolic >100
2 Treat those with systolic 140–159 or diastolic 90–99 with evidence of
  (a) Target organ damage
  (b) Cardiovascular disease
  (c) Diabetes
  (d) Or 10-year cardiovascular risk > 20%
3 Target < 140 systolic < 90 diastolic or 130/75 for diabetics and those
  with renal impairment

VALVULAR HEART DISEASE

Mitral stenosis

1 Causes
  (a) Rheumatic fever
  (b) Congenital
  (c) Infective endocarditis
  (d) Carcinoid
  (e) SLE
  (f) RA
2 Symptoms
  (a) Breathlessness
  (b) Haemoptysis
  (c) Palpitations
  (d) Recurrent chest infections
  (e) Acute pulmonary oedema
3 Clinical signs
  (a) Malar flush
  (b) AF
  (c) Tapping undisplaced apex
  (d) Opening snap (mobile valve)
  (e) Mid-diastolic murmur
  (f) Evidence of pulmonary hypertension (TR, RV heave, RHF)
4 CXR
  (a) Enlarged LA
  (b) Calcification of the MV
  (c) Upper lobe diversion and enlarges pulmonary arteries
  (d) Pulmonary oedema

5 Treatments
   (a) Treat AF (rate control and anticoagulation)
   (b) Endocarditis prophylaxis
   (c) Treat heart failure
   (d) Valvuloplasty
   (e) Open/closed valvulotomy
   (f) MVR
6 Indications for valvuloplasty/valvotomy/MVR
   (a) Heart failure unresponsive to medical management
   (b) Moderate to severe MS (NYHA 3 or 4) with
       (i) PA pressure > 50 mmHg or
       (ii) Valve area < 1.5 cm^2

Mitral regurgitation

1 Causes
   (a) 'Functional', due to LV dilatation
   (b) Rheumatic fever
   (c) Mitral valve prolapse
   (d) IHD (post MI, papillary muscle ischaemia)
   (e) Endocarditis/myocarditis/cardiomyopathy
   (f) Connective tissue disorders
   (g) Collagen disorders (Marfan's syndrome etc.)
2 Signs
   (a) AF
   (b) Displaced hyperdynamic apex (thrusting)
   (c) PSM radiates to axilla
   (d) S3
   (e) Signs of pulmonary hypertension
3 Treatments
   (a) Endocarditis prophylaxis
   (b) MVR
       (i) Indications
           (1) Acute MR with CCF/cardiogenic shock
           (2) Endocarditis
           (3) NYHA 3 or 4
           (4) Ejection fraction < 55%
           (5) Dilated LV

Aortic stenosis

1 Causes
   (a) Congenital
   (b) Congenitally bicuspid valve
   (c) Degenerative calcification
   (d) Rheumatic fever
2 Symptoms
   (a) Breathlessness
   (b) Chest pain (despite normal coronaries)
   (c) Syncope
   (d) PND
3 Signs
   (a) Slow rising pulse (narrow pulse pressure)
   (b) Heaving undisplaced apex
   (c) Single S2
   (d) ESM radiates to carotids
4 Treatment
   (a) AVR
      (i) Indications
         (1) Symptomatic AS
         (2) Moderate or severe when CABG planned
         (3) Asymptomatic
            (a) LV systolic dysfunction
            (b) Abnormal response to exercise
            (c) Marked LVH
            (d) VT
            (e) Valve area < 0.6 cm^2

Aortic regurgitation

1 Causes
   (a) Congenital (bicuspid or otherwise abnormal valve)
   (b) Rheumatic fever
   (c) Infective endocarditis
   (d) Marfan's syndrome
   (e) Syphilis
   (f) Aortic dissection
   (g) Trauma
   (h) SLE
   (i) Hypertension

    (j) Ankylosing spondylitis
2 Symptoms
    (a) Breathlessness
    (b) PND
    (c) Pulmonary oedema
3 Signs
    (a) Collapsing pulse
    (b) Hyperdynamic undisplaced apex (thrusting)
    (c) EDM at LSE
    (d) ESM ($\uparrow$ systolic flow over valve)
    (e) Austin Flint murmur (MDM)
    (f) Corrigan's sign (prominent carotid pulsation)
    (g) De Musset's sign (head nodding)
    (h) Quincke's sign (pulsating nail beds)
    (i) Pistol-shot femorals
4 Treatment
    (a) Endocarditis prophylaxis
    (b) ACEI
    (c) AVR
        (i) Severe symptomatic AR (NYHA 3 or 4)
        (ii) Endocarditis
        (iii) Aortic root disease
        (iv) LV dilatation
        (v) LV impairment

Tricuspid regurgitation

1 Causes
    (a) RV dilatation (pulmonary hypertension, cor pulmonale)
    (b) Infective endocarditis (intravenous drug users)
    (c) Rheumatic fever
    (d) Right ventricular infarction
    (e) Carcinoid syndrome
    (f) Ebstein's anomoly
2 Signs
    (a) Giant V waves in JVP
    (b) RV heave
    (c) Pulsatile hepatomegaly
    (d) PSM at LSE (increases on inspiration)
    (e) Ascites

CARDIOLOGY

3 Treatment
  (a) Diuretics
  (b) Surgery (rare)

INFECTIVE ENDOCARDITIS

Predisposing factors

1 Rheumatic heart disease
2 Degenerative heart disease
3 Mitral valve prolapse
4 Intravenous drug use
5 Prosthetic valves
6 Congenital heart disease (bicuspid aortic valve is most common)
7 Hypertrophic cardiomyopathy

Microbiology

1 *Viridans* streptococci
2 *Streptococcus bovis* (can indicate underlying bowel cancer)
3 *Staphylococcus aureus* (IVDU)
4 Enterococci
5 Gram-negative organisms
6 HACEK group
7 *Coxiella burnetti*
8 Fungal
9 Culture negative (5%)

Clinical features

1 Fever (90%)
2 Anorexia and weight loss
3 New or changing murmur
4 Splinter haemorrhages
5 Clubbing
6 Splenomegaly
7 Petechiae
8 Osler's nodes
9 Janeway lesions
10 Roth spots

11 Systemic emboli (infarction or abscess in end organ)
12 Haematuria
13 Glomerulonephritis

CONGENITAL HEART DISEASE

Causes of cyanotic congenital heart disease

Right to left shunt

1 Tetralogy of Fallot
2 Complete transposition of the great vessels
3 Severe Ebstein's anomaly

Without a shunt

1 Tricuspid atresia
2 Pulmonary atresia
3 Severe pulmonary stenosis
4 Hypoplastic left heart

Reversal of a previous left to right shunt

1 Eisenmenger's syndrome

Causes of acyanotic congenital heart disease

Left to right shunt

1 Ventricular septal defect
2 Atrial septal defect
3 Patent ductus arteriosus

Without a shunt

1 Congenital aortic stenosis
2 Coarctation of the aorta

Associations of congenital heart disease

Table 2

Cause	Defect
Chromosomal defects	
Down's	ASD, VSD, Fallot's
Turner's	coarctation, bicuspid AV, PS
Drugs	
Alcohol	VSD
Lithium	Ebstein's anomaly, tricuspid atresia
Connective tissue disorders	
Marfan's	Aortic root dilatation, AR, MR
Kartagener's	Dextrocardia
Holt–Oram	ASD
Rubella	PDA, ASD, PS

Atrial septal defect (10%)

1 Ostium secundum (70%)
  (a) Defect of fossa ovale
  (b) Associated with MVP
  (c) Partial RBBB and RAD, prolonged PR interval on ECG
  (d) May develop AF
  (e) Low risk of endocarditis
2 Ostium primum (15%):
  (a) Usually detected earlier in childhood
  (b) Associated with
    (i) MR
    (ii) Down's
    (iii) Klinefelter's
    (iv) Noonan's
  (c) ECG shows RBBB, LAD, first-degree heart block
3 Sinus venosus (15%)
  (a) Defect in upper part of septum
  (b) Associated with anomalous pulmonary venous drainage
4 Clinical features
  (a) Wide fixed splitting of the second heart sound
  (b) Loud P2
  (c) Pulmonary systolic flow murmur
  (d) Tricuspid diastolic murmur if shunt is large

5 CXR
  (a) Cardiomegaly
  (b) Small aorta
  (c) Enlarged pulmonary artery
  (d) Pulmonary plethora
6 Complications
  (a) AF
  (b) Pulmonary hypertension
  (c) Eisenmenger's syndrome
  (d) TR
  (e) Cardiac failure
  (f) Infective endocarditis

Ventricular septal defect (25–30%)

1 Leads to left to right shunt
2 Maladie de Roger is a small defect with a loud murmur
3 Clinical features
  (a) Parasternal thrill
  (b) Single S2 (absent A2)
  (c) Pansystolic murmur throughout precordium but loudest at LSE
4 Cardiac associations
  (a) PDA
  (b) AR
  (c) PS
  (d) ASD
  (e) Tetralogy of Fallot
  (f) Coarctation of the aorta
5 Complications
  (a) AF
  (b) Ventricular arrhythmias
  (c) SBE
  (d) Pulmonary hypertension and Eisenmenger's syndrome
  (e) Cardiac failure

Patent ductus arteriosus (15%)

1 Persistent ductus arteriosus between aorta and pulmonary artery
2 More common in women
3 More common in those born at altitude
4 May be closed with indomethacin

5 Can be kept open with prostaglandins (some cyanotic heart diseases)
6 Collapsing pulse and continuous machinery murmur
7 Complications
   (a) 'Endocarditis' of the ductus
   (b) Eisenmenger's syndrome

Tetralogy of Fallot (10%)

1 Usually presents after 6 months of age
2 Four components
   (a) Pulmonary stenosis
   (b) Right ventricular hypertrophy
   (c) VSD (right to left shunt due to the pulmonary stenosis)
   (d) Overriding of the VSD by the aorta
3 Clinical features
   (a) Cyanotic attacks (due to pulmonary infundibular spasm) with syncope (associated with squatting to reduce them)
   (b) Clubbing
   (c) Parasternal heave from RVH
   (d) ESM in pulmonary area
   (e) Single S2
   (f) RVH on ECG
4 CXR
   (a) Boot-shaped heart
   (b) Small pulmonary artery
   (c) Large aorta
   (d) Pulmonary oligaemia
5 Complications
   (a) Cerebral abscess
   (b) Endocarditis
   (c) Paradoxical embolus
   (d) Polycythaemia
   (e) Coagulopathy
   (f) Ventricular arrhythmias

Coarctation of the aorta (5%)

1 Congenital stenosis of aorta (most distal to the left subclavian artery)
2 More common in males

3 Associations
  (a) Berry aneurysms
  (b) Turner's syndrome
  (c) Bicuspid aortic valve
  (d) PDA
  (e) VSD
  (f) Mitral valve disease
4 Clinical features
  (a) Often asymptomatic
  (b) Hypertension in upper part of body
  (c) Radiofemoral delay
  (d) Absent or weak femoral pulses
  (e) Systolic murmur (infraclavicular or posterior)
  (f) Collateral artery formation (around scapulae or below ribs posteriorly)
  (g) May lead to 'endocarditis'
5 CXR
  (a) Double aortic knuckle
  (b) Rib notching
6 Complications
  (a) Headaches
  (b) CVA
  (c) LVH
  (d) Premature IHD
  (e) Aortic dissection

Eisenmenger's syndrome

1 Reversal of left to right shunt owing to development of pulmonary hypertension
2 Occurs in
  (a) VSD
  (b) ASD
  (c) PDA
3 Clinical features
  (a) Central cyanosis
  (b) Clubbing
  (c) Decreasing intensity of murmurs (reduced flow)
  (d) Pulmonary hypertension
  (e) Single S2 (loud P2)
  (f) Graham Steell murmur (PR)

4 ECG shows RVH
5 CXR
   (a) Enlarged pulmonary vessels
   (b) Peripheral pruning
6 Complications
   (a) Cor pulmonale
   (b) Syncope
   (c) Angina
   (d) Massive haemoptysis
   (e) Cerebral abscess/embolus
   (f) Endocarditis

Causes of syncope

1 Cardiac
   (a) Sinus node disease
   (b) Atrioventricular disease
   (c) Tachycardia
   (d) Bradycardia
   (e) Myocardial ischaemia
   (f) Aortic stenosis
   (g) Hypertrophic cardiomyopathy
   (h) Pulmonary embolus
   (i) Aortic dissection
2 Neurogenic
   (a) Epilepsy
   (b) Vertebrobasilar ischaemia
3 Others
   (a) Hypoglycaemia
   (b) Vasovagal syncope
   (c) Postural hypotension
      (i) Elderly
      (ii) Vasodilator drugs
      (iii) Parkinson's disease
      (iv) Autonomic neuropathy
   (d) Micturition and cough syncope

CARDIOMYOPATHIES

Dilated cardiomyopathy

1 Global ventricular dilatation and dysfunction
2 Causes
  (a) Hereditary (30%) (X-linked, AD)
  (b) Alcohol
  (c) IHD and hypertension
  (d) Following myocarditis
  (e) Viruses, eg Coxsackie, influenza, HIV
  (f) Connective tissue disorders
  (g) Pregnancy
  (h) Thiamine deficiency
  (i) Friedreich's ataxia

Restrictive cardiomyopathy

1 Stiff, rigid ventricles lead to impaired diastolic filling
2 Causes
  (a) Idiopathic
  (b) Amyloidosis
  (c) Endomyocardial fibrosis
  (d) Eosinophilic endomyocarditis (Loeffler's syndrome)
  (e) Sarcoidosis
  (f) Haemochromatosis
  (g) Glycogen storage diseases
  (h) Malignancy (metastases, carcinoid, radiotherapy)
  (i) Drugs (doxorubicin)

Diagnosis and treatment

1 Diagnosis
  (a) Echo (chamber size, wall thickness, function)
  (b) Angiography to exclude ischaemia
  (c) Endomyocardial biopsy
2 Treatment
  (a) Family screening
  (b) Treat heart failure
  (c) Amiodarone for arrhythmia
  (d) Anticoagulation (many develop intracardiac thrombi)
  (e) Heart transplantation

Hypertrophic cardiomyopathy

1 AD (more than 50 mutations described)
2 Asymmetric hypertrophy of left or right ventricle, or both
3 Often septum involved, leading to outflow obstruction
4 Clinical features
   (a) Breathlessness
   (b) Chest pains
   (c) Collapse/syncope (due to ↓ cardiac output or arrhythmias)
   (d) Palpitations (AF, SVT, VT)
   (e) Orthopnoea and PND
   (f) Sudden death
5 Signs
   (a) Jerky pulse with double impulse
   (b) Forceful apex
   (c) Ejection systolic murmur (increased by squatting)
   (d) Prominent a wave in JVP
   (e) Fourth heart sound (not AF)
6 ECG changes
   (a) ST–T-wave changes
   (b) LVH
   (c) Axis deviation (L or R)
   (d) Bundle branch block
   (e) Arrhythmias
7 Echo findings
   (a) Elevated flow across LV outflow tract
   (b) Diastolic dysfunction
   (c) Systolic anterior wall motion of the anterior mitral valve
   (d) Asymmetrical septal wall hypertrophy
   (e) MR
8 Treatment
   (a) Beta blockers
   (b) Verapamil
   (c) Amiodarone (↓ risk of VT)
   (d) Anticoagulation (AF)
   (e) Pacemakers
   (f) Catheter septal ablation (reduce septal thickening)
   (g) Implantable cardioverter defibrillator

PERICARDIAL DISEASES

Acute pericarditis

1 Post MI (Dressler's syndrome)
   (a) Occurs 2 weeks to 2 months post MI or cardiac surgery
   (b) Fever, pleurisy and pericarditis
   (c) Antibodies to heart muscle
   (d) Treat with NSAIDs
2 Infective
   (a) Viral (most common): Coxsackie B, Echo, rubella
   (b) Bacterial (eg staphylococcal)
   (c) TB
3 Hypothyroidism
4 Severe uraemia
5 Neoplasia (primary and secondary)
6 Radiotherapy
7 Trauma/postcardiotomy
8 Autoimmune (SLE, RA, rheumatic fever, systemic sclerosis, PAN)

Causes of constrictive pericarditis

1 Post-infective
2 Recurrent pericarditis
3 Connective tissue disease
4 Haemopericardium
5 TB
6 Radiotherapy
7 Uraemic pericarditis

Clinical features of constrictive pericarditis and restrictive cardiomyopathy

Table 3

Clinical features	Constrictive pericarditis	Restrictive cardiomyopathy
History	Previous pericarditis or condition causing pericarditis	History of systemic disease
Heart sounds	Pericardial knock Pericardial rub No murmurs	Third heart sound MR, TR
CXR	Pericardial calcification	Normal or large heart
Echo	Normal-sized ventricles and atria, pericardial thickening	Non-dilated normally contracting non-hypertrophied ventricle with dilated atria
Catheterisation		
RVEDP/LVEDP	< 5 mmHg difference	> 5 mmHg difference
RVSP	< 50 mmHg	> 50 mmHg

Drugs and the heart

[See Table 4, opposite]

Table 4

Drug	Mode of action	Indications	Side effects
Aspirin	Cyclo-oxygenase inhibitor ↓ Platelet aggregation	Primary/secondary prevention of MI/CVA/PVD	Bleeding peptic ulcer Rash
Clopidogrel	ADP receptor antagonist ↓ Platelet aggregation	Primary/secondary prevention of MI if intolerant of aspirin. Secondary prevention of NSTEMI with aspirin Coronary stent insertion	Bleeding Rash Neutropenia
Streptokinase tPA	Activates plasmin to degrade fibrin	Thrombolysis of MI	Bleeding Anaphylaxis (streptokinase) Hypotension (streptokinase)
GP11b/111a blockers Abciximab Tirofiban eptifibatide	Glycoprotein 11b/111a blocker ↓ Platelet aggregation Inhibits fibrinogen binding to platelets	PTCA Unstable angina NSTEM when early angiography planned	Bleeding Thrombocytopenia
Beta-blockers Atenolol Metoprolol Bisoprolol Carvedilol	↓ Sympathetic activity Negatively inotropic Negatively chronotropic Class 2 antiarrhythmic	Secondary prevention of MI Antianginal Antihypertensive Antiarrhythmic (AF, SVT, VT) Heart failure	Fatigue Bradycardia Bronchospasm Heart failure Sleep disturbance Cold extremities
Sotalol	Beta blocker Also has class 3 antiarrhythmic activity Lengthens cardiac action potential	AF termination AF prophylaxis WPW prophylaxis VT prophylaxis	Bradycardia QT prolongation Negative inotrope Bronchospasm

continued

CARDIOLOGY

Table 4 (cont.)

Drug	Mode of action	Indications	Side effects
Calcium antagonists	Block calcium channels on smooth muscle in the heart and arteries		
Cardioselective			
Verapamil	Vasodilate	Antianginal	Ankle swelling
Smooth muscle selective	Verapamil and diltiazem	Antihypertensive	Negative inotrope
Nifedipine	slows conduction through AV	Antiarrythmic (AF, SVT) –	Hypotension
Amlodipine	and SA nodes – class 4	verapamil and diltiazem	Headache
Intermediate	antiarrhythmic activity		Constipation
Diltiezem			
Amiodarone	Prolongs cardiac action potential	AF treatment + prophylaxis	Thyroid $\downarrow\uparrow$
	Class 1–4 antiarrhythmic activity	VT treatment + prophylaxis	Photosensitivity
	Very long $T_{1/2}$ 50 days	WPW	Alveolitis
		HCM	Hepatitis
			Skin pigmentation
			Peripheral neuropathy
			Corneal microdeposits
			Long QT
Digoxin	Cardiac glycoside	Rate control in AF (will not	Any arrhythmia
	Na/K ATPase inhibitor	cardiovert)	Nausea and vomiting
	Slows AV conduction	Heart failure	Gynaecomastia
	positive inotrope		Diarrhoea
			Confusion
			Yellow vision

Drug	Mode of action	Indications	Side effects
Lignocaine	Membrane stabiliser Class 1b antiarrythmic Blocks Na channels Shortens cardiac action potential	Antiarrhythmic (VT)	Fits ↓ LV function
Adenosine	Transient AV block	SVT termination	Chest pain Bronchospasm Prolonged asystole if administered with dipyridamole
Flecainide	Membrane stabiliser Class 1c antiarrythmic Inhibits Na channels No effect on cardiac action potential	AF termination/prophylaxis WPW prophylaxis Don't use in IHD	Proarrhythmic Negative inotrope
Atropine	Anticholinergic	Bradycardia Asystole	Dry mouth
Nitrates	Release NO to relax smooth muscle Venodilators	Antianginal Heart failure	Headache Hypotension
Nicorandil	K channel activator Arterial and venous dilator	Angina	Headache Flushing
Thiazides Bendrofluazide Metolazone Indapamide	↓ Na reabsorption in the distal convoluted tubule Inhibits Na/Cl transporter	Diuretic Antihypertensive	↓ Na ↓ K ↓ Mg ↑ urate ↑ Ca Postural hypotension Hypochloraemic alkalosis Hyperglycaemia Impotence

continued

CARDIOLOGY

Table 4 (cont.)

Drug	Mode of action	Indications	Side effects
Loop diuretics Frusemide Bumetanide	↓ Na reabsorption in Loop of Henle Inhibits Na/K/2Cl transporter in the thick ascending loop	Diuretic Heart failure	Renal failure ↓ K ↓ Ca ↓ Mg Deafness Postural hypotension Hypochloraemic alkalosis
ACE inhibitors Ramipril Captopril Lisinopril	Inhibit angiotensin-converting enzyme	Heart failure (all grades) Primary/secondary prevention of MI/CVA Hypertension Diabetic nephropathy Asymptomatic LV dysfunction	Renal failure Hypotension Cough (↑ bradykinin) Angio-oedema ↑ K Nephrotic syndrome Rash
ARBs Losartan Valsartan	Inhibit angiotensin-2 receptors	Hypertension Heart failure (when intolerant of ACEI) Diabetic nephropathy	Renal failure Hypotension Angio-oedema ↑ K Rash
Spironolactone	Aldosterone antagonist	Diuretic Heart failure Ascites	↑ K Gynaecomastia Impotence

Clinical Pharmacology

DRUG METABOLISM AND PHARMACOKINETICS

Important liver enzyme inducers

Of cytochrome P450, > 200 inducers known
PC BRASS
1 **P**henytoin
2 **C**arbamazepine
3 **B**arbiturates
4 **R**ifampicin
5 **A**lcohol (chronic)
6 **S**ulphonylureas
7 **S**moking

Important drugs whose metabolism is affected by enzyme inducers

Those metabolised by cytochrome P450, leads to **increased** metabolism of the drug
1 Warfarin ($\downarrow$ INR)
2 OCP (pregnancy)
3 Corticosteroids ($\downarrow$ effect)
4 Ciclosporin ($\downarrow$ immunosuppression)
5 Theophyllines ($\downarrow$ effect)
6 All of the enzyme inducers themselves ($\downarrow$ effect)

Important liver enzyme inhibitors

Leads to **reduced** metabolism of the drug and toxicity
OAAK DEVVICCES

1 **O**meprazole
2 **A**miodarone
3 **A**llopurinol
4 **K**etoconazole (and fluconazole)
5 **D**isulfiram
6 **E**rythromycin
7 **V**alproate
8 **V**erapamil
9 **I**soniazid
10 **C**iprofloxacin
11 **C**imetidine
12 **E**thanol (acute)
13 **S**ulphonamides

Important drugs affected by liver enzyme inhibitors

1 Warfarin ($\uparrow$ INR)
2 Phenytoin (toxicity)
3 Carbamazepine (toxicity)
4 Theophylline (toxicity)
5 Ciclosporin (toxicity)

Some other clinically important drug interactions

[See Table 5, opposite]

Drugs exhibiting zero-order kinetics (saturation kinetics)

1 Alcohol
2 Phenytoin
3 Fluoxetine

Drugs exhibiting partial agonist activity

1 Oxprenolol
2 Buprenorphine
3 Methysergide
4 Tamoxifen
5 Pentazocine

Table 5

Drug	Drug	Effect
Azathioprine	Allopurinol	Xanthine oxidase inhibition leads to azathioprine toxicity
	Cyclophosphamide	Reduced clearance of cyclophosphamide leading to ↑ toxicity
Alcohol	Metronidazole	Flushing, hypotension
	Chlorpropamide	
MAOIs	Tyramine	Acute hypertensive crisis
	Alpha agonists	CNS excitation
	Amphetamines	
	Pethidine	
ACE inhibitors	Potassium-sparing diuretics	Hyperkalaemia
	NSAIDs	Reduced effect of ACEI
Digoxin	Thiazides	Digoxin toxicity by ↓ protein binding/renal excretion
	Loop diuretics	
	Amiodarone	
	Nifedipine	
	Verapamil	
	Antacids	↓ Absorption
	Cholestyramine	
Beta blockers	Verapamil	Hypotension and asystole
Lithium	Thiazides	Lithium toxicity (↓ excretion)
Adenosine	Dipyridamole	Prolonged half-life of adenosine leading to asystole
Statins	Fibrates	Increased incidence of myopathy and rhabdomyolysis
	Ciclosporin	
Aminoglycosides	Loop diuretics	Increased nephrotoxicity and ototoxicity

Some examples of prodrugs (need to be metabolised before having an effect)

1 Enalapril
2 Azathioprine
3 L-Dopa
4 Aciclovir
5 Spironolactone
6 Zidovudine (AZT)
7 Cyclophosphamide

Examples of drugs that cause their effect by inhibiting enzymes

Table 6

Drug	Enzyme
ACE inhibitors	ACE
Aciclovir	DNA polymerase
Allopurinol	Xanthine oxidase
Zidovudine (AZT)	Reverse transcriptase
Disulfiram	Aldehyde dehydrogenase
MAOIs	MAO
Methotrexate/trimethoprim	Dihydrofolate reductase
Neostigmine	Cholinesterases
Aspirin/NSAIDs	Cyclooxygenase (COX)
Penicillins	Transpeptidase
Vigabatrin	GABA transaminase

Drugs for which therapeutic monitoring is useful

Good correlation between blood concentration and therapeutic effect
1 Digoxin
2 Lithium
3 Aminoglycosides
4 Vancomycin
5 Phenytoin
6 Carbamazepine
7 Theophylline
8 Ciclosporin
9 Phenobarbitone

Drugs in the elderly

1 Gastric pH ↑, gastric emptying ↓, ↓ blood flow – affects absorption of drugs
2 Absorption from im injections slower owing to ↓ muscle mass and ↓ blood flow to muscles
3 Reduced hepatic extraction and metabolism
4 Half-life of some drugs prolonged (eg benzodiazepines)
5 Greater volume of fat leads to increased volume of distribution for lipid-soluble drugs

6 GFR reduced in the elderly, leading to accumulation of renally excreted drugs (lithium, digoxin etc.)
7 Changes in homoeostatic responses make the elderly more susceptible to side effect of some drugs
8 Polypharmacy leads to more interactions

DRUGS AND THE KIDNEY

Drugs causing direct nephrotoxicity

Generally avoid these drugs in renal impairment unless there is a specific indication, eg ACEIs
1 Glomerular damage
   (a) Penicillamine
   (b) Gold
   (c) Captopril
2 Change renal vascular dynamics
   (a) ACEIs
   (b) NSAIDs
   (c) Ciclosporin
3 Tubular damage
   (a) Amphotericin
   (b) Aminoglycosides
   (c) Cisplatin
   (d) Demeclocycline
   (e) Lithium
   (f) Thiazides
4 Interstitial damage
   (a) NSAIDs
   (b) Sulphonamides
   (c) 5-ASA drugs
   (d) Vancomycin

Drugs excreted unchanged by the kidney

1 Atenolol
2 Antibiotics
   (a) Penicillins
   (b) Cephalosporins
   (c) Aminoglycosides
   (d) Tetracycline

3 Frusemide
4 Thiazides
5 Digoxin
6 Lithium
7 Chlorpropamide
8 Metformin
9 H$_2$ blockers
10 Aspirin (in overdose)

Drugs to use with caution in renal failure (or ↓ dose)

1 Aciclovir
2 ACEIs
3 Aminoglycosides
4 Allopurinol
5 Cephalosporins
6 Digoxin
7 H$_2$ blockers
8 Penicillins
9 Sulphonylureas
10 Vigabatrin

Drugs to avoid in renal failure

1 Chlorpropamide
2 Retinoids
3 Metformin
4 Nitrofurantoin
5 Methotrexate
6 Tetracyclines
7 Amphotericin
8 NSAIDs
9 Lithium
10 Gold
11 Penicillamine
12 Vancomycin

DRUGS AND THE LIVER

Drugs undergoing major hepatic metabolism

1 Beta blockers
  (a) Propranolol
  (b) Labetolol
  (c) Metoprolol
2 Beta agonists
  (a) Salbutamol
  (b) Terbutaline
3 Rifampicin
4 Erythromycin
5 Spironolactone
6 Cardiac drugs
  (a) GTN
  (b) Verapamil
  (c) Nifedipine
  (d) Lignocaine
  (e) Digitoxin (cf. digoxin)
  (f) Prazosin
7 CNS drugs
  (a) Chlormethiazole
  (b) TCAs
  (c) Phenothiazines
  (d) Benzodiazepines
  (e) Barbiturates
  (f) L-Dopa
8 Analgesics
  (a) Paracetamol
  (b) Pethidine
  (c) Aspirin

Drugs causing jaundice (See page 163)

GENETIC POLYMORPHISMS DETERMINING DRUG TOXICITY

Essential features of acetylator status

1 Toxic effects of some drugs depend on speed of acetylation and metabolism
2 Slow acetylators (50%) and fast acetylators – genetic
3 Diseases associated with slow acetylator status
   (a) Gilbert's syndrome
   (b) Sjögren's syndrome
   (c) Arylamine-induced bladder cancer

Table 7

	Slow	Fast (increased toxic metabolites)
Isoniazid	Neuropathy (glove & stocking) Drug-induced SLE ↑ Phenytoin toxicity ↑ Carbamazepine toxicity ↑ Rifampicin	Failure of TB therapy Hepatitis
Sulphasalazine	↑ Toxicity: headaches, leukopenia ↑ Haemolysis in G6PD-deficient patients	
Hydralazine	Drug-induced SLE	↓ BP control
Procainamide	Drug-induced SLE	
Dapsone	↑ Haemolysis in G6PD-deficient patients	↓ Benefit in dermatitis herpetiformis

Essential features of G6PD deficiency

1 X-linked dominant
2 Present in 5–10% of black males
3 Predisposes to haemolytic anaemia
4 Heterozygotes have increased resistance to malaria
5 Drugs causing haemolysis in these patients:
   (a) Primaquine
   (b) Sulphonamides
   (c) Sulphasalazine
   (d) Dapsone

(e) Quinolones (ciprofloxacin etc)
(f) Nitrofurantoin
(g) Nalidixic acid

Other drugs causing haemolytic anaemia (immune mediated)

1 Penicillins
2 Methyldopa
3 Quinine
4 Quinidine
5 Sulphonylureas

Important drugs that precipitate acute attacks of porphyria

1 All enzyme inducers (See page 51)
2 ACEIs
3 Erythromycin
4 Sulphonamides
5 Frusemide
6 OCPs
7 Calcium channel blockers

Some drugs that are safe in porphyria

1 Aspirin
2 Beta blockers
3 Penicillin
4 Morphine + codeine
5 Paracetamol
6 Metformin

Other genetic polymorphisms

Table 8

Polymorphism	Toxicity
Pseudocholinesterase deficiency (AR)	Suxamethonium toxicity, Prolonged apnoea post anaesthesia
Malignant hyperthermia (AD)	Hypercatabolic response to halothane, suxamethonium, TCAs, MAOIs
Steroid-induced glaucoma (AR)	5% population
Sulphonylurea flushing (AD)	30% population
Warfarin resistance (AD)	Rare
Cytochrome P-450 polymorphisms	Leads to altered metabolism
Omeprazole	2%
Nortriptyline	10%
Metoprolol	10%

DRUGS IN PREGNANCY AND BREASTFEEDING

Physiological changes affecting drug metabolism in pregnancy

1 ↑ GFR
2 ↑ Metabolism by P-450 enzymes (induction)
3 ↑ Volume of distribution
4 ↓ Protein binding
5 ↓ Gastric emptying

Drugs causing teratogenesis (first trimester)

[See Table 9, opposite]

Drugs affecting the fetus during intrauterine life and the neonatal period

[See Table 10, overleaf]

Drugs contraindicated in breastfeeding

1 Amiodarone (thyroid anomalies)
2 Aspirin (Reye's syndrome, hypoprothrombinaemia, impaired platelet function)

Table 9

Agent	Effect
Thalidomide	Phocomelia, heart defects
Anticonvulsants	
Carbamazepine	Neural tube defects
Phenytoin	Cleft palate, microcephaly, retardation
Valproate	Neural tube defects
Cytotoxics (including folic acid antagonists)	Hydrocephalus, neural tube defects, cleft palate
Alcohol	Fetal alcohol syndrome
Warfarin	Retarded growth, limb defects, saddle nose
Stilboestrol	Adenocarcinoma of vagina (20 yrs later)
Oestrogens	Testicular atrophy in males
Anabolic steroids	Masculinisation of female
ACE inhibitors	Oligohydramnios, renal failure
Retinoids	Hydrocephalus, neural tube defects
Lithium	Heart defects

3 Indomethacin (seizures)
4 ACEIs
5 Cytotoxics
6 Benzodiazepines (sedation, respiratory depression)
7 Ergotamine (ergotism)
8 Lithium (involuntary movements)
9 Phenytoin
10 Retinoids
11 Sex hormones (feminisation of males, masculinisation of females)
12 Tetracyclines (tooth discoloration)
13 Gold (renal impairment, haematological reactions)
14 Vitamin A (toxicity)
15 Vitamin D (hypercalcaemia)

Some drugs that are relatively safe in pregnancy

1 Heparin
2 Insulin
3 Thyroxine
4 Antibiotics
  (a) Penicillins
  (b) Cephalosporins
  (c) Erythromycin

(d) Ethambutol
(e) Isoniazid
5 Inhaled salbutamol
6 Methyldopa
7 Hydralazine
8 Paracetamol
9 Metoclopramide
10 Cyclizine

Table 10

Drug	Effect
Antibiotics	
Tetracyclines	Tooth discoloration
Aminoglycosides	Eighth-nerve damage
Sulphonamides	Jaundice, kernicterus, neonatal haemolysis and methaemoglobinaemia
Chloramphenicol	Cardiovascular collapse of the newborn 'Grey baby syndrome'
Antithyroid drugs	
Iodides	Neonatal hypothyroidism, goitre
Carbimazole	
Anticoagulants	
Warfarin	Fetal and neonatal haemorrhage
Hypoglycaemics	
Sulphonylureas	Fetal and neonatal hypoglycaemia
Cardiovascular	
Beta agonists	Fetal tachycardia, delayed labour
Beta antagonists	Fetal and neonatal bradycardia, neonatal hypoglycaemia, IUGR
CNS drugs	
Alcohol	CNS depression, withdrawal syndromes
Barbiturates	
Narcotics	
Benzodiazepines	
Lithium	Neonatal hypothyroidism, goitre
Corticosteroids and sex hormones	Fetal and neonatal adrenal suppression, virilisation of female fetus
NSAIDs	
Aspirin	Premature closure of ductus arteriosus, delayed labour, increased blood loss, impaired platelet function
Indomethacin	

DRUG SIDE EFFECTS

Peripheral neuropathy

1 TCAs
2 Amiodarone
3 Metronidazole
4 Nitrofurantoin
5 Zidovudine
6 Vinca alkaloids
7 Isoniazid (pyridoxine prevents)
8 Phenytoin

Drugs causing convulsions

1 Penicillins
2 Ciprofloxacin
3 Chlorpromazine
4 TCAs
5 Halothane
6 Lignocaine
7 IV contrast media
8 Pethidine
9 Lithium
10 Cimetidine
11 Chloroquine
12 All antiepileptics

Drugs causing agranulocytosis/neutropenia

1 Carbimazole
2 Zidovudine (AZT)
3 Clozapine
4 Mianserin
5 NSAIDs
6 Sulphonylureas
7 Sulphonamides
8 Azathioprine
9 Cytotoxics
10 Captopril
11 Cephalosporins

13 Chloramphenicol
14 Dapsone
15 Penicillins
16 Sulphonamides

Drugs causing bronchoconstriction

1 Adenosine
2 Beta blockers
3 NSAIDs
4 ACEIs
5 Muscle relaxants
6 Some opioids

Drugs causing pulmonary oedema

1 Adrenaline (epinephrine)
2 Heroin
3 Hydrochlorothiazide
4 IV fluids
5 IV β blockers
6 Methadone
7 Naloxone
8 Salicylate overdose
9 TCA overdose

Drugs causing pulmonary eosinophilia

1 Carbamazepine
2 Phenytoin
3 Sulphonamides
4 Dantrolene
5 Nitrofurantoin
6 Penicillin
7 Erythromycin
8 Chlorpropamide

Drugs causing gout (See page 429)

Drugs causing pulmonary fibrosis (See page 408)

Drugs causing photosensitivity (See page 94)

Drugs causing hyperprolactinaemia (See page 112)

Drugs causing gynaecomastia (See page 116)

Drugs causing gum hypertrophy (See page 127)

SOME DRUGS THAT COMMONLY APPEAR IN EXAMS

Phenytoin (See also page 337)

1 Voltage-activated Na blocker – stabilises membrane
2 Zero-order kinetics
3 Enzyme inducer
4 Useful for partial and generalised seizures but not absence
5 Toxic effects
   (a) Ataxia
   (b) Nystagmus
   (c) Vertigo
   (d) Tremor
   (e) Dysarthria
   (f) Coma
   (g) Arrhythmias
6 Side effects
   (a) Gum hypertrophy
   (b) Hirsutism
   (c) Megaloblastic anaemia
   (d) Seizures
   (e) Coarse facies
   (f) Osteomalacia
   (g) Lupus
   (h) Erythema nodosum
   (i) Hepatitis
   (j) Dupuytren's contracture
   (k) IgA deficiency

Ciclosporin

1 Calcineurin inhibitor
2 Powerful immunosuppressive which inhibits lymphocytes
3 Affects cell-mediated and antibody-mediated reactions
4 Main effect is inhibition of cytotoxic T cells via IL-2
5 **No** bone marrow suppression
6 Uses
   (a) Transplant rejection
   (b) RA
   (c) Psoriasis
   (d) Atopic dermatitis
7 Adverse effects
   (a) Nephrotoxicity
   (b) Hypertension
   (c) Gum hypertrophy
   (d) Hepatotoxicity
   (e) Tremor
   (f) Paraesthesiae of hands and feet
   (g) Hypertrichosis
   (h) Increased risk of skin cancers and lymphoproliferative malignancies

Retinoids (isotretinoin)

1 Vitamin A derivatives
2 Uses
   (a) Psoriasis
   (b) Acne
   (c) Acute promyelocytic leukaemia
3 Side effects
   (a) Mucosal dryness
   (b) Alopecia
   (c) Hypertriglyceridaemia
   (d) Thrombocytopenia
   (e) Reduced night vision
   (f) Photosensitivity
   (g) Mood changes
   (h) Hepatitis
   (i) Teratogenicity
   (j) Benign intracranial hypertension
   (k) Skeletal hyperostosis (high dose)

Tamoxifen

1 Anti-oestrogen drug used for oestrogen-positive breast tumours
2 60% of oestrogen receptor-positive respond, whereas only 10% of oestrogen receptor-negative respond
3 Partial agonist
4 Delays metastases and prolongs survival
5 Should be continued for 5 years
6 Adverse effects
  (a) Thromboembolism
  (b) Tumour flare
  (c) Hypercalcaemia
  (d) Amenorrhoea
  (e) Hot flushes
  (f) Endometrial hyperplasia and cancer
  (g) Alopecia
  (h) Leukopenia
  (i) Visual disturbance

Carbimazole

1 Inhibits peroxidase, thereby reducing iodination of tyrosil residues on thyroglobulin
2 May be immunosuppressive
3 Takes several weeks to work
4 Crosses the placenta and is present in breast milk
5 Adverse effects
  (a) Agranulocytosis (reversible by stopping the drug)
  (b) Rashes common (up to 25%)
  (c) Arthralgia
  (d) Jaundice
  (e) N+V

Interferons

1 Uses
  (a) Alpha
    (i)   Hepatitis B (chronic)
    (ii) Hepatitis C (chronic)
    (iii) Hairy cell leukaemia
    (iv) AIDS-related Kaposi's sarcoma

    (v)   Condylomata acuminata
    (vi) Renal cell carcinoma
    (vii) CML
    (viii) Some lymphomas
  (b) Beta
    (i)   MS
  (c) Gamma
    (i)   To reduce risk of infection in chronic granulomatous
       disease
2 Side effects
  (a) Nausea
  (b) Influenza-like symptoms
  (c) Lethargy
  (d) Depression
  (e) Hypersensitivity
  (f) Myelosuppression

SOME NEWER DRUGS

TNF-α antagonists

1 Infliximab (chimeric IgG monoclonal antibody which inhibits TNF-α)
2 Etanercept (recombinant molecule that inactivates TNF-α and -β)
3 Uses
  (a) RA (severe)
  (b) Juvenile chronic arthritis
  (c) Ankylosing spondylitis
  (d) Crohn's disease/UC (severe not responded to conventional
     therapy)
  (e) Crohn's fistulae
4 Adverse effects
  (a) Infusion-related effects (fever, pruritus, urticaria, hypotension)
  (b) ANA or dsDNA antibodies develop in some patients
  (c) Drug-induced lupus
  (d) Infections
  (e) Reactivation of TB
  (f) Leukopenia
  (g) Avoid in pregnancy and breastfeeding

GM-CSF

1 Haematopoietic growth factor
2 Enhances survival of cells committed to the granulocytic and macrophage lineages and stimulates their proliferation
3 Enhances neutrophil, monocyte and eosinophil counts
4 Used to treat life-threatening neutropenia
5 Side effects
  (a) Pericardial effusion and pericarditis
  (b) Fluid retention
  (c) Peritonitis
  (d) Serum enzyme rises
  (e) GI disturbances

Leukotriene antagonists (montelukast, zafirlukast)

1 Blocks the cysteinyl leukotriene 1 receptor
2 Add on therapy for mild to moderate asthma
3 Beneficial in exercise-induced asthma
4 Should not be used for treatment of an acute attack
5 Metabolised by cytochrome P450
6 May cause or aggravate Churg–Strauss syndrome
7 Side effects
  (a) Headaches
  (b) GI disturbance
  (c) Hypersensitivity (including angio-oedema)
  (d) Hepatitis

Low molecular weight heparins (LMWH)

1 Are at least as effective as unfractionated heparin (UFH) in the prevention of DVT and subsequent embolism and the treatment of unstable angina and PE
2 Act by selectively inhibiting factor Xa
3 Longer duration of action than UFH
4 Monitoring not required (do not prolong APTT)
5 Cannot be effectively reversed by protamine
6 Duration of action is prolonged in renal failure
7 Safe in pregnancy

8 Side effects
   (a) Thrombocytopenia
   (b) Bleeding
   (c) Osteoporosis (less than UFH)

Bupropion (Zyban)

1 Atypical antidepressant
2 Aid to smoking cessation
3 More effective than placebo and nicotine patches
4 Most effective when combined with nicotine patches and counselling

Sildenafil (Viagra)

1 Phosphodiesterase inhibitor (PDE5 receptor) inhibiting the breakdown of cGMP and leading to smooth muscle relaxation
2 Used for erectile dysfunction
3 Metabolised by cytochrome P450 (significantly interacts with inhibitors)
4 Reduce dose in cirrhosis and severe renal impairment
5 Nitrates contraindicated, as together severe hypotension occurs
6 Adverse effects
   (a) Hypotension
   (b) Priapism
   (c) Headache
   (d) Cardiovascular events post intercourse (?drug, ?sexual activity)

Sumatriptan

1 $5HT_{1D}$ receptor agonist
2 Used for acute treatment of migraine and cluster headaches (effective in 80%)
3 Maintains vasoconstriction in cranial arteries, preventing the vasodilator phase (headache) of migraine
4 Tablets, injection and nasal spray
5 Contraindicated in hemiplegic migraine, IHD, CVA and PVD
6 Adverse effects
   (a) Coronary artery spasm
   (b) Paraesthesiae
   (c) Tightness sensation over body
   (d) Hypertension

Donepezil

1 Reversible inhibitor of acetylcholinesterase
2 Used for mild to moderate Alzheimer's disease
3 50% of patients show a slower rate of cognitive decline
4 Patient should be assessed at 3 months and only continue if MMSE improves or has not deteriorated and functional ability has improved

COX-2 inhibitors (celecoxib, rofecoxib)

1 Selective inhibitors of COX-2 (COX-2 is induced at sites of inflammation)
2 As effective as diclofenac
3 Risk of serious GI bleeding reduced (but not excluded)
4 Shares side effects of other NSAIDs
5 Used for RA and OA in patients with high risk of GI bleeding
6 Rofecoxib recently withdrawn owing to increased risk of cardiovascular death
7 Increased risk of cardiovascular death (contraindicated in IHD)
8 Combination with low-dose aspirin leads to loss of reduction in GI bleeding

Anastrazole

1 Aromatase inhibitor
2 Used in treatment of postmenopausal oestrogen receptor-positive breast cancer
3 Prevents conversion of androgens to oestrogens outside the ovaries
4 Less menopausal side effects than tamoxifen
5 May be more effective than tamoxifen in reducing recurrence (not mortality)
6 Side effects: menopausal symptoms and fractures

Ezetimibe

1 Inhibits intestinal absorption of cholesterol
2 Used to treat hypercholesterolaemia
3 Reduces total cholesterol, LDL, TG, and increases HDL
4 Used with diet ± statin
5 Side effects
  (a) Diarrhoea
  (b) Abdominal pain

(c) Rash
(d) Angio-oedema

Sibutramine

1 Noradrenaline (norepinephrine) and serotonin reuptake inhibitor
2 Reduces food intake that leads to weight loss
3 Indicated for those with BMI > 30 and other risk factors
4 Side effects
   (a) Hypertension
   (b) Hepatotoxicity

Adefovir

1 Antiviral for the treatment of chronic hepatitis B with evidence of viral replication or hepatitis and fibrosis
2 Less viral resistance than lamivudine
3 Effective in lamivudine-resistant disease
4 Side effects
   (a) Diarrhoea
   (b) Lactic acidosis
   (c) Hepatotoxicity
   (d) Nephrotoxicity

Strontium renelate

1 Treatment of osteoporosis
2 Inhibits bone resorption and stimulates formation
3 Increases bone density and reduces vertebral and non-vertebral fractures
4 Side effects
   (a) Nausea
   (b) Diarrhoea

Linezolid

1 Oxazolidinone antibacterial agent
2 Useful in Gram-positive infection (poor for Gram-negatives)
3 Indicated for MRSA and vancomycin-resistant enterococci
4 Linezolid is a reversible monoamine oxidase inhibitor (interactions!)

5 Side effects
   (a) Thrombocytopenia, leukopenia and pancytopenia
   (b) Diarrhoea
   (c) Hypertension

Bosentan

1 Endothelin-1 antagonist
2 Treatment of primary pulmonary hypertension (WHO class 3 or 4)
3 Increases exercise capacity in patients
4 Side effects
   (a) Hepatotoxicity
   (b) Flushing
   (c) Hypotension

SOME ALTERNATIVE REMEDIES

St John's wort

1 Herb *Hypericum perforatum*
2 Used to treat depression
3 Better than placebo and equal to conventional antidepressants for mild to moderate depression
4 Cytochrome P450 inducer, so may interact with numerous drugs

Glucosamine

1 May be effective in osteoarthritis
2 May aggravate diabetes
3 Should not be given to those allergic to shellfish

Garlic

1 May reduce total cholesterol
2 May increase bleeding in patients on warfarin and aspirin

POISONING

Antidotes

Table 11

Drug	Antidote
Benzodiazepines	Flumazenil
Beta blockers	Atropine
	Glucagon (7 mg)
	Pacing
Calcium antagonists	Anticholinergics
	Calcium
Carbon monoxide	Oxygen
	Hyperbaric oxygen
Cyanide	Dicobalt edetate
	Sodium thiosulphate
	Sodium nitrite
Digoxin	Digoxin-binding antibody
Methanol and ethylene glycol	Ethanol infusion
	Fomepizole
Iron	Desferrioxamine
Paraquat	Fuller's earth
	IV Vitamin E
Opiates	Naloxone
Organophosphorous insecticides	Atropine
	Pralidoxime
Paracetamol	N-acetylcysteine
	Methionine
Warfarin	Vitamin K
	FFP
Lead	DMSA
	Penicillamine
Arsenic and mercury	Dimercaprol
Thallium	Prussian blue

Specific drugs

Paracetamol

1 Physiology
  (a) In overdose paracetamol oxidised to NAPQI
  (b) Glutathione required to inactivate this toxic metabolite
  (c) In overdose glutathione levels rapidly deplete

(d) Toxic liver injury occurs from NAPQI
(e) 12 g or more potentially serious
(f) Patients with pre-existing liver disease, alcoholism, anorexia nervosa, or those on enzyme-inducing drugs are at higher risk as they have lower glutathione stores

2 Features
(a) N+V
(b) Most asymptomatic for 24 hrs
(c) Lactic acidosis (< 12 hrs)
(d) Liver damage not detectable until 18 hrs
(e) Hepatic tenderness and abdominal pain on second day
(f) Maximal liver damage 72–96 hrs
(g) Renal failure (ATN) 25%
(h) Hypo-/hyperglycaemia
(i) Arrhythmias
(j) Pancreatitis
(k) Cerebral oedema
(l) GI bleeding

3 Important prognostic markers
(a) PT > 20 s at 24 hrs significant liver damage
(b) pH < 7.3 after 24 hrs = 15% survival
(c) Creatinine > 300 = 23% survival
(d) PT > 180 s = 8% survival

4 Indications for liver transplant
(a) pH < 7.3 at 36 hrs
(b) PT >100 s
(c) Creatinine > 300
(d) Grade 3 encephalopathy

5 Management
(a) Gastric lavage up to 4 hrs
(b) N-acetyl cysteine (6% rash and bronchospasm)
(c) Methionine
(d) Liver transplant

Salicylates

1 Features
(a) Mild to moderate (< 700 mg/l)
    (i) Deafness
    (ii) Tinnitus

      (iii) N+V
      (iv) Hyperventilation
      (v) Sweating
      (vi) Vasodilatation
      (vii) Tachycardia
      (viii) Respiratory alkalosis
      (ix) Metabolic acidosis

(b) Severe (> 700 mg/l)
      (i) Those above
      (ii) Delirium
      (iii) Hypotension
      (iv) Cardiac arrest

(c) Rare complications:
      (i) Non-cardiogenic pulmonary oedema
      (ii) Cerebral oedema
      (iii) Convulsions
      (iv) Coma
      (v) Encephalopathy
      (vi) Renal failure
      (vii) Tetany
      (viii) Hyperpyrexia
      (ix) Hypoglycaemia

2 Treatments
  (a) Gastric lavage
  (b) Activated charcoal
  (c) Urine alkalisation with bicarbonate (not forced alkaline diuresis, as this may induce pulmonary oedema)
  (d) Haemodialysis
  (e) Supportive measures

Tricyclic antidepressants (TCAs)

1 Features
  (a) Anticholinergic (dry mouth, drowsiness, sinus tachycardia, urinary retention)
  (b) Pyramidal signs (brisk reflexes, extensor plantars)
  (c) Coma
  (d) Convulsions
  (e) Respiratory depression and hypoxia
  (f) Hypotension

(g) Prolonged QT interval and arrhythmias (aggravated by acidosis)
(h) Respiratory and metabolic acidosis
(i) Hypothermia
(j) Skin blisters
2 Management
(a) Gastric lavage (up to 12 hrs due to gastroparesis)
(b) Activated charcoal
(c) Arrhythmias treated with bicarbonate (ie treat acidosis)
(d) Treat convulsions with diazepam

Lithium

1 Overdosage (> 1.5 mmol/l)
(a) Tremor
(b) Ataxia
(c) Dysarthria
(d) Nystagmus
(e) Renal impairment
(f) Convulsions
2 Overdosage (> 2 mmol/l)
(a) Above +
(b) Hyperreflexia
(c) Toxic psychosis
(d) Oliguria
(e) Circulatory failure
(f) Coma
(g) Death
3 Treat with
(a) Stop lithium
(b) Stop diuretics and NSAIDs
(c) Gastric lavage (within 6–8 hrs)
(d) Forced diuresis
(e) Haemodialysis

Carbon monoxide

1 Physiology
(a) Carboxyhaemoglobin formed so ↓ Hb for O_2 to bind to
(b) Dissociation curve shifts to left, impairing O_2 liberation
2 Acute features
(a) Headache

(b) Dizziness
(c) N+V
(d) ↓ Consciousness
(e) Hyperventilation
(f) Hypotension
(g) ↑ Muscle tone and reflexes
(h) Metabolic acidosis
(i) Rhabdomyolysis
(j) MI
(k) Pulmonary oedema
(l) Papilloedema
(m) Cerebral oedema
3 Delayed complications
(a) Parkinsonism
(b) Cortical blindness
(c) Mutism
(d) Hemiplegia
(e) Peripheral neuropathy
4 Management
(a) High-flow oxygen
(b) Dantrolene (to ↓ muscle activity)
(c) Hyperbaric oxygen

Ethylene glycol (antifreeze)

1 Physiology
(a) Metabolised by alcohol dehydrogenase to glycoaldehyde (CNS symptoms), glycocholate (main cause of acidosis), oxalate and lactic acid
2 Features
(a) Inebriation but no alcohol on breath
(b) N+V
(c) Haematemesis
(d) Coma
(e) Convulsions
(f) Papilloedema
(g) Nystagmus and ophthalmoplegia
(h) Hyporeflexia
(i) Fifth, sixth and seventh cranial nerve palsies
(j) Tachypnoea and pulmonary oedema
(k) ATN

3 Management
 (a) Ethanol infusion (competitively inhibits alcohol dehydrogenase)
 (b) Fomepizole
 (c) Dialysis

Iron

1 Features
 (a) Vomiting and diarrhoea
 (b) Abdominal pain
 (c) GI bleeding
 (d) Drowsiness
 (e) Coma
 (f) Convulsions
 (g) Metabolic acidosis
 (h) Circulatory failure
 (i) Jaundice and liver failure
 (j) Gastric stricture/pyloric stenosis (late)
2 Management
 (a) Gastric lavage
 (b) Supportive measures
 (c) Desferrioxamine
 (d) Dialysis
 (e) Exchange transfusion

Lead

1 Features
 (a) Lethargy
 (b) Abdominal pain (diffuse and colicky)
 (c) Vomiting
 (d) Encephalopathy
 (e) Motor peripheral neuropathy
 (f) Reversible tubular dysfunction
 (g) Blue discoloration of gums
 (h) Haemolytic anaemia
2 Investigations
 (a) Haemolysis
 (b) ↑ Delta aminolaevulinic acid
 (c) Basophilic stippling of RBCs
3 Management
 (a) DMSA

Theophylline

1 Features
  (a) N+V
  (b) Abdominal pain
  (c) Diarrhoea
  (d) GI bleeding
  (e) Hypokalaemia (marked)
  (f) Hyperglycaemia
  (g) Respiratory alkalosis
  (h) Metabolic acidosis
  (i) Arrhythmias (all)
  (j) Hypotension
  (k) Rhabdomyolysis
  (l) ARF
  (m) Restlessness
  (n) Headache
  (o) Convulsions
  (p) Coma
2 Management
  (a) Activated charcoal
  (b) K supplements
  (c) Beta blockers (not COPD) for arrhythmias
  (d) Diazepam for seizures
  (e) Haemoperfusion

Paraquat

1 Features
  (a) N+V
  (b) Oral and oesophageal ulcers
  (c) Oliguric renal failure
  (d) Dyspnoea
  (e) ARDS
  (f) Pulmonary fibrosis (second week)
2 Management
  (a) Gastric lavage with Fuller's earth
  (b) Oral administration of repeat-dose activated charcoal
  (c) Haemoperfusion/filtration
  (d) IV vitamin E

Dermatology

HAIR

Causes of diffuse non-scarring alopecia

1 Endocrine
   (a) Androgenic alopecia
   (b) Hypothyroidism
   (c) Hypopituitarism
2 Nutritional
   (a) Iron deficiency
3 Chronic disease
   (a) Liver disease
   (b) Renal disease
   (c) HIV
   (d) Malignancy
4 Skin diseases
   (a) Alopecia areata
   (b) Psoriasis
   (c) Erythroderma
5 Others
   (a) Pregnancy
   (b) Severe systemic illness or major surgery
   (c) Starvation
   (d) Emotional stress
6 Drugs
   (a) Cytotoxics
   (b) Warfarin
   (c) Retinoids and vitamin A
   (d) OCPs
   (e) Carbimazole
   (f) Valproate
   (g) Carbamazepine
   (h) Lithium

(i)   Allopurinol
(j)   Colchicine

Causes of scarring alopecia

1 Infection
    (a) Tinea capitis
    (b) Staphylococcal folliculitis
    (c) Syphilis
    (d) Lupus vulgaris (TB)
    (e) HSV and VZV
2 Skin disease
    (a) Lichen planus
    (b) BCC
    (c) Pemphigoid
3 Trauma
    (a) Burns
    (b) Radiotherapy
4 Systemic disorders
    (a) Sarcoid
    (b) SLE
    (c) Scleroderma
    (d) Metastatic carcinoma

Causes of hirsutism (excess hair occurs in androgen-dependent areas)

1 Polycystic ovarian disease
2 Ovarian tumours
3 Congenital adrenal hyperplasia
4 Adrenal tumours
5 Cushing's syndrome
6 Acromegaly
7 Prolactinoma
8 Androgen therapy
9 Corticosteroids
10 Phenytoin
11 Idiopathic

Causes of hypertrichosis (excess hair in non androgenic areas)

1 Hypothyroidism
2 Malnutrition
3 Anorexia nervosa (lanugo hair)
4 Porphyria
5 Underlying malignancy
6 Drugs
   (a) Ciclosporin
   (b) Corticosteroids
   (c) Minoxidil
   (d) Diazoxide
   (e) Penicillamine

NAILS

Causes of clubbing

1 Lung
   (a) Carcinoma of bronchus
   (b) Chronic suppurative lung disease
      (i) Bronchiectasis
      (ii) Lung abscess
      (iii) Empyema
      (iv) CF
   (c) TB
   (d) Mesothelioma
   (e) Fibrosing alveolitis (idiopathic pulmonary fibrosis)
   (f) Asbestosis
2 Heart
   (a) Congenital heart disease (cyanotic)
   (b) Bacterial endocarditis
   (c) Atrial myxoma
3 GI
   (a) Crohn's/UC
   (b) Cirrhosis
   (c) Tropical sprue
   (d) Malabsorption

4 Thyroid
   (a) Acropachy
5 Familial

Causes of nail changes

[See Table 12, opposite]

PIGMENTATION

Causes of hyperpigmentation

1 Endocrine
   (a) Addison's disease
   (b) Cushing's syndrome
   (c) Acromegaly
   (d) Nelson's syndrome
   (e) Pregnancy
   (f) Porphyria
2 Renal failure
3 Cirrhosis
4 Haemochromatosis
5 Nutritional
   (a) Vitamin B_{12} deficiency
   (b) Pellagra
6 Amyloid
7 Acanthosis nigricans
8 Lymphoma
9 Peutz–Jeghers' syndrome (perioral)
10 Drugs
   (a) Amiodarone
   (b) OCPs
   (c) Minocycline

Causes of hypopigmentation

1 Localised
   (a) Vitiligo
   (b) Pityriasis versicolor
   (c) Postinflammatory

Table 12

Nail change	Causes
Pitting	Psoriasis
	Eczema
	Alopecia areata
	Lichen planus
Ridges	Psoriasis
Dystrophy	Psoriasis
	Raynaud's phenomenon
	Arterial disease
	Lichen planus
	Onychomycosis (fungal nail infection)
White spots	Trauma
Black spots	Trauma
	Naevi
	Melanoma
Red spot	Glomus tumour
Onycholysis	Psoriasis
	Onychomycosis
	Hypothyroidism
	Hyperthyroidism
	Trauma
Grooves	Acute illness (Beau's lines)
	Psoriasis
White bands	Arsenic poisoning
	Hypoalbuminaemia
Leukonychia	Cirrhosis
	DM
	CCF
	Anaemia
Yellow nails	Yellow nail syndrome
Blue nails	Wilson's disease
	Melanoma
	Subungal haematoma
Koilonychia	Iron deficiency anaemia
Splinter haemorrhages	Trauma
	Bacterial endocarditis
	CTDs
Nailfold telangiectasia	CTDs

(d) Tuberous sclerosis
(e) Leprosy
2 Generalised
(a) Hypopituitarism
(b) Albinism
(c) Phenylketonuria

Disorders associated with vitiligo

1 Thyroid disease
2 Pernicious anaemia
3 Addison's disease
4 Diabetes mellitus
5 Myasthenia gravis
6 Alopecia areata
7 Malignant melanoma

REACTION PATTERNS

Causes of orogenital ulceration

1 Stevens–Johnson syndrome
2 Reiter's disease
3 Crohn's disease
4 UC
5 Syphilis
6 Gonococcal infection
7 HCV
8 Behçet's disease
9 Lichen planus
10 HIV
11 Pemphigus
12 Pemphigoid

Common causes of urticaria and angio-oedema

1 Drugs
(a) Penicillins
(b) Cephalosporins
(c) ACEIs

(d) NSAIDs
(e) Opiates
(f) X-ray contrast media
(g) Blood products
2 Foods
   (a) Azo dyes
   (b) Benzoate preservatives
3 Arthropod reactions
4 Physical stimuli
   (a) Light pressure (dermographism)
   (b) Cold
   (c) Increase in body temperature (cholinergic)
   (d) Light
5 Plants
6 Systemic diseases
   (a) Viral infections (hepatitis B)
   (b) SLE
   (c) Vasculitides
7 Animal saliva (in atopics)
8 Inhalants
   (a) Grass pollens
   (b) House dust
9 C1 esterase inhibitor deficiency – angio-oedema

Causes of erythroderma

Generalised exfoliative dermatitis involving > 90% of the skin

1 Eczema (40%)
2 Psoriasis (25%)
3 Mycosis fungoides (15%)
4 Reactions to sunlight
5 Toxic erythroderma
6 Toxic shock syndrome
7 Scalded skin syndrome
8 Toxic epidermal necrolysis
9 Infestations
10 Congenital

11 Drugs (10%)
   (a) Sulphonamides
   (b) Phenytoin
   (c) Carbamazepine
   (d) Isoniazid
   (e) Lithium
   (f) Captopril
   (g) Allopurinol
   (h) Gold
   (i) Chloroquine
   (j) Methyldopa

Causes of livedo reticularis

1 Idiopathic
2 Physiological
3 Vasculitis
4 Hyperviscosity
5 Thrombocythaemia
6 Cryoglobulinaemia
7 Heart failure
8 Drugs (amantadine)

Causes of pyoderma gangrenosum

1 Idiopathic (50%)
2 UC
3 Crohn's
4 RA
5 Wegener's granulomatosis
6 Myeloma
7 Paraproteinaemia
8 Leukaemia

Causes of erythema nodosum

1 Systemic diseases
   (a) Sarcoidosis
   (b) UC
   (c) Crohn's
   (d) Leukaemia
   (e) Hodgkin's disease
   (f) Behçet's disease

2 Infections
   (a) *Streptococcus*
   (b) TB
   (c) Leprosy
   (d) EBV
   (e) Histoplasmosis
   (f) *Yersinia*
   (g) Lymphogranuloma venereum
   (h) Cat scratch disease
   (i) Blastomycosis
   (j) Coccidiodomycosis
3 Drugs
   (a) Sulphonamides
   (b) OCPs
   (c) Penicillins
   (d) Tetracyclines
   (e) Sulphonylureas

Causes of erythema multiforme (severe systemic form – Stevens–Johnson syndrome)

1 Idiopathic (50%)
2 Infections
   (a) HSV
   (b) EBV
   (c) *Mycoplasma*
   (d) *Streptococcus*
   (e) Histoplasmosis
   (f) Typhoid
3 SLE
4 PAN
5 UC
6 Carcinoma
7 Lymphoma
8 Sarcoidosis
9 Pregnancy
10 Drugs
   (a) Penicillins
   (b) Sulphonamides
   (c) Co-trimoxazole

(d) Phenytoin
(e) Salicylates
(f) Barbiturates
(g) Carbamazepine
(h) Rifampicin
(i) Sulphonylureas
(j) Gold

Causes of the Koebner phenomenon (develops at site of trauma)

1 Psoriasis
2 Lichen planus
3 Vitiligo
4 Viral warts
5 Molluscum contagiosum
6 Bullous pemphigoid

SKIN MANIFESTATIONS OF SYSTEMIC DISEASE

Causes of leg ulceration

1 Trauma
2 Infections
3 Venous insufficiency
4 Peripheral vascular disease
5 DM
6 Neuropathy
7 Pressure sores
8 Neoplasia
9 Vasculitis
10 Bullous disorders
11 Necrobiosis lipoidica
12 Pyoderma gangrenosum
13 Leishmaniasis
14 Tropical ulcer
15 Haemoglobinopathy

Associations with internal malignancy

1 Ichthyosis (lymphoma)
2 Acanthosis nigricans (AN; usually gastric adenocarcinoma)
   Other associations of AN include:
   (a) Obesity
   (b) Inherited
   (c) DM
   (d) Lipodystrophy
   (e) Cushing's syndrome
   (f) Acromegaly
   (g) PCOS
   (h) Hypothyroidism
3 Acanthosis palmaris (bronchial cancer)
4 Erythema gyratum repens (bronchial cancer)
5 Acquired hypertrichosis (Hodgkin's lymphoma)
6 Superficial migratory thrombophlebitis (cancer of the pancreas)
7 Necrolytic migratory erythema (glucagonoma)
8 Dermatomyositis (bronchial, breast and ovarian)
9 Bullous pyoderma gangrenosum (leukaemia, lymphoma)
10 Pemphigoid
11 Tylosis (familial plantar and palmar keratosis associated with oesophageal cancer)

Skin changes in DM

1 Cutaneous infections
2 Neuropathic ulcers
3 Necrobiosis lipoidica
4 Diabetic dermopathy
5 Disseminated granuloma annulare
6 Bullosis diabeticorum
7 Acanthosis nigricans
8 Xanthomas and xanthelasma
9 Lipoatrophy (porcine insulins)
10 Lipohypertrophy (highly purified human insulins)
11 Vitiligo

Skin features of sarcoidosis

1 Erythema nodosum
2 Lupus pernio
3 Scar sarcoid
4 Plaques and subcutaneous nodules
5 Scarring alopecia

Causes of generalised pruritus (without diagnostic skin lesions)

1 Endocrine
  (a) Thyroid disease (hypo- and hyper-)
  (b) DM
  (c) DI
2 Haematological
  (a) Iron deficiency
  (b) Polycythaemia rubra vera
  (c) Lymphoma
  (d) Leukaemia
  (e) Myeloma
3 Others
  (a) Obstructive biliary disease
  (b) Pregnancy
  (c) Chronic renal failure
  (d) Scabies
  (e) Intestinal parasites
  (f) Senile pruritus
  (g) Psychogenic
4 Drugs
  (a) Opiates
  (b) Gold
  (c) Alcohol
  (d) Hepatotoxic drugs
  (e) OCPs

Cutaneous features of some congenital disorders

[See Table 13, opposite]

Table 13

Syndrome	Skin features	Other manifestations
Xeroderma pigmentosa (AR) Defect in DNA repair	Photosensitivity, pigment changes, keratoses, skin cancers	
Tuberous sclerosis (AD) See also Genetics, page 176	Angiofibromas, periungual fibromas, shagreen patches, ash leaf patches	Epilepsy, mental retardation
Neurofibromatosis (AD) See also Genetics, page 176	Café au lait spots, axillary freckling, neurofibromas	Acoustic neuromas, sarcoma, retinal Lisch nodules, epilepsy
Hereditary haemorrhagic telangiectasia (AD)	Facial and mucosal telangiectasia	Epistaxis, GI bleeding
Pseudoxanthoma elasticum (AD+AR) Defective elastin	'Chicken skin'	Angioid retinal streaks, MVP, IHD, cerebral haemorrhage, GI bleeding
Peutz–Jeghers syndrome (AD) See also GI, page 150	Perioral hyperpigmentation	Multiple GI polyps, intussusception, GI malignancy
Ehlers–Danlos (AD+AR) Defective collagen	Skin fragility, tissue paper scars, hyperelasticity	Bruising, hyperextensible joints
Cutis laxa	Lax pendulous skin, premature ageing	
Sturge–Weber syndrome	Facial port wine stain	Epilepsy, cortical haemangioma, cortical calcification, glaucoma

DRUGS AND THE SKIN

Causes of fixed drug eruptions

1 Phenytoin
2 Sulphonamides
3 Barbiturates
4 Dapsone
5 Quinine
6 NSAIDs
7 Tetracyclines

Drugs leading to photosensitivity

1 Amiodarone
2 Thiazides
3 Frusemide
4 ACEIs
5 NSAIDs
6 Nalidixic acid
7 Tetracyclines
8 Ciprofloxacin
9 Isoniazid
10 Sulphonamides
11 Griseofulvin
12 Sulphonylureas
13 Phenothiazines (chlorpromazine etc)
14 Chlordiazepoxide
15 Chloroquine

Drugs causing a vasculitic rash

1 Allopurinol
2 Thiazides
3 Phenytoin
4 NSAIDs
5 Sulphonamides
6 Hydralazine
7 Quinidine
8 Captopril

Drugs causing a lichen planus-like eruption

1 Gold
2 Penicillamine
3 Streptomycin
4 Tetracycline
5 Chloroquine
6 Quinine
7 Isoniazid
8 Ethambutol
9 Thiazides
10 Frusemide
11 Captopril
12 Sulphonylureas
13 Phenothiazines

DERMATITIS

Common causes of contact dermatitis (patch testing useful)

1 Nickel (jewellery)
2 Cobalt
3 Chromate (leather, engineering processes)
4 Epoxy resin (glue)
5 Paraphenylenediamine (hair dyes)
6 Rubber antioxidants (gloves and shoes)
7 Preservatives
8 Lanolin (cosmetics)
9 Perfumes
10 Plants (primula, poison ivy)
11 Topical drugs
    (a) Neomycin
    (b) Antihistamines
    (c) Sulphonamides
    (d) Local anaesthetics
12 Sticking plasters

Aetiological factors in atopic dermatitis (eczema)

1 Atopy
2 Skin irritants
3 Contact allergens
4 Friction
5 UV light
6 Low humidity
7 Infections
8 Drugs and foods
9 Venous stasis
10 Ichthyosis

PSORIASIS

Essential features of psoriasis

1 Associated with HLA-Cw6 (B27 joint disease)
2 35% have family history
3 More common in smokers and heavy alcohol drinkers
4 Scaly, erythematous plaques affecting any part of the skin
5 Epidermal cell hyperplasia
6 Epidermal turnover time reduced from 28 days to 4 days
7 Aetiology unknown
8 Exhibits Koebner's phenomenon (develops at sites of trauma)
9 Arthropathy seen in 8–10% of patients (See page 440)
10 Multiple variants
   (a) Chronic plaque
   (b) Guttate
   (c) Palmoplantar pustular
   (d) Generalised pustular
   (e) Erythrodermic
   (f) Flexural and genital
   (g) Scalp
   (h) Facial
   (i) Nails (pitting, ridging, onycholysis, dystrophy, subungual keratosis)
11 Treatments
   (a) Topical
      (i) Tar

(ii)   Dithranol
(iii) Steroids
(iv) Calcipotriol (vitamin D analogue)
(v)   UVB
(b) Systemic
(i)   PUVA (psoralens and UVA)
(ii)   Methotrexate
(iii) Acitretin (retinoid)
(iv) Ciclosporin
(v)   Hydroxyurea
(vi) Sulphasalazine

BLISTERING SKIN DISORDERS

Causes of blistering

1 Genetic
   (a) Epidermolysis bullosa
2 Physical
   (a) Heat and cold
   (b) Irradiation (sun)
   (c) Contact with irritants
   (d) Friction
   (e) Oedema
3 Inflammatory
   (a) Infections
      (i)   Staphylococcal – bullous impetigo, scalded skin syndrome
      (ii)   Streptococcal – including necrotizing fasciitis
      (iii) HSV
      (iv) Herpes zoster
      (v)   Hand, foot and mouth disease (Coxsackie)
      (vi) Fungal
   (b) Eczema
   (c) Erythema multiforme
   (d) Insect bites
4 Invasion
   (a) Carcinoma
   (b) Amyloidosis
5 Immunological

(a) Bullous pemphigoid
(b) Pemphigus
(c) Dermatitis herpetiformis
(d) Pemphigoid gestationalis
(e) Linear IgA disease
(f) Epidermolysis bullosa
(g) SLE
(h) Lichen planus
(i) Porphyria cutanea tarda
6 Drug reactions

Essential features of pemphigoid

1 Autoimmune disorder of the elderly
2 Lesions are large tense blisters (up to 3 cm) with an erythematous base (subepidermal)
3 Usually on limbs, trunk and mucous membranes
4 Specific antibody (IgG) to the basement membrane of the epidermis in 70%
5 Associated with malignancy
6 Treat with high-dose prednisolone (60–80 mg/day)
7 Complete remission in 1 year common

Essential features of pemphigus

1 Autoimmune blistering condition of the epidermis
2 Associated with HLA A-10, DR4
3 IgG autoantibodies to intracellular material of the epidermis (*cf.* pemphigoid – basement membrane) in 90%
4 Penicillamine can cause pemphigus
5 Very fragile blisters which rupture easily (pemphi*gus* lesions b*ust*)
6 Any site may be affected and blistering is usually widespread
7 Mucous membranes often involved – lesions painful
8 Treatment with prednisolone 80–100 mg/day
9 Azathioprine, methotrexate, ciclosporin and iv immunoglobulin also used
10 Disease persists for life
11 Mortality 15–20%

Essential features of dermatitis herpetiformis

1 Intense pruritic vesicular rash on the buttocks and extensor aspect of the elbows and knees
2 Associated with coeliac disease, HLA B8, DR3 and DQ2 (See page 142)
3 IgA deposited in the basement membrane zone
4 Treated with dapsone
5 Gluten-free diet results in slow improvement of rash (1–2 yrs)
6 Increased risk of lymphoma (reduced by gluten-free diet)

Causes of skin tumours

1 UV light
2 Thermal injury
3 X-irradiation
4 Hydrocarbons
5 Arsenic
6 Immunosuppression (renal transplantation)
7 HPV
8 HTLV-1
9 HHV-8 (Kaposi's sarcoma)
10 Genetic predisposition (xeroderma pigmentosum)
11 Long-standing skin disease (chronic leg ulcers)

Endocrinology

THYROID HORMONES

1 TRH – thyrotrophin-releasing hormone
2 TSH – thyroid-stimulating hormone
3 T_4/T_3 – thyroxine/triiodothyronine

Thyroid hormone physiology

Table 14

	TRH	TSH	T_4/T_3
Type	Peptide	Peptide	Amine (acts like steroid)
From	Hypothalamus	Anterior pituitary (basophils)	Thyroid
Acts at/via	Intracellular Ca^{2+}	Cyclic AMP	Nuclear binding
Pregnancy	↑	↑	↑
Illness		↓	↓

1 Thyroid peroxidase iodinates thyroglobulin to T_3 and T_4
2 Mainly T_4 is released by thyroid
3 T_4 is converted to T_3 in the tissues and liver
4 Free T_3 is active thyroid hormone
5 Thyroid hormones bound to thyroid-binding globulin (TBG) and thyroid-binding prealbumin (TBPA)
6 TSH measurement is most accurate in diagnosis and monitoring of treatment
7 Total T_3 and T_4 are inaccurate measures of thyroid status as levels are affected by TBG levels
8 Free T_3 and T_4 are more accurate
9 Causes of ↑ TBG and hence ↑ total T_4
   (a) Oestrogens
   (b) Chronic liver disease

(c) Acute intermittent porphyria

(d) Pregnancy

10 Causes of ↓ TBG and hence ↓ total T_4

   (a) Acromegaly

   (b) Protein loss (malabsorption and nephrotic syndrome)

   (c) Androgens and steroids

11 Drugs displacing T_4/T_3 from TBG

   (a) Aspirin

   (b) Phenytoin

   (c) Frusemide

Causes of goitre

1 Types

   (a) Multinodular

   (b) Diffuse

2 Causes

   (a) Physiological

      (i) Puberty

      (ii) Pregnancy

   (b) Autoimmune thyroid disease

      (i) Graves' disease

      (ii) Hashimoto's thyroiditis

   (c) Thyroiditis

   (d) Iodine deficiency

   (e) Tumours

   (f) Cysts

Hyperthyroidism

1 Causes

   (a) Hyperthyroidism associated with overactive gland (increased uptake of radioiodine tracer)

      (i) Graves' (50–60%)

      (ii) Hot nodule

      (iii) Toxic multinodular goitre

      (iv) Pituitary tumour (rare)

      (v) Drugs, eg amiodarone

   (b) Hyperthyroidism with normal gland (decreased/absent uptake of radioiodine tracer)

      (i) De Quervain's thyroiditis

    (ii) Postpartum thyroiditis

    (iii) Ectopic thyroid

    (iv) Thyroxine overdose

2 Symptoms and signs (below)

3 Diagnosis

    (a) Low TSH (high in pituitary)

4 Treatment

    (a) Symptomatic with β blockers (reduces sympathetic symptoms)

    (b) Carbimazole (See page 67)

    (c) Radioactive iodine (usually leads to hypothyroid state)

    (d) Subtotal thyroidectomy

Graves' disease

1 Autoimmune hyperthyroidism

    (a) Thyroid-stimulating immunoglobulins

    (b) Antithyroperoxidase antibodies

2 Associated with other organ-specific autoimmune diseases

3 Diffusely enlarged gland with bruit

4 Associated with HLA DRw3 and B89

5 Thyroid eye disease (See pages 104 and 371)

Hypothyroidism

1 Causes

    (a) Autoimmune

        (i) Antimicrosomal antibodies in 90%

        (ii) Antithyroglobulin antibodies in 60%

    (b) Previous thyroid surgery or radioactive iodine

    (c) Drugs

        (i) Carbimazole

        (ii) Propylthiouracil

        (iii) Lithium

        (iv) Amiodarone

    (d) Dietary iodine deficiency

    (e) Congenital (agenesis of thyroid, inborn error of thyroid metabolism, TSH receptor defect, iodine deficiency)

    (f) Pituitary hypothyroidism

2 Symptoms and signs (below)

3 Diagnosis

    (a) High TSH (peak levels are in evening)

4 Treatment
  (a) Replace thyroxine
  (b) Aim for normalisation of TSH level
  (c) Increase dose every 6 weeks by 25–50 µg
  (d) Reduced dose in elderly or IHD

Clinical features of thyroid disease

Table 15

Features of hyperthyroidism	Features of hypothyroidism
Heat intolerance	Cold intolerance
Sweating	Dry skin
Weight loss	Weight gain
Hair loss	Hair loss
Amenorrhoea	Menorrhagia
Diarrhoea	Constipation
Tremor	Periorbital puffiness
Microcytic anaemia	Macrocytic anaemia
Leukopenia	
Proximal myopathy	Myotonia
Intermittent periodic paralysis	Cerebellar degeneration
Atrial fibrillation	Ischaemic heart disease
Cardiac failure	Hypercholesterolaemia
Shortness of breath	Effusions

Eye signs of hyperthyroidism

Table 16

	Graves'	Non-Graves'
Lid lag	✓	✓
Lid retraction	✓	✓
Periorbital oedema	✓	✗
Proptosis and exophthalmos	✓	✗
Diplopia	✓	✗
Optic nerve compression	✓	✗

Thyroid carcinoma

1 Most commonly presents with a lump in the neck
2 Hoarseness may indicate recurrent laryngeal nerve involvement
3 10% of thyroid nodules malignant
4 Rarely causes hyperthyroidism
5 Radiation exposure increases risk of thyroid cancer
6 Diagnosed with FNA of nodule
7 Types
  (a) Papillary
    (i) Commonest (80%)
    (ii) Least aggressive
    (iii) Spreads locally to cervical nodes (one-third at presentation)
    (iv) Histology may show psammoma bodies
  (b) Follicular
    (i) Moderately aggressive
    (ii) Distant metastases more common
  (c) Anaplastic
    (i) Very aggressive
    (ii) Uncommon
    (iii) Rapid local growth can lead to tracheal obstruction
  (d) Medullary carcinoma
    (i) Arises from C cells.
    (ii) 25% familial
    (iii) Associated with MEN 11 and *RET* oncogene (See page 110)
    (iv) Calcitonin levels raised
  (e) Lymphoma
8 Treatment
  (a) Thyroidectomy
  (b) Radiotherapy with ^{131}I

CORTISOL PHYSIOLOGY

1 CRH – corticotrophin-releasing hormone
2 ACTH – adrenocorticotrophic hormone
3 Cortisol bound to corticosteroid-binding hormone (CBG) – 10% free in plasma is active fraction

Table 17

	CRH	ACTH	Cortisol
Type	Peptide	Peptide	Steroid
From	Hypothalamus	Anterior pituitary (basophils)	Adrenal zona fasciculata
Acts via	cAMP	cAMP	Nuclear binding

Cushing's syndrome/disease

1 Causes
  (a) Pituitary tumour (Cushing's disease) – 75–80%
  (b) Adrenal tumour – 15%
  (c) Ectopic ACTH (small cell carcinoma, carcinoid) – 5–10%
  (d) Ectopic CRH (very unusual)
  (e) Exogenous steroids
2 Clinical features
  (a) Obesity and moon face
  (b) Buffalo hump
  (c) Hirsutism
  (d) Acne
  (e) Thin skin
  (f) Bruising
  (g) Hypertension
  (h) Hyperglycaemia
  (i) Hypokalaemic alkalosis
  (j) Osteoporosis
  (k) Proximal weakness
  (l) Psychosis
  (m) Amenorrhoea
3 Diagnosis
  [See Fig. 1, opposite]
4 Treatment
  (a) Removal of tumour (pituitary/adrenal/ectopic)
  (b) Bilateral adrenalectomy
    (i) Patients may develop Nelson's syndrome
    (ii) Pituitary enlargement
      (1) Pigmentation due to melanocyte stimulation by MSH which is derived from the precursor to ACTH, pro-opiomelanocortin

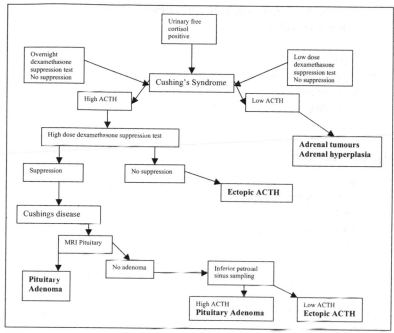

Figure 1 Cushing's syndrome diagnosis

(c) Ketoconazole, metyrapone and aminoglutethimide (inhibits steroidogenesis)

Conn's syndrome

1 Causes
   (a) Adrenal adenoma
   (b) Bilateral adrenal hyperplasia
2 Clinical features
   (a) Hypertension
   (b) Metabolic alkalosis
   (c) Hypokalaemia
   (d) Hypernatraemia
3 Diagnosis
   (a) Typical biochemistry
   (b) Low renin
   (c) High aldosterone

(d) Aldosterone/renin ratio > 20 (off diuretics, ACEI, ARBs)
(e) Adrenal imaging
4 Treatment
  (a) Adrenalectomy
  (b) Sodium restriction
  (c) Spironolactone
  (d) Thiazides
  (e) ACEI

Hypoadrenalism

1 Causes
  (a) Autoimmune – Addison's
  (b) TB
  (c) Metastasis
  (d) Sarcoidosis
  (e) HIV
  (f) Haemorrhage (Friderichsen–Waterhouse secondary to meningococcus)
  (g) Congenital adrenal hyperplasia
  (h) Pituitary failure
      (i) Drugs
      (i) Withdrawal of long-term steroids
      (ii) Ketoconazole
      (iii) Metyrapone
      (iv) Aminoglutethimide
2 Clinical features
  (a) Pigmentation
  (b) Vitiligo (autoimmune)
  (c) Weakness and lethargy
  (d) Weight loss
  (e) Hypotension
  (f) Dehydration
  (g) Abdominal pain
  (h) Hypoglycaemia
  (i) Hyponatraemia
  (j) Hyperkalaemia
  (k) Hypercalcaemia
  (l) Normocytic anaemia with lymphocytosis or eosinophilia
  (m) Mild metabolic acidosis

3 Diagnosis
  (a) Random cortisol
  (b) Synacthen test
  (c) Adrenal cortex antibodies (to 21-hydroxylase)
  (d) Imaging of adrenals
4 Treatment
  (a) Hydrocortisone (increase with intercurrent infection)
  (b) Fludrocortisone (to replace mineralocorticoids)

Congenital adrenal hyperplasia

1 21-Hydroxylase deficiency (90%)
2 11-Hydroxylase deficiency (5%)
3 Autosomal recessive
4 Low levels of mineralocorticoid and cortisol produced due to enzyme deficiency
5 High ACTH
6 All steroid precursors driven into androgen production, causing virilisation, genital ambiguity etc.
7 Treated with hydrocortisone and fludrocortisone

Phaeochromocytoma

1 Tumour of adrenal medulla
2 Release of catecholamines leads to symptoms
3 10% familial
4 10% bilateral
5 10% malignant
6 10% outside adrenals
7 Features
  (a) Persistent or intermittent hypertension
  (b) Tachycardia and palpitations
  (c) Bradycardia
  (d) Postural hypotension
  (e) Pallor or flushing
  (f) Hyperglycaemia and glycosuria
  (g) Weight loss
  (h) Change in bowel habit
  (i) Raynaud's phenomenon
8 Investigation
  (a) Urinary metanephrins
  (b) CT scan

(c) MRI (T_2-weighted)
(d) MIBG scan
9 NB invasive procedures or radiocontrast studies need α and β blockade to prevent hypertensive crisis

Multiple endocrine neoplasia (MEN)

1 All autosomal dominant
2 MEN I (chromosome 11)
   (a) **P**arathyroid
   (b) **P**ancreas including
      (i) Insulinoma
      (ii) Gastrinoma
      (iii) Glucagonoma
      (iv) VIPoma
      (v) PPoma
   (c) **P**ituitary (60% prolactinoma)
3 MEN IIA (chromosome 10)
   (a) Medullary carcinoma of thyroid (MCT)
   (b) Phaeochromocytoma
   (c) Parathyroid
4 MEN IIB
   (a) MCT
   (b) Phaeochromocytoma
   (c) Parathyroid
   (d) Marfanoid
   (e) Mucosal neuromas
5 MEN II have 100% risk of MCT therefore should have a prophylactic thyroidectomy
6 Syndrome associated with *RET* oncogene on chromosome 6 (can be tested for with PCR to screen relatives)

PITUITARY

Important anatomical associations

1 Optic chiasm (bitemporal hemianopia)
2 Cavernous sinus containing branches of III, IV, V (ophthalmic only) and VI
3 Sphenoidal sinus (surgery)

Pituitary tumours

1 Microadenoma < 1 cm, macroadenoma > 1 cm
2 Nearly always benign, but can get metastases from breast cancers
3 50% of all tumours are non-secreting
4 Prolactinoma is the most common hormone-secreting tumour
5 Macroadenomas may present with bitemporal hemianopia or cranial nerve palsy (above)
6 Some tumours present with hormonal effects
7 Diagnosis
  (a) MRI pituitary
  (b) Hormone levels
  (c) Visual field testing

Panhypopitutarism

1 Deficiency of all pituitary hormones
  (a) Adrenal insufficiency
  (b) Hypothyroidism
  (c) Hypogonadism
  (d) GH deficiency
  (e) Diabetes insipidus
2 Causes
  (a) Pituitary tumours (including metastases)
  (b) Craniopharyngiomas
  (c) Infiltration
    (i) TB
    (ii) Sarcoidosis
    (iii) Histiocytosis X
  (d) Sheehan's syndrome (pituitary infarction with postpartum haemorrhage)
  (e) Empty sella syndrome
  (f) Encephalitis
  (g) Syphilis
  (h) Trauma
3 Treatment
  (a) Replace all deficient hormones

Prolactin

1 Anterior pituitary hormone

2 Under negative control of hypothalamus by dopamine, ie **increased** dopamine results in **decreased** prolactin
3 Causes of raised prolactin
   (a) Prolactinoma
   (b) Stress, eg epileptic fit
   (c) Pregnancy
   (d) Oestrogens (ie oral contraceptive)
   (e) Dopamine antagonist drugs, ie metoclopramide, phenothiazines
   (f) Polycystic ovary
   (g) Damage to hypothalamus or pituitary stalk
   (h) Renal or hepatic failure
2 Clinical features of high prolactin
   (a) Galactorrhoea
   (b) Secondary hypogonadism
3 Causes of low prolactin
   (a) Dopamine and dopamine agonists, ie bromocriptine

Prolactinoma

1 25% of all pituitary tumours
2 Usually large in men, small in women
3 May be part of MEN I
4 Diagnosis
   (a) MRI pituitary
   (b) Hormone levels
5 Treatment
   (a) Bromocriptine
   (b) Pergolide
   (c) Cabergoline
   (d) Pituitary irradiation
   (e) Pituitary surgery

Growth hormone

1 Peptide hormone from anterior pituitary
2 Under control of growth hormone-releasing hormone (GHRH) from hypothalamus, and somatostatin
3 Secreted in pulsatile fashion mainly at night – levels may be undetectable in between
4 Acts directly and via stimulation of IGF-1 production in liver
5 Causes of GH deficiency

(a) Pituitary tumours
(b) Parapituitary tumour, ie craniopharyngioma
(c) Trauma, ie surgery
(d) Infarction (pituitary apoplexy – bleed into tumour)
(e) Pituitary infection (abscess, TB)
6 Features of GH deficiency
(a) Decreased energy and exercise tolerance
(b) Decreased bone density
(c) Reduced muscle mass
(d) Increased body fat
(e) Increased lipids
(f) Reduced cardiac output

Acromegaly

1 95% due to pituitary tumour
2 12% of all pituitary tumours secrete GH. Of these, 90% are macroadenomas
3 Rarely due to ectopic GHRH from carcinoid
4 Diagnosis
(a) Failure of GH to suppress with oral glucose load – may get paradoxical rise
(b) Raised serum IGF-1 levels
(c) Visual fields
(d) MRI pituitary
5 Features of acromegaly
(a) Symptoms of mass effect from tumour
(b) Coarse facial appearance
(c) Large tongue
(d) Large hands/feet
(e) Enlarged lower jaw
(f) Hypertension
(g) Diabetes mellitus
(h) Increased cardiovascular mortality
(i) Obstructive sleep apnoea
(j) Carpal tunnel syndrome
(k) Hyperhidrosis
(l) Arthropathy
(m) Renal stones
(n) Increased risk of colonic malignancy

    (o) LVH and cardiomyopathy
6 Treatment
    (a) Pituitary surgery
    (b) Octreotide (somatostatin analogue)
    (c) Pituitary irradiation
    (d) Bromocriptine

Vasopressin (ADH)

1 Peptide hormone
2 Secreted by hypothalamus
3 Stored in posterior pituitary
4 Cranial diabetes insipidus caused by damage to hypothalamic
  nuclei by
    (a) Pituitary tumours
    (b) Parapituitary tumour, eg craniopharyngioma
    (c) Trauma and surgery
    (d) Infiltration of hypothalamus by sarcoid, histiocytosis X
    (e) Idiopathic

SEX HORMONES

1 LH – luteinizing hormone
2 FSH – follicle-stimulating hormone
3 Under control of GnRH (positive) and inhibin (reduces FSH secretion)
4 Testosterone and oestrogen circulate bound to sex hormone-binding
  globulin
5 Men
    (a) LH stimulate Leydig cells to produce testosterone
    (b) FSH stimulates testicular growth
6 Women
    (a) LH stimulates oestrogen and progesterone production and surge
       of LH mid cycle causes ovulation
    (b) FSH controls the development of the follicle
7 Primary gonadal failure will lead to increased FSH and LH levels
8 Low levels of FSH and LH lead to hypogonadism
  (hypogonadotrophic or secondary)

Hypogonadism

Table 18

	Causes	Features

♂	Hypopituitarism
	Selective gonadal deficiency
	Hyperprolactinaemia
	Primary congenital gonadal disease
	  • Klinefelter's, anorchia
	Primary acquired gonadal disease
	  • Torsion, castration, radiotherapy
	  • Renal failure, liver failure
	Androgen receptor deficiency
		Loss of libido
		Increasing pitch of voice
		Loss of male pattern of hair
		Decreased testicular size
		Loss of erectile and ejaculatory function
		Failure of spermatogenesis
		Loss of muscle bulk

♀	Ovarian failure (total)
	  • Dysgenesis
	  • Steroid biosynthetic defect
	  • Oophorectomy
	  • Radio/chemotherapy
	Ovarian failure (partial)
	  • Polycystic ovary syndrome
	  • Resistant ovary syndrome
	Gonadotrophin failure
	  • Hypothalamopituitary disease
	  • Kallmann's syndrome
	  • Anorexia
	  • Systemic illness
	Hypothyroidism
		Thinning and loss of pubic hair
		Small atrophic breasts
		Vaginal dryness and dyspareunia
		Atrophy of vulva and vagina
		Osteoporosis
		Infertility
		Amenorrhoea

Polycystic ovarian syndrome

1 Multiple ovarian cysts
2 Raised androgen levels
3 High LH, normal FSH
4 Clinical features
  (a) Obesity
  (b) Hirsutism
  (c) Oligomenorrhoea
  (d) Infertility (some)
  (e) Peripheral insulin resistance and diabetes
5 Treatment
  (a) Metformin improves insulin resistance and increases ovulation

   (b) Diet and exercise increases sex hormone-binding globulin and androgens
   (c) Antiandrogens, such as spironolactone

Precocious puberty

1 True, ie gonadotrophin-dependent causes
   (a) Idiopathic
   (b) CNS/hypothalamic disease (tumour, trauma, infection)
2 Gonadotrophin-independent causes
   (a) CAH
   (b) Excess testosterone
   (c) Adrenal or ovarian tumour
   (d) Oestrogen therapy
   (e) Severe hypothyroidism

Delayed puberty

1 Overt/occult systemic disease
2 Anorexia
3 Genetic disorders, eg Turner's, Klinefelter's, Noonan's, androgen insensitivity

Causes of gynaecomastia

1 Physiological
   (a) Neonate
   (b) Puberty
   (c) Old age
2 Pathological
   (a) Chronic liver disease
   (b) Hyper-/hypothyroidism
   (c) Tumours producing oestrogen (adrenal, testicular)
   (d) Tumours producing HCG (lung, testis)
   (e) Acromegaly
   (f) Starvation
3 Drugs
   (a) Oestrogens
   (b) Digoxin
   (c) Spironolactone
   (d) Cimetidine
   (e) Cyproterone

(f) Gonadotrophins
(g) Cytotoxics
(h) Diamorphine
(i) Cannabis

INSULIN

1 Peptide hormone
2 Synthesised as proinsulin in pancreatic β cells
3 On secretion, cleaved to form insulin and C-peptide
4 Short plasma half-life
5 Acts via receptor tyrosine kinases
6 Stimulates hepatic glycogen and fat synthesis
7 Stimulates muscle to synthesise glycogen and protein
8 Stimulates adipose tissue to synthesise triglycerides
9 Stimulates uptake of glucose and amino acids by muscle
10 Stimulates cellular uptake of potassium
11 Regulators of blood glucose
    (a) Lower blood glucose
        (i) Insulin
    (b) Raise blood glucose
        (i) Glucagon
        (ii) Adrenaline
        (iii) Cortisol
        (iv) GH

Diabetes

WHO definitions

All based on venous plasma values of glucose during oral glucose tolerance test

[See Table 19, overleaf]

or
Single fasting glucose ≥ 7.0 and characteristic diabetic symptoms
or
Fasting glucose of ≥ 7.0 on two separate occasions without characteristic symptoms

Table 19

	Plasma glucose (mmol/l)	
	Fasting	2 hours post glucose load
Diabetes mellitus	≥ 7.0	≥ 11.1
Impaired glucose tolerance	< 7.0	7.8–11.0
Normal	< 7.0	< 7.8

Aetiology

1 Type 1 diabetes mellitus
   (a) 10% of cases
   (b) Juvenile onset
   (c) Insulin dependent (low levels of insulin and C-peptide)
   (d) Antibodies to islet cells in pancreas cause autoimmune destruction of insulin-producing cells
   (e) 60–90% have islet cell antibodies (mainly glutamic acid decarboxylase) at diagnosis
   (f) Some have anti-insulin antibodies
   (g) 50% concordance in identical twins
   (h) 10–20% risk to child if both parents have DM
   (i) HLA DR3/4 associated in 95%
   (j) HLA DR2 protective
   (k) Commonest in Caucasians
2 Type 2 diabetes mellitus
   (a) 85% of cases
   (b) Maturity onset
   (c) Non-insulin dependent
   (d) Peripheral cell resistance to insulin
   (e) No associated autoantibodies
   (f) Identical twins
   (g) 70–100% risk if both parents have
   (h) No HLA association
   (i) Commonest in blacks and Asians
3 Secondary diabetes (5%)
   (a) Due to pancreatic disorders causing insulin deficiency
       (i) Pancreatitis
       (ii) Carcinoma of the pancreas
       (iii) Cystic fibrosis

(iv) Haemochromatosis
(v) Pancreatectomy
(b) Due to insulin resistance
(i) Endocrine causes
(1) Cushing's syndrome
(2) Thyrotoxicosis
(3) Acromegaly
(4) Phaeochromocytoma
(5) Polycystic ovarian syndrome
(6) Glucagonoma
(ii) Drugs
(1) Steroids
(2) Thiazides
(iii) Genetic causes
(1) Congenital lipodystrophy
(2) Friedreich's ataxia

Management

1 Type 1
(a) Insulin therapy
2 Type 2
(a) Weight loss
(b) Oral hypoglycaemics (below)
(c) Insulin
3 All
(a) Good glycaemic control (HbA$_{1c}$ < 7)
(b) Low-sugar, low-fat diet
(c) Avoid smoking
(d) Aggressive blood pressure control (< 130/80) – ACEI first line
(e) Aggressive lipid control
(f) Monitoring renal function and proteinuria
(g) Regular podiatry
(h) Retinal screening
(i) Aspirin

Oral hypoglycaemic agents

1 Metformin
(a) Reduces glucose absorption from gut and increases insulin sensitivity

ENDOCRINOLOGY

(b) No hypoglycaemia
(c) Used in overweight type 2 diabetics as it causes weight loss
(d) May be used with sulphonylureas or glitazones
(e) Duration of action 12–20 hrs
(f) Excreted unchanged in urine
(g) Side effects
   (i) Anorexia
   (ii) Diarrhoea and abdominal pain
   (iii) Contraindicated in renal/hepatic/cardiac failure
   (iv) May cause lactic acidosis

2 Sulphonylureas [See Table 20]
(a) Increase insulin secretion, both basal and stimulated
(b) Reduce peripheral resistance to insulin
(c) Albumin bound, so may be displaced by other drugs
(d) Contraindicated in pregnancy
(e) Effects may be reduced by steroid or thiazide diuretic therapy

Table 20

Name	Duration of action (hours)	Excretion/ metabolism	Side effects
Tolbutamide	6–8	Hepatic	Hypoglycaemia – may be prolonged in drugs with long half-life; skin rashes
Gliclazide	10–12	Hepatic and renal	
Glibenclamide	12–20	Hepatic and renal	
Chlorpropamide	36–48	Renal	Hypoglycaemia, facial flushing with alcohol, cholestatic jaundice, SIADH

3 Thiazolidinedione (glitazones)
(a) Insulin sensitiser
(b) Activate peroxisome proliferator-activated receptor (PPAR-γ)
(c) Used with other oral hypoglycaemics
(d) Hyperinsulinaemia, hyperglycaemia, hypertriglyceridaemia and HbA$_{1c}$ levels improved
(e) May induce cytochrome P450
(f) Side effects: weight gain, oedema, worsening of heart failure and hepatotoxicity

4 Alpha-glucosidase inhibitors, i.e. acarbose
(a) Slow carbohydrate absorption
(b) Not complicated by hypoglycaemia

Diabetic emergencies

Diabetic ketoacidosis (DKA)

1 Usually type 1 DM, may be first presentation
2 State of uncontrolled catabolism due to insulin deficiency
3 Usually due to insulin omission or intercurrent illness
4 Symptoms
  (a) Vomiting
  (b) Polyuria
  (c) Dehydration and thirst
  (d) Abdominal pain
  (e) Kussmaul breathing (acidosis)
  (f) Reduced conscious level
5 Biochemical findings
  (a) Ketonuria
  (b) Hyperglycaemia
  (c) Metabolic acidosis
  (d) Hyperkalaemia
  (e) Renal failure
6 Treatment
  (a) Rehydration (with saline and KCl)
  (b) Insulin
  (c) Low molecular weight heparin
  (d) Treat underlying precipitant

Hyperosmolar non-ketotic state (HONK)

1 Usually type 2 DM
2 Insidious onset
3 May be due to glucose overload or steroid/thiazide treatment in undiagnosed diabetic
4 Profound dehydration and hyperglycaemia
5 Vomiting, acidosis and hyperkalaemia infrequent
6 Raised osmolality
7 Treatment with rehydration; may have dramatic glucose fall with only small amount of insulin

Hypoglycaemia

Causes in diabetes

1 Excess insulin/sulphonylurea treatment
2 Inadequate carbohydrate intake

Causes unrelated to diabetes

1 Insulinoma
2 Malignancy (due to IGF-2)
3 Adrenal failure
4 Pituitary failure
5 Hepatic failure
6 End stage renal failure
7 Chronic alcohol abuse
8 Sepsis
9 Inherited metabolic disorder
10 Post gastrectomy (dumping syndrome)

Insulinoma

1 Pancreatic islet cell tumour
2 Episodic secretion of insulin leading to recurrent hypoglycaemia
3 Diagnosis
   (a) Low fasting glucose with high insulin and high C-peptide
   (b) MRI pancreas

NB Insulin overdose will have high insulin but low C-peptide

Complications of diabetes

Macrovascular

1 Increasing risk of (in increasing size of risk) cerebrovascular disease, ischaemic heart disease and myocardial infarction and peripheral vascular disease
2 Independent of glycaemic control and HbA$_{1c}$
3 Multifactorial: increased age, duration of diabetes, systolic hypertension, hyperlipidaemia and proteinuria. Proteinuria strong risk factor for IHD

Microvascular

1 Progress dependent on degree of glycaemic control

Retinopathy (See Ophthalmology, page 369)

1 Affects 90% at some time
2 Commonest cause of blindness in under 60s
3 Background (early) vs proliferative (late)
4 After 20 years, proliferative retinopathy in 60% of type 1 DM and 20% of type 2

Neuropathy

1 Affects 70–90% at some time
2 Huge range of presentations and severity
3 May be due to ischaemia in vasa nervorum
4 Erectile dysfunction

Autonomic neuropathy

1 General and gustatory sweating
2 Postural hypotension
3 Gastroparesis
4 Diarrhoea
5 Cardiac arrhythmias
6 Charcot joints

Nephropathy (See page 369)

1 Affects 30–40% at some time
2 Commonest cause of death in young diabetics
3 Microalbuminuria = 25–250 mg/day
4 Macroalbuminuria > 250 mg/day
5 With persistent proteinuria, progression to ESRF is likely in 8–10 years
6 ACE inhibitors beneficial

Pregnancy and diabetes

1 Poorly controlled diabetes in the mother is associated with
   (a) Fetal macrosomia (fetal hyperinsulinaemia secondary to hyperglycaemia)

(b) Intrauterine death
(c) 4–8-fold increase in fetal malformation
  (i) Especially poor control weeks 3–6
  (ii) If HbA$_{1c}$ < 7 normal risk
(d) Polyhydramnios
(e) Pre-eclampsia
(f) Neonatal respiratory distress syndrome
(g) Neonatal hypoglycaemia
2 DKA carries 50% mortality
3 Close monitoring important

Gestational diabetes

1 Glucose intolerance during pregnancy which remits after delivery
2 Usually asymptomatic
3 Treatment with diet, but most will need insulin (oral agents may harm fetus)
4 Likely to recur in subsequent pregnancies
5 Increased incidence of type 2 DM later

Gastroenterology

GI PHYSIOLOGY

Gut hormones

Originate from enterochromaffin cells in the epithelium of the GI tract

[See Table 21, overleaf]

Stimulators of acid secretion

1 Vagus
   (a) Direct: stimulates acetylcholine receptors on the parietal cell
   (b) Indirect: increases gastrin secretion
2 Gastrin
3 Histamine (H_2 receptors)

Inhibitors of acid secretion

1 Higher centres
2 Low pH
3 CCK
4 Somatostatin
5 GIP
6 Secretin
7 Protaglandin E_2 (misoprostol)
8 H_2 receptor antagonists (ranitidine, cimetidine)
9 Proton pump inhibitors (omeprazole etc)

Table 21

Hormone	Source	Stimulus	Action
Gastrin	G cells in antrum	Gastric distension Amino acids in antrum Vagal stimulation	↑ Pepsin ↑ Gastric acid ↑ Intrinsic factor ↑ Mucosal blood flow ↑ Gastric motility
Cholecystokinin (CCK)	Duodenum and jejunum	Fats and amino acids in the small bowel	↑ Pancreatic secretion ↑ Gallbladder contraction ↓ Gastric emptying ↑ Insulin and glucagon
Secretin	S cells in duodenum and jejunum	Acid in the small bowel	↑ Pancreatic bicarbonate secretion ↓ Gastric emptying
Motilin	Duodenum and jejunum	Acid in the small bowel	↑ Motility
Vasoactive intestinal peptide (VIP)	Small intestine	Neural stimulation	↓ Gastric acid and pepsin secretion ↑ Secretion by intestine and pancreas
Gastric inhibitory peptide (GIP)	Duodenum and jejunum	Glucose, fats and amino acids	↓ Gastric acid secretion ↑ Insulin secretion ↓ Motility
Somatostatin	D cells in pancreas	Vagal and beta adrenergic stimulation	↓ Gastric and pancreatic secretion Regulates insulin and glucagon secretion
Substance P	Brain and endocrine cells of GI tract	Vagal stimulation	↑ Motility ↑ Gallbladder contraction ↑ Pancreatic secretion
Pancreatic polypeptide	PP cells in pancreas	Protein-rich meal	↓ of pancreatic and biliary secretion

MOUTH

Causes of mouth ulcers

1 Local causes
  (a) Aphthous
  (b) Carcinoma (squamous, adenocarcinoma)
  (c) Trauma
  (d) Denture gingivitis
  (e) Infections
      (i) Herpes simplex (HSV 1)
      (ii) Coxsackie A
      (iii) *Fusobacterium fusiformis*
      (iv) *Borrelia vincenti*
2 Systemic diseases
  (a) GI
      (i) Crohn's
      (ii) Coeliac disease
  (b) Rheumatoid conditions
      (i) Behçet's disease
      (ii) Reiter's syndrome
      (iii) Wegener's granulomatosis
      (iv) SLE
  (c) Infections
      (i) Glandular fever
      (ii) Tuberculosis
      (iii) Syphilis
  (d) Dermatological conditions
      (i) Pemphigus vulgaris
      (ii) Pemphigoid
      (iii) Erythema multiforme and Stevens–Johnson syndrome
      (iv) Lichen planus
  (e) Others
      (i) Cytotoxic drugs
      (ii) Radiotherapy
      (iii) Leukaemia

Causes of gum hypertrophy

1 Scurvy
2 Pregnancy

3 Acute promyelocytic leukaemia
4 Drugs
  (a) Phenytoin
  (b) Nifedipine
  (c) Ciclosporin

Causes of white oral plaques

1 Candidiasis
2 Squamous cell carcinoma
3 Leukoplakia (premalignant condition)
4 Oral hairy leukoplakia (EBV)
5 Frictional keratosis
6 Condylomata lata of secondary syphilis

Causes of pigmentation of oral mucosa

1 Addison's disease
2 Peutz–Jeghers' disease (perioral freckling)
3 Smoker's melanosis
4 Malignant melanoma
5 Acanthosis nigricans
6 Lead poisoning (usually gums)
7 Arsenic poisoning
8 Drugs
  (a) Chloroquine
  (b) Minocycline
  (c) Cyclophosphamide

Causes of glossitis

1 Nutritional deficiency
  (a) B_{12}
  (b) Iron
  (c) Riboflavin
  (d) Niacin
  (e) Pyridoxine
2 Syphilis
3 Inhalation burns
4 Ingestion of corrosive materials

Causes of macroglossia

1 Primary
2 Amyloidosis
3 Acromegaly
4 Hypothyroidism
5 Tongue haemangiomas
6 Neurofibromatosis

Essential features of tongue cancer

1 Squamous cell carcinoma
2 Risk factors
  (a) Smoking
  (b) Alcohol
  (c) Chilli consumption
  (d) Betel nut consumption
  (e) HIV
  (f) HPV-16 infection
3 Leukoplakia and submucosal fibrosis are precancerous lesions
4 Presents as non-resolving lump or oral ulcer
5 Metastasises to submandibular and upper cervical nodes
6 Treatment by excision

Causes of parotid swelling

1 Usually unilateral
  (a) Bacterial parotitis
  (b) Parotid tumours
2 Usually bilateral
  (a) Alcoholism and cirrhosis
  (b) Sarcoidosis
  (c) Sjögren's syndrome
  (d) Lymphoma
  (e) Amyloidosis
  (f) Mumps
  (g) Anorexia nervosa
  (h) Malabsorption
  (i) Acromegaly
  (j) Drugs
    (i) Lead

(ii) Iodides
(iii) Propylthiouracil

Causes of xerostomia (↓ saliva)

1 Dehydration
2 Sjögren's syndrome
3 Granulomatous disease (sarcoid, TB, leprosy)
4 DM
5 Amyloidosis
6 Graft versus host disease
7 Mumps
8 HIV
9 Radiotherapy
10 Drugs
   (a) Anticholinergics
   (b) Neuroleptics
   (c) Antihistamines
   (d) Antidepressants

UPPER GI TRACT

Causes of upper GI bleeding

1 Common
   (a) Duodenal ulcer – 35%
   (b) Gastric ulcer – 20%
   (c) Gastric erosions – 18%
   (d) Mallory–Weiss tear – 10%
2 5% or less
   (a) Duodenitis
   (b) Oesophageal varices
   (c) Oesophagitis
   (d) Upper GI neoplasia
3 1% or less
   (a) Angiodysplasia
   (b) Hereditary haemorrhagic telangiectasia
   (c) Portal hypertensive gastropathy
   (d) Watermelon stomach (gastric antral vascular ectasia)
   (e) Mesenteric ischaemia

(f) Munchausen's syndrome
(g) Aortoduodenal fistula

Causes of dysphagia

1 Obstructive
   (a) Oesophageal cancer
   (b) Peptic strictures
   (c) Oesophageal web or ring
   (d) Gastric cancer
   (e) Pharyngeal cancer
   (f) Plummer–Vinson (Paterson–Brown–Kelly) syndrome –
        oesophageal web, iron deficiency anaemia and oesophageal
        cancer
   (g) Extrinsic pressure from
        (i)   Lung cancer
        (ii)   Mediastinal cancers
        (iii) Retrosternal goitre
        (iv)   Enlarged left atrium
        (v)   Lymphadenopathy
2 GORD and oesophagitis
3 Hiatus hernia
4 Motility disorders
   (a) Neurological
        (i)   Stroke
        (ii)   Bulbar palsy (MND)
        (iii) Pseudobulbar palsy
        (iv)   Myasthenia gravis
        (v)   Parkinson's disease
   (b) Oesophageal
        (i)   Achalasia
        (ii)   Diffuse oesophageal spasm (nutcracker oesophagus,
               corkscrew oesophagus)
        (iii) Systemic sclerosis
        (iv)   Chagas' disease
5 Pharyngeal pouch
6 Oesophageal diverticula
7 Oesophageal candidiasis
8 Herpes simplex oesophagitis
9 Globus hystericus

Essential features of oesophageal cancer

1 Squamous (sq) – usually upper or middle third
2 Adenocarcinoma (ad) – usually lower third (arises from Barrett's epithelium)
3 Incidence increasing
4 50% have metastases at diagnosis
5 Currently 14% overall 5-year survival
6 Risk factors:
   (a) Smoking (sq, ad)
   (b) Alcohol (sq)
   (c) Achalasia (sq)
   (d) Barrett's oesophagus (ad)
   (e) Tylosis (sq) – autosomal dominant palmar and plantar keratosis
   (f) Paterson–Brown–Kelly syndrome (Plummer–Vinson) (sq)
   (g) GORD (ad)
   (h) Caustic injury (sq)
7 Symptoms
   (a) Dysphagia (74%) for solids then liquids
   (b) Weight loss (57%)
   (c) Pain and dyspepsia
   (d) Haematemesis and melaena
8 Diagnosis
   (a) Endoscopy
   (b) Barium swallow
   (c) CT, EUS and laparoscopy for staging
9 Treatment
   (a) Surgery
   (b) Endoscopy and stenting
   (c) Radiotherapy
   (d) Chemotherapy (cisplatin and 5-fluorouracil)

Essential features of Barrett's oesophagus

1 Complication of long-term gastro-oesophageal reflux
2 Present in 11% of patients symptomatic of GORD
3 Lower oesophageal squamous mucosa replaced with columnar specialised intestinal metaplasia in response to acid
4 Predisposes to adenocarcinoma (0.5% per year if ≥ 3 cm segment)
5 Patients with dysplasia are at highest risk of developing carcinoma
6 Treatment with long term PPIs (but this will not reverse it)

7 Screening for carcinoma in patients with Barrett's has been advocated – no evidence of lives saved yet

Essential features of hiatus hernia

1 Herniation of proximal stomach into the thoracic cavity
2 Sliding (80%) or rolling (20%)
3 Common 30% > 50 yrs
4 50% have GORD
5 Diagnosis by gastroscopy or barium meal
6 Treatment
   (a) Weight loss
   (b) Antacids
   (c) PPIs
   (d) Surgery

Essential features of gastro-oesophageal reflux disease and oesophagitis

1 Very common
2 Symptoms
   (a) Chest pain – retrosternal discomfort
   (b) Dysphagia
   (c) Waterbrash
   (d) Nocturnal cough and wheeze
   (e) Eructation (belching)
3 Complications
   (a) Oesophagitis/ulcer
   (b) Stricture
   (c) Iron deficiency anaemia
   (d) Barrett's oesophagus
   (e) Pulmonary aspiration
4 Aggravating factors
   (a) Obesity
   (b) Smoking
   (c) Alcohol
   (d) Coffee
   (e) Large meals
   (f) Hiatus hernia
   (g) Pregnancy
   (h) Systemic sclerosis

   (i) Fatty foods
   (j) Chocolate
   (k) Drugs – nitrates, anticholinergics, NSAIDs, bisphosphonates, K$^+$
5 Investigation
   (a) Symptoms do not correlate with endoscopic appearance
   (b) 24 hr pH monitoring (symptoms correlate with low pH)
6 Treatment
   (a) Lifestyle changes
   (b) Antacids
   (c) H$_2$ antagonists
   (d) PPIs
   (e) Promotility agents – metoclopramide, domperidone
   (f) Fundoplication (open/laparoscopic/endoscopic)

Essential features of achalasia

1 Lack of relaxation of lower oesophageal sphincter (LOS), abnormal peristalsis and dilated oesophagus proximal to sphincter
2 Loss of ganglia from myenteric plexus
3 Symptoms
   (a) Dysphagia – solids and liquids from onset
   (b) Regurgitation
   (c) Chest pain
   (d) Weight loss
   (e) Aspiration pneumonia
4 Diagnosis by barium swallow or oesophageal manometry
5 Complications: squamous carcinoma, aspiration
6 Treatment
   (a) Endoscopic dilatation
   (b) Surgical myotomy
   (c) Botulinum toxin to LOS

Helicobacter pylori

1 Spiral, flagellate, Gram-negative, microaerophilic bacteria
2 Cag A-positive *H. pylori* are pathogenic
3 Produces urease, which hydrolyses urea to ammonia to neutralise the surrounding area
4 More common in low socioeconomic groups and gastroenterologists!

5 Diseases associated
  (a) Acute gastritis (some patients have an acute illness when infected)
  (b) Chronic gastritis
    (i) Pangastritis – leads to atrophic gastritis
    (ii) Antral gastritis – may lead to DU
    (iii) Gastritis of corpus – may lead to GU and adenocarcinoma
  (c) DU (95% HP-positive)
  (d) GU (80% HP-positive)
  (e) Gastric adenocarcinoma
  (f) Gastric lymphoma – MALToma
6 Methods of detection:
  (a) Rapid urease test at endoscopy (95% specificity, 95% sensitivity)
  (b) Histology (100% specificity, 85% sensitivity)
  (c) Culture (100% specificity, 95% sensitivity – useful for sensitivities to antibiotics)
  (d) Urea breath test (95% specificity, 97% sensitivity)
  (e) Serology (50–90% specificity, 70–90% sensitivity)
  (f) Stool antigen tests (90% specificity, 89–98% sensitivity)
7 Eradicate with triple therapy, e.g. omeprazole, metronidazole and clarithromycin

Causes of gastritis

1 *H. pylori*
2 Atrophic gastritis
3 Pernicious anaemia
4 NSAIDs
5 Alcohol
6 Stress
7 Infections in the immunocompromised
  (a) CMV
  (b) HSV
  (c) *Candida*
  (d) TB
8 Gastric ischaemia
9 Radiation
10 Corrosive substances
11 Ménétrièr's disease
12 Eosinophilic gastritis
13 Granulomatous gastritis

Risk factors for peptic ulcer disease

1 *H. pylori*
2 High alcohol intake
3 NSAID use
4 High-dose steroids
5 Male gender
6 Smoking
7 Zollinger–Ellison syndrome
8 Stress (Curling's ulcer)
9 Head trauma (Cushing's ulcer)
10 Blood group O (duodenal)

Risk factors for gastric carcinoma

1 Japanese
2 *H. pylori*
3 Pernicious anaemia
4 Chronic atrophic gastritis
5 Male gender
6 Blood group A
7 Gastric resection (increased bile reflux)
8 Nitrosamines in diet
9 Adenomatous polyps > 2 cm in stomach

Essential features of gastrinoma

1 Leads to Zollinger–Ellison syndrome
2 Usually pancreatic (also stomach, duodenum or adjacent tissues)
3 50–60% malignant
4 10% multiple
5 Associated with MEN 1 (30%)
6 Signs
   (a) Single ulcer (most common endoscopic finding)
   (b) Multiple peptic ulcers
   (c) Steatorrhoea and diarrhoea (40%)
7 Diagnosis
   (a) High serum fasting gastrin with little further increase with
      pentagastrin
   (b) CT/EUS/MRI to find tumour (40% < 1 cm) and assess for
      metastases

(c) Somatostatin receptor scintigraphy (most sensitive non-invasive method for localising primary and metastases)

8 Treatment
   (a) High-dose omeprazole 80–120 mg daily
   (b) Surgery to resect adenoma
   (c) Octreotide to reduce diarrhoea

Causes of hypergastrinaemia

1 Achlorhydria
2 PPI therapy
3 Zollinger–Ellison syndrome
4 *H. pylori*
5 Antral G-cell hyperplasia
6 CRF
7 Gastric outlet obstruction

Complications of gastrectomy

1 Early satiety
2 Abdominal fullness
3 Dumping syndrome (40%)
4 Postprandial hypoglycaemia
5 Bile reflux
6 Weight loss and malnutrition
7 Iron deficiency anaemia (common)
8 Malabsorption and bacterial overgrowth
9 B_{12} deficiency
10 Osteoporosis/osteomalacia
11 Gallstones
12 Anastomotic ulcers
13 May predispose to carcinoma in the gastric remnant

Causes of vomiting

1 GI irritation
   (a) Enteritis
   (b) Drugs – NSAIDs, alcohol
   (c) Poisons
   (d) Gastritis
   (e) Gastric ulcer

2 Obstruction
   (a) Atresia
   (b) Stricture or stenosis – malignant, benign
   (c) Adhesions
   (d) Intussusception
   (e) Volvulus
   (f) Hernia
   (g) Paralytic ileus
3 Intra-abdominal inflammation
   (a) Hepatitis
   (b) Pancreatitis
   (c) Appendicitis
   (d) Pyelonephritis
   (e) Cholecystitis
4 Metabolic and endocrine
   (a) Diabetic ketoacidosis/hypoglycaemia
   (b) Pregnancy
   (c) Uraemia
   (d) Hypoadrenalism
   (e) Hypercalcaemia
5 CNS
   (a) Psychogenic
   (b) Severe pain
   (c) Drugs (opioids, chemotherapeutic drugs)
   (d) Migraine
   (e) Motion sickness
   (f) Meningitis
   (g) Menière's disease
   (h) Labyrinthitis
   (i) Raised ICP (benign, malignant)
6 Miscellaneous
   (a) Acute dilatation of the stomach
   (b) Cyclical vomiting
   (c) Radiation sickness

SMALL BOWEL DISORDERS

Causes of malabsorption

Conditions within the gut lumen

1 Lack of pancreatic enzymes
   (a) Chronic pancreatitis
   (b) Cystic fibrosis
   (c) Pancreatic carcinoma
   (d) Genetic pancreatic insufficiency
2 Lack of bile salts
   (a) Obstructive jaundice
   (b) Cholestatic liver disease
   (c) Bile salt loss
   (d) Bacterial overgrowth
3 Infective
   (a) Travellers' diarrhoea
   (b) Intestinal TB
   (c) Parasitic disease (especially *Giardia*)/helminthic
   (d) HIV
   (e) Tropical sprue
4 Inadequate mixing and motility disorders
   (a) Post gastrectomy
   (b) Thyrotoxicosis
   (c) Diabetes (autonomic neuropathy)
   (d) Systemic sclerosis

Conditions in the gut mucosa

1 Coeliac disease
2 Disaccharidase deficiency (lactase, sucrase–isomaltase deficiency)
3 Postinfectious malabsorption
4 Whipple's disease
5 Immunodeficiency (hypogammaglobulinaemia)
6 Crohn's disease
7 Cows' milk sensitivity in infants

Structural disorders

1 Intestinal/gastric resection
2 Radiation enteritis

3 Mesenteric arterial insufficiency
4 Small intestinal lymphoma or other malignancy
5 Amyloidosis

Conditions outside the gut mucosa

1 Intestinal lymphangiectasia

Drugs

1 Alcohol
2 Neomycin
3 Metformin
4 Cholestyramine
5 Colchicine

Some useful tests for malabsorption

Table 22

Test	Use
Iron/ferritin	↓ in proximal small bowel disease
Folate	↓ in proximal small bowel disease
	↑ in bacterial overgrowth
B_{12}	↓ PA
	↓ in bacterial overgrowth
	↓ in terminal ileal disease
	↓ in chronic pancreatitis
	Shilling's test useful to differentiate
Faecal fat	Steatorrhoea
^{14}C triolein breath test	↓ in fat malabsorption
Stool α_1-antitrypsin	↑ in protein losing enteropathy
D-xylose test	↓ in small bowel disease
	Normal in pancreatic disease
PABA test	↓ in pancreatic disease
Pancreolauryl test	
Faecal elastase	
Hydrogen breath test	↑ in bacterial overgrowth
^{14}C glycocholate breath test	
Duodenal biopsy	Histological diagnosis, eg coeliac
Jejunal aspirate	Bacterial overgrowth
Barium follow-through/small bowel enema	Structural defects in the small bowel, eg terminal ileal stricture, diverticulae
SeHCAT	Bile acid malabsorption

Causes of non-infective diarrhoea (See Infective diarrhoea, page 251)

1 Colonic
   (a) IBS
   (b) Colonic neoplasia
   (c) Inflammatory bowel disease
   (d) Microscopic/lymphocytic/collagenous colitis
2 Small bowel
   (a) Coeliac disease
   (b) Crohn's
   (c) Disaccharidase deficiency
   (d) Small bowel bacterial overgrowth
   (e) Mesenteric ischaemia
3 Bile acid malabsorption
   (a) Giardiasis
   (b) Intestinal lymphoma
   (c) Whipple's disease
   (d) Tropical sprue
   (e) Amyloidosis
4 Pancreatic
   (a) Chronic pancreatitis
   (b) Pancreatic carcinoma
   (c) Cystic fibrosis
5 Endocrine
   (a) Thyrotoxicosis
   (b) Diabetes (autonomic neuropathy)
   (c) Adrenal insufficiency
   (d) Carcinoid syndrome
   (e) VIPomas
   (f) Gastrinomas
   (g) Medullary carcinoma of thyroid
6 Others
   (a) Post vagotomy/gastrectomy
   (b) Small bowel resections/fistulae
   (c) Laxative abuse
   (d) HIV
   (e) Immunoglobulin deficiency
7 Drugs
   (a) Antibiotics

(b) Mg-based antacids
(c) Lansoprazole
(d) Metformin
(e) Alcohol

Causes of bacterial overgrowth

1 ↓ Acid
   (a) Atrophic gastritis
   (b) Vagotomy
   (c) PPIs and H_2 blockers
2 Blind loops
3 Diverticulae
4 Fistulae
5 Obstruction
   (a) Adhesions
   (b) Strictures
6 Disordered motility
   (a) Systemic sclerosis
   (b) Diabetic autonomic neuropathy
   (c) Amyloid
7 Hypogammaglobulinaemia
8 Cirrhosis

Essential features of coeliac disease

1 Sensitivity to gluten (gliadin fraction) leads to inflammatory injury to the small intestine
2 0.5% of population (recent ↑ diagnosis due to serology)
3 HLA DQ2 in 95%
4 Inappropriate T-cell response against ingested gluten, with the enzyme tissue transglutamase the target of autoimmune response
5 Definite associations are: DM, autoimmune thyroid disease, Sjögren's, RA, microscopic colitis, Down's, IgA nephropathy
6 Clinical features
   (a) Diarrhoea
   (b) Anaemia (iron, folate, B_{12})
   (c) Weight loss
   (d) Steatorrhoea (vitamin A, D, E, K deficiency)
   (e) Growth retardation
   (f) Oral aphthous ulcers

(g) Increased incidence of all GI malignancy (esp. small bowel lymphoma)
(h) Reduced incidence of breast and lung cancer
(i) Dermatitis herpetiformis
(j) Hyposplenism
(k) ↓ Ca/osteomalacia/osteoporosis
(l) IgA deficiency (5%)

7 Diagnosis
(a) Duodena/jejunal biopsy – ↑ intraepithelial lymphocytes, villous atrophy
(b) Tissue transglutaminase (tTG Abs) – most accurate
(c) Endomysial Ab
(d) Antigliadin Ab and antireticulin Ab – poorly specific

8 Treatment with gluten-free diet – 3-month recovery of villous atrophy

Essential features of Whipple's disease

1 Infection with *Tropheryma whippleii* (Gram-positive actinomycete)
2 Associated with HLA B27
3 Clinical features
(a) Diarrhoea
(b) Malabsorption
(c) Arthropathy
(d) Lymphadenopathy
(e) Finger clubbing
4 Diagnosis is histological – jejunal biopsy shows macrophages containing PAS-positive granules within the villi
5 Treatment with penicillin, erythromycin or cephalosporin (long-term recommended)

Causes of villous atrophy

1 Coeliac disease
2 Dermatitis herpetiformis
3 Whipple's disease
4 Hypogammaglobulinaemia
5 Lymphoma
6 Tropical sprue

Essential features of carcinoid tumours

1 Carcinoid tumours present in 1% of postmortems – rarely metastasise
2 Carcinoid syndrome (very rare) – liver metastases lead to systemic release of serotonin
3 Tumours arise from enterochromaffin cells in the lamina propria
4 Appendix is most common site (also bronchial, rectal and ovarian)
5 Can present with intestinal obstruction
6 Clinical features (carcinoid syndrome)
  (a) Flushing of head and upper thorax
  (b) Bronchoconstriction
  (c) Diarrhoea
  (d) Right valvular stenosis (left if an ASD is present or bronchial carcinoid)
  (e) Can lead to pellagra due to tumour uptake of tryptophan
7 Diagnosis
  (a) 5-Hydroxyindoleacetic acid (5-HIAA) detected in the urine.
  (b) CT/EUS/MRI to find primary
8 Treatment
  (a) Surgical resection
  (b) Chemotherapy
  (c) Embolisation of hepatic metastases
  (d) Octreotide
  (e) Cyproheptadine – $5HT_2$ antagonist

Essential features of VIPoma

1 Neuroendocrine tumour, produces VIP (90% pancreatic)
2 50% malignant
3 Clinical features
  (a) Secretory diarrhoea (large volume: > 3 l/day)
  (b) Severe hypokalaemia and acidosis (K^+ and HCO_3 loss)
  (c) Severe dehydration
  (d) Hypotension
  (e) Abdominal colic
  (f) Flushing
  (g) Weight loss
4 Diagnosis
  (a) ↑ VIP
  (b) CT/MRI/EUS to find tumour

(c) ^{123}I – VIP receptor scintigraphy
5 Treatment
   (a) Resection
   (b) Octreotide (reduces diarrhoea)
   (c) Chemotherapy

Protein-losing enteropathy

1 Excessive loss of protein from the GI tract, leading to hypoalbuminaemia
2 Causes
   (a) Ulcerative/erosive mucosal diseases
      (i)   Ileitis
      (ii) Ulcerative colitis
      (iii) Mucosal neoplasia
      (iv) GVHD
      (v) Pseudomembranous colitis (*Clostridium difficile*)
   (b) Lymphatic obstruction or ↑ interstitial pressure
      (i)   Intestinal lymphangiectasia
      (ii) Constrictive pericarditis
   (c) Non-erosive GI diseases
      (i)   Coeliac disease
      (ii) Tropical sprue
      (iii) Whipple's disease
      (iv) Ménétrièr's disease (Giant hypertrophy of gastric rugae)
      (v) Eosinophilic gastroenteropathy
   (d) Diagnosis:
      (i)   ↑ Stool α_1-antitrypsin
      (ii) Rate of loss of protein into the intestine with radiolabelled ^{51}Cr-albumin
      (iii) Diagnosis of underlying disease
   (e) Treatment: correct underlying cause

Features of Crohn's disease and ulcerative colitis

[See Table 23, overleaf]

Table 23

Crohn's disease	Ulcerative colitis
• Patchy transmural inflammation that may affect any part of the GI tract • Commonly terminal ileum, colon, anorectum • 'Skip lesions' of normal mucosa between affected areas	• Diffuse mucosal inflammation limited to the colon • Usually involves rectum and extends confluently into the colon (occasional rectal sparing) • Terminal ileum may be affected by 'backwash ileitis'

Pathology

• Transmural inflammation • Non-caseating granuloma (65%) – most reliable • Fissuring ulcers • Lymphoid aggregates • Neutrophil infiltrates	• Mucosa and submucosa only involved, leading to ulceration • Neutrophil infiltrate • Crypt abscesses • Loss of goblet cells

Clinical features

• Abdominal pain prominent and fever
• Diarrhoea +/- blood PR
• Mouth ulcers
• Weight loss
• Anal/perianal/oral lesions
• Fistulae
• Stricturing common, resulting in obstructive symptoms
• Anaemia (Fe, B_{12} or folate deficiency)
• ↑ Incidence in smokers
• Extraintestinal features
  o Erythema nodosum
  o Pyoderma gangrenosum
  o Uveitis/episcleritis
  o Arthropathy
  o Sacroileitis
  o Cholelithiasis
  o Clubbing
	• Diarrhoea, often with blood and mucus
	• Urgency and tenesmus
	• Weight loss
	• Fever
	• Abdominal pain less prominent
	• Iron deficiency anaemia
	• ↓ Incidence in smokers
	• ↑ Incidence of primary sclerosing cholangitis
	• Other systemic manifestations less common than in Crohn's disease
	• Hyposplenism
	• pANCA (70%)

Diagnosis

• Colonoscopy/ileoscopy and biopsy
• Barium studies
  o Cobblestoning of mucosa
  o Rose thorn ulcers
  o Skip lesions
  o Strictures
	• Sigmoidoscopy/colonoscopy and biopsy
	• Barium studies:
	  o Pseudopolyps
	  o Loss of haustral pattern
	  o Featureless shortened colon

Table 23 (cont.)

Crohn's disease	Ulcerative colitis

- Isotope leukocyte scans useful to diagnose active small bowel disease
- Capsule endoscopy

Complications

Crohn's disease
- Fistulae
  - o Enteroenteral
  - o Enterovesical
  - o Enterovaginal
  - o Perianal
- Carcinoma – slightly increased incidence of colonic malignancy and small bowel lymphoma
- Abscess formation
- B_{12} deficiency (terminal ileal disease)
- Osteomalacia/osteoporosis
- Amyloidosis

Ulcerative colitis
- Toxic megacolon (urgent indication for colectomy)
- Increased incidence of carcinoma – risk ↑ after 8–10yrs of disease
- Preventative colectomy of value
- Iron deficiency anaemia

Treatment

Active CD
- Stop smoking
- 5-ASA
- Steroids (oral/IV)
- Azathioprine
- Methotrexate
- Infliximab
- Surgery
- Nutritional support
- Elemental diets

Perianal disease
- Metronidazole
- Ciprofloxacin
- Azathioprine
- Infliximab
- Surgery

- **Maintenance of remission**
- Stop smoking
- 5-ASA
- Azathioprine
- Methotrexate
- Infliximab

Active UC
Extensive colitis
Mild to moderate
- 5-ASA (mesalazine, balsalazide)
- Steroids (enemas)

Severe
- Steroids (oral/IV)
- Surgery

Refractory
- Steroids
- Ciclosporin
- Azathioprine
- Infliximab
- Surgery

Distal colitis
- Rectal 5-ASA (first-line)
- Rectal steroids
- Oral 5-ASA
- Oral steroids if fail to respond

- **Maintenance of remission**
- Oral 5-ASA (will also ↓ risk of colorectal cancer)
- Azathioprine
- Steroids do not reduce relapse

LARGE BOWEL DISORDERS

Causes of lower GI bleeding

1 Haemorrhoids
2 Anal fissure
3 Diverticular disease
4 Lower GI neoplasia – adenomatous polyps, carcinomas
5 Inflammatory bowel disease (UC/Crohn's)
6 Infective enterocolitis – *Salmonella*, *Shigella*, *E. coli*, amoebiasis
7 Ischaemic colitis
8 Rectal varices
9 Angiodysplasia
10 Meckel's diverticulum
11 Iatrogenic (endoscopy)

Causes of constipation

1 Inadequate dietary fibre
2 Dehydration
3 Immobility
4 Obstruction
   (a) Colonic neoplasm
   (b) Crohn's disease (strictures)
   (c) Volvulus
   (d) Pelvic mass
5 Disordered motility
   (a) Functional constipation (IBS)
   (b) Diverticular disease
   (c) Chronic pseudo-obstruction
   (d) Hirschsprung's disease
6 Endocrine
   (a) Hypercalcaemia
   (b) Hypothyroidism
   (c) Pregnancy
7 Neurological
   (a) Spinal cord and sacral nerve disease
   (b) Parkinson's disease
   (c) Diabetic neuropathy
8 Drugs
   (a) Opiates

(b) Iron
(c) Anticholinergics
(d) TCAs
(e) Calcium antagonists

Essential features of colorectal cancer (CRC)

1 Adenocarcinoma arising from tubular or villous adenomatous polyps
2 Multiple genetic mutations occur in the transition from normal to carcinoma, eg APC, K-*ras*, p53.
3 Commonest in rectum (30%) and sigmoid (30%)
4 Risk factors
    (a) Male gender
    (b) Colitis (UC, Crohn's)
    (c) Strong family history
        (i) Familial polyposis coli (AD)
        (ii) Hereditary non-polyposis colon cancer (AD)
    (d) Dietary (low fibre, high in fat and red meat)
    (e) Alcohol and smoking
    (f) Ureterosigmoidostomy
    (g) PSC
    (h) Acromegaly
    (i) NSAIDs may be protective
5 Clinical features
    (a) Weight loss
    (b) Altered bowel habit
    (c) Abdominal pain
    (d) Abdominal mass
    (e) Right-sided
        (i) Iron deficiency anaemia
    (f) Left-sided
        (i) Blood PR
        (ii) Altered bowel habit
        (iii) Obstruction
        (iv) Tenesmus
6 Treatment
    (a) Surgical resection (including partial hepatectomy in metastases confined to one lobe and no distant metastases)
    (b) Radiotherapy
    (c) Adjuvant chemotherapy for Duke's B and C

(d) Carcinoembryonic antigen (CEA) can be used to monitor for recurrence.

Duke's staging of CRC

Table 24

Stage	5-yr survival
A – confined to mucosa and submucosa	80%+
B – extends through muscularis propria	60–70%
C – regional lymph nodes involved	30–40%
D – distant spread	0%

Inherited GI syndromes that predispose to CRC

1 Familial adenomatous polyposis
  (a) AD
  (b) Hundreds of adenomatous polyps in colon
  (c) 100% risk of CRC
  (d) Mutation of APC gene
  (e) Treatment with colectomy
2 Hereditary non-polyposis colorectal cancer
  (a) Develop adenomatous polyps
  (b) 80% develop CRC
  (c) Defect in mismatch repair genes *MLH1*, *MSH2*, *MSH6*
  (d) Patients have strong family history of CRC at young age
  (e) Family members need screening
3 Peutz–Jegher's syndrome
  (a) Perioral freckling
  (b) Multiple hamartomatous polyps throughout GI tract
  (c) Mutation of STK11 gene
  (d) 40% risk of CRC
  (e) Need to undergo screening colonoscopy

Essential features of IBS

1 Diagnosed by Rome II criteria
  (a) 12 weeks or more in the last 12 months of abdominal discomfort that has two of the following three features
    (i) Relieved by defecation
    (ii) Associated with a change in frequency of stool
    (iii) Associated with a change in consistency of stool

2 Treatment
  (a) Dietary modification
  (b) ↑ or ↓ fibre
  (c) TCAs (can aggravate constipation)
  (d) Loperamide or codeine if diarrhoea
  (e) Laxatives if constipation
  (f) Antispasmodics
  (g) Anticholinergics
  (h) Psychotherapy
  (i) 5HT$_3$ and 5HT$_4$ antagonists have shown promise, but there is risk of ischaemic colitis

Causes of acute intestinal pseudo-obstruction

1 Postoperative
2 Liver failure
3 Acute pancreatitis
4 Acute cholecystitis
5 Intestinal ischaemia
6 Retroperitoneal haematoma
7 Idiopathic
8 Metabolic
  (a) Hypokalaemia
  (b) Hyper-/hypocalcaemia
  (c) Hypomagnesaemia
  (d) Hypothyroidism

LIVER DISORDERS

Causes of jaundice

Prehepatic

1 Congenital hyperbilirubinaemia (below)
2 Haemolysis (See page 192)

Hepatic

1 Alcohol
2 Hepatitis viruses
  (a) A–E viruses (See page 153)

    (b) Non A–E
    (c) EBV
    (d) CMV
    (e) HIV
3 Drugs (See page 163)
4 Autoimmune
    (a) Primary biliary cirrhosis
    (b) Autoimmune (lupoid) hepatitis
    (c) Primary sclerosing cholangitis
    (d) SLE
    (e) Scleroderma
5 Hereditary
    (a) Wilson's disease
    (b) Haemochromatosis
    (c) $Alpha_1$-antitrypsin deficiency
    (d) Cystic fibrosis
6 Neoplastic
    (a) Hepatocellular carcinoma
    (b) Liver metastases
7 Non-alcoholic steatohepatitis
8 Pregnancy (See page 170)
9 Right heart failure/constrictive pericarditis
10 Budd–Chiari syndrome
11 Other infections
    (a) Schistosomiasis (*Schistosoma japonicum*)
    (b) Leptospirosis
    (c) Toxoplasmosis
    (d) Amoebiasis
    (e) Malaria

Posthepatic

Benign

1 Gallstones in bile duct
2 Ascending cholangitis
3 Acute and chronic pancreatitis
4 Post-traumatic stricture
5 Sclerosing cholangitis
6 Biliary atresia
7 Choledochal cyst

8 Retroperitoneal fibrosis
9 Haemobilia
10 Helminthic infections
11 Mirizzi's syndrome

Malignant

1 Pancreatic carcinoma
2 Cholangiocarcinoma
3 Carcinoma of the gallbladder
4 Carcinoma of the ampulla of Vater
5 Carcinoma of duodenum
6 Hilar lymphadenopathy

Essential features of congenital hyperbilirubinaemia

[See Table 25, overleaf]

Essential features of viral hepatitis

[See Table 26, overleaf]

HBV serology

1 HBsAg – present in acute infection; if present for more than 6 months = chronic hepatitis
2 HBeAg – present in acute or chronic infection; signifies high infectivity (absent in precore mutant)
3 HBcAg – present in acute or chronic infection; found only in liver tissue; present for life
4 AntiHBs – signifies immunity after vaccination or acute infection
5 AntiHBe – signifies declining infectivity and resolving infection
6 AntiHBc IgM – signifies recent acute infection; lasts less than 6 months
7 AntiHBc IgG – a lifelong marker of past acute or chronic infection; does not signify immunity or previous vaccination

[See Table 27, page 156]

Table 25

Syndrome	Genetics	Defect	Clinical features	Treatment
Gilbert's	AD	Defect in conjugation	Raised unconjugated bilirubin Asymptomatic or jaundice (increases with fasting)	None
Crigler–Najjar type 1	AR UGT-1 gene	Defect in conjugation	Neonatal kernicterus and death	Fatal untreated Liver transplant
Crigler–Najjar type 2	AD UGT-1 gene	Defect in conjugation	Jaundice as a neonate/child, survive into adulthood	Phenobarbitone reduces jaundice
Dubin–Johnson	AR CMOAT gene	Defect in hepatic excretion	Raised conjugated bilirubin Jaundice with RUQ pain and malaise	None benign
Rotor	AD	Defect in uptake and storage of bilirubin	Raised conjugated bilirubin	None benign

Table 26

	Spread	Virus	Clinical	Management	Incubation
A	F-O	RNA	Anorexia Jaundice Nausea Joint pains Fever	Supportive Benign condition Fulminant hepatitis in 0.2% No chronicity	15–40 days
B	Blood, sexual, vertical	DNA	Asymptomatic (70%) Jaundice Acute fever Arteritis Glomerulonephritis Arthropathy	Supportive <1% fulminant hepatitis 5–10% remain chronic HBV (risk of cirrhosis and HCC) – treatment below	50–180 days
C	Blood, sexual	RNA	Asymptomatic (95%) Jaundice Malaise	Fulminant hepatitis rare 60–80% chronic HCV (risk of cirrhosis and HCC) – treatment below	40–55 days
D	Blood (depending on concurrent HBV infection for replication)	Incomplete	Exacerbates HBV infection and increases risk of hepatic failure and cirrhosis	Supportive Increases incidence of cirrhosis in chronic HBV	
E	F-O	RNA	Acute self-limiting illness In pregnancy mortality (fetal and maternal) of 25%	Supportive No chronicity	30–50 days

Table 27

	HB surface Ag	HB core IgM	HBBe Ag	HBe Ab	Hb core Ab (total)	Hb surface Ab
Active infection with HBV	+	+	+	–	+	–
Chronic carrier of high infectivity	+	–	+	–	+	–
Chronic carrier of intermediate infectivity	+	–	–	–	+	–
Chronic carrier of low infectivity	+	–	–	+	+	–
Infection with HBV sometime in the past	–	–	–	–/+	+	–
Natural immunity to HBV	–	–	–	–/+	+	+
Vaccine-induced immunity to HBV	–	–	–	–	–	+

Treatment of chronic viral hepatitis

HBV

[See Table 28, opposite]

HCV

1 Pegylated interferon and ribavirin
2 Genotype 1 or 4 – 50% sustained viral response rate with 48 weeks' treatment

Table 28

Characteristic	Chronic hepatitis B	Inactive HBsAg carrier
HBsAg	Pos (> 6 months)	Pos (> 6 months)
ALT	Raised (> 2 × upper limit normal)	Normal
Serum HBV DNA	> 10^5	< 10^5
Liver biopsy (histological activity)	≥ 4	≤ 3
Risk of HCC	↑↑	↑
Treatment	Yes *Options* Interferon (16 weeks) 30% response (viral and histological) Lamivudine – 21% response at 1yr Risk of viral resistance – YMDD mutation Long-term will reduce risk of HCC and hepatic decompensation Adefovir – can be used when viral resistance a problem Liver transplant	No – slow progression

3 Genotype 2 or 3 – 80% sustained viral response rate with 24 weeks' treatment
4 Side effects
   (a) IFN – fever, headache, myelosuppression, depression, development of autoantibodies
   (b) Ribavirin – haemolytic anaemia, teratogenicity

Essential features of primary biliary cirrhosis (PBC)

1 Progressive inflammation and destruction of small bile duct, leading to cirrhosis
2 Probably autoimmune
3 90% are female
4 Associations
   (a) HLA DR8

   (b) Scleroderma
   (c) CREST syndrome
   (d) Sjögren's syndrome
   (e) Seropositive and seronegative arthritis
   (f) Thyroiditis
   (g) Renal tubular acidosis
   (h) Coeliac disease
   (i) Pulmonary fibrosis
5 Clinical features
   (a) Asymptomatic
   (b) Cholestatic jaundice
   (c) Pruritus
   (d) Xanthelasma (hypercholesterolaemia)
   (e) Skin pigmentation
   (f) Clubbing
   (g) Hepatosplenomegaly
   (h) Portal hypertension
   (i) Osteomalacia/osteoporosis
6 Diagnosis
   (a) Antimitochondrial antibodies in 95%
   (b) Predominantly raised ALP (cholestatic picture)
   (c) Raised IgM
   (d) Liver biopsy – portal tract inflammation, destruction of
        interlobular ducts, small duct proliferation, fibrosis and cirrhosis
7 Treatment
   (a) Symptomatic therapy
   (b) Transplantation
   (c) Ursodeoxycholic acid may reduce time to transplantation

Essential features of autoimmune hepatitis

1 Female predominance 4:1
2 Associations: other autoimmune disorders and HLA DR3 and DR4
3 Clinical features
   (a) Present with acute hepatitis, chronic hepatitis or cirrhosis
   (b) Epigastric pain
   (c) Arthralgia
   (d) Myalgia
   (e) Fluctuating jaundice
   (f) Cushingoid appearance

4 Diagnosis
  (a) Raised IgG
  (b) Hepatitic LFTs
  (c) 80% ANA or SMA positive (type 1)
  (d) 3–4% liver/kidney/microsomal Abs positive (type 2)
  (e) Anti-SLA Abs (type 3)
  (f) Liver biopsy is required for diagnosis – interface hepatitis
5 Treatment
  (a) Steroids to induce remission and azathioprine to maintain it
  (b) Liver transplant

Essential features of primary sclerosing cholangitis (PSC)

1 Obliterative inflammatory fibrosis of the biliary tract
2 Generalised beading of and stenosis of the biliary tract
3 Aetiology: unknown
4 Complications
  (a) Cirrhosis
  (b) Cholangiocarcinoma 15% (CA19-9 useful to screen)
  (c) Cholangitis
  (d) ↑ Risk of colorectal carcinoma
5 Associations
  (a) Inflammatory bowel disease (mainly UC (95%))
  (b) HLA DR2
6 Diagnosis
  (a) ↑ ALP
  (b) Bilirubin raised late in disease
  (c) ERCP or MRCP for diagnosis
  (d) Liver biopsy
  (e) pANCA positive in 80%
  (f) Smooth muscle antibody (30%)
  (g) ANA positive in 30%
7 Treatment
  (a) Symptomatic
  (b) Ursodeoxycholic acid
  (c) Dilatation or stenting of dominant strictures
  (d) Liver transplant (second most common reason for transplant in UK)

Fatty liver

1 Non-alcoholic fatty liver (NAFL)
   (a) Benign steatosis without inflammation of fibrosis
2 Non-alcoholic steatohepatitis (NASH) – 20%
   (a) Necroinflammation and pericellular fibrosis
   (b) Can progress to cirrhosis
   (c) Major cause of cryptogenic cirrhosis
   (d) Can lead to HCC
   (e) Associations
      (i) Central obesity
      (ii) Type 2 diabetes
      (iii) Syndrome X
      (iv) PCOS
      (v) TPN
      (vi) Drugs
         (1) Amiodarone
         (2) Tamoxifen
         (3) Methotrexate
   (f) Treatment
      (i) > 10% loss in weight and exercise
      (ii) Metformin and glitazones have shown promise in early trials

Essential features of hepatocellular carcinoma

1 Rare (incidence increasing)
2 Predisposing factors
   (a) HBV
   (b) HCV
   (c) Alcohol
   (d) Haemochromatosis
   (e) Cirrhosis (any cause)
   (f) Aflatoxin (carcinogen from the mould *Aspergillus flavus*)
   (g) Thorotrast
3 Diagnosis
   (a) ↑ AFP (80%) > 500 – high probability
   (b) USS liver
   (c) Liver biopsy (can cause seeding of the tumour)
   (d) CT/MRI/angiography

4 Treatment
   (a) Local tumour ablation (ethanol, radiofrequency ablation)
   (b) Chemoembolisation
   (c) Liver resection
   (d) Liver transplant

Essential features of liver abscess

1 Usually occurs with underlying biliary tract pathology
2 Usually multiple
3 Most frequent organisms
   (a) *Escherichia coli*
   (b) *Klebsiella*
   (c) *Streptococcus milleri*
   (d) *Proteus*
   (e) *Pseudomonas*
   (f) Anaerobes
4 Presents with spiking fevers and RUQ pain
5 Investigations
   (a) ↑ WCC
   (b) ↑ ESR
   (c) Abnormal LFTs
   (d) Diagnosis on ultrasound or CT
   (e) Aspiration and culture grows an organism in 90%
6 Treatment
   (a) Antibiotics – broad spectrum and guided by culture results
   (b) Aspiration
   (c) Occasionally surgery

Essential features of amoebic liver abscess

1 Caused by *Entamoeba histolytica*
2 Presents with fever and RUQ pain
3 < 10% have bloody diarrhoea
4 Usually single
5 More common in the right lobe
6 Diagnosed by US, CT or serology (↑ IgG)
7 Aspiration not required but is like 'anchovy paste'
8 Treatment with metronidazole and diloxanide to eradicate luminal organisms

Hydatid liver cysts

1 Caused by the ingestion of *Echinococcus granulosus* eggs (from dogs and cattle)
2 Eggs hatch in the intestine and migrate to the liver
3 Forms septated calcified cysts (daughter cysts) in the liver
4 Presents with fever, hepatomegaly and eosinophilia
5 Diagnosis with US, CT and serology
6 Ruptured cysts can cause anaphylactic reactions
7 Treatment with albendazole and surgery

Causes of Budd–Chiari syndrome (thrombosis of the hepatic veins)

1 Thrombophilic disorders
2 Tumours
   (a) HCC
   (b) Renal cell
   (c) Stomach
   (d) Pancreas
   (e) Adrenal
3 Drugs
   (a) OCPs
   (b) Cytotoxics
4 Infections
   (a) Amoebic abscess
   (b) Aspergillosis
   (c) Hydatid cysts
   (d) Schistosomiasis
   (e) Syphilis
5 Trauma
6 Miscellaneous
   (a) IBD
   (b) Nephrotic syndrome
   (c) Sarcoidosis
   (d) Protein-losing enteropathy
   (e) Behçet's

Drugs that cause jaundice

Hepatitis

1 Antibiotics
   (a) Rifampicin
   (b) Isoniazid
   (c) Pyrizinamide
   (d) Nitrofurantoin
2 Antiepileptics
   (a) Valproate
   (b) Phenytoin
3 Analgesics
   (a) Paracetamol
   (b) Diclofenac
4 Others
   (a) Methyldopa
   (b) HMG CoA reductase inhibitors (statins)
   (c) Amiodarone
   (d) Halothane
   (e) Methotrexate
   (f) Tamoxifen

Cholestasis

1 Antibiotics
   (a) Erythromycin
   (b) Penicillins
   (c) Clavulanic acid
2 Chlorpromazine
3 Carbamazepine
4 Sulphonylureas
5 Oestrogens
6 Anabolic steroids
7 Cimetidine
8 Hydralazine

Granulomas

1 Sulphonamides
2 Phenylbutazone
3 Allopurinol

Malignancy

1 Anabolic steroids
2 OCPs

Fibrosis (activate stellate cells)

1 Methotrexate
2 Vitamin A
3 Retinoids

Causes of cirrhosis

1 Alcohol
2 Chronic HBV and HCV infection
3 Obesity/diabetes/NASH
4 Drugs
5 Autoimmune
  (a) PBC
  (b) Autoimmune hepatitis
  (c) PSC
6 Hereditary
  (a) Haemochromatosis
  (b) Wilson's disease
  (c) Alpha$_1$-antitrypsin deficiency
7 Biliary obstruction
8 Cardiac failure
9 Cryptogenic
10 Rare
  (a) Budd–Chiari syndrome
  (b) Sarcoidosis
  (c) Syphilis
  (d) Indian childhood cirrhosis
  (e) Cystic fibrosis
  (f) Glycogen storage disease
  (g) Galactosaemia
  (h) Abetalipoproteinaemia
  (i) Porphyria

Causes of hepatic granuloma

Infective

1 Viral
   (a) EBV
   (b) CMV
   (c) HAV
   (d) HCV
2 Bacterial
   (a) Mycobacteria
   (b) Brucellosis
   (c) *Yersinia*
   (d) Whipple's disease
   (e) Syphilis
3 Fungal
   (a) Histoplasmosis
   (b) Blastomycosis
   (c) *Cryptococcus*
4 Protozoal
   (a) Leishmaniasis
   (b) Toxoplasmosis
   (c) Schistosomiasis

Metals

1 Beryllium
2 Copper

Immunological disorders

1 Sarcoidosis
2 PBC
3 IBD (UC/Crohn's)
4 HIV
5 Hypogammaglobulinaemia
6 SLE
7 Polymyalgia rheumatica
8 BCG vaccine

Idiopathic

1 Granulomatous hepatitis

Enzyme defects

1 Chronic granulomatous disease in children

Neoplasia

1 Lymphoma
2 Carcinoma

Clinical signs of chronic liver disease

1 General
   (a) Jaundice
   (b) Spider naevi
   (c) Bruising
   (d) Gynaecomastia
   (e) Testicular atrophy
   (f) Loss of body hair
   (g) Encephalopathy
   (h) Peripheral oedema
   (i) Fetor hepaticus
2 Hands
   (a) Finger clubbing
   (b) Leukonychia
   (c) Palmar erythema
   (d) Liver flap
3 Abdomen
   (a) Ascites
   (b) Hepatosplenomegaly
   (c) Caput medusae

Clinical signs of chronic liver disease secondary to alcohol

1 Tremor
2 Parotid enlargement
3 Dupuytren's contracture
4 Pseudo-Cushing's
5 Proximal myopathy

6 Peripheral neuropathy
7 Central neurological signs – Wernicke's encephalopathy/Korsakoff's syndrome
8 Cognitive impairment

Other effects of alcohol abuse

Neuromuscular

1 Epilepsy
2 Polyneuropathy
3 Myopathy
4 Withdrawal

Cardiovascular

1 Cardiomyopathy (dilated)
2 Beri beri
3 Arrhythmias – AF
4 Hypertension

Metabolic

1 Gout
2 Hyperlipidaemia – triglycerides
3 Hypoglycaemia
4 Obesity

Respiratory

1 Chest infections
2 TB
3 Aspiration pneumonia

Haematological

1 Macrocytosis
2 Thrombocytopenia
3 Leukopenia

Bone

1 Osteoporosis
2 Osteomalacia

Factors that may precipitate hepatic encephalopathy

1 Infection/spontaneous bacterial peritonitis
2 Oral protein load
3 Upper GI haemorrhage
4 Constipation
5 Diuretic therapy
6 Paracentesis
7 Diarrhoea and vomiting
8 Hypoglycaemia
9 Hypotension
10 Hypoxia
11 Anaemia
12 Sedative/hypnotic drugs
13 Surgery

Hepatic encephalopathy

1 Grade 1
   (a) Mild confusion
   (b) Agitation
   (c) Sleep disorder
2 Grade 2
   (a) Drowsiness
   (b) Lethargy
   (c) Asterixis
   (d) Dysarthria
3 Grade 3
   (a) Somnolent but rousable
   (b) Asterixis
   (c) Extensor plantars
   (d) Increased reflexes
4 Grade 4
   (a) Coma

Causes of ascites

Venous hypertension

1 Cirrhosis
2 Congestive heart failure
3 Constrictive pericarditis

4 Budd–Chiari syndrome
5 Portal vein thrombosis

Hypoalbuminaemia

1 Nephrotic syndrome
2 Malnutrition
3 Protein-losing enteropathy

Malignant disease

1 Secondary carcinomatosis
2 Lymphoma and leukaemia
3 Primary mesothelioma

Infections

1 Tuberculous peritonitis
2 Fungal (*Candida*, *Cryptococcus*)
3 Parasitic (*Strongyloides*, *Entamoeba*)

Miscellaneous

1 Chylous
2 Bile
3 Pancreatic
4 Urinary
5 Ovarian disease
6 Myxoedema
7 Pseudomyxoma peritonei
8 Eosinophilic peritonitis

Treatments for oesophageal varices

1 Primary prophylaxis against bleeding in patients with known varices
   (a) Propranolol
   (b) Nitrates
   (c) Banding if intolerant of above
2 Treatment of bleeding varices
   (a) Resuscitation
   (b) Banding or sclerotherapy
   (c) Terlipressin
   (d) Octreotide

   (e) Balloon tamponade (temporary)
   (f) TIPS
   (g) Surgical shunt
   (h) Liver transplant

Physiological changes in the liver in pregnancy

1 Hepatic blood flow remains constant despite an increase in cardiac output, so proportion of cardiac output is reduced from 35% to 29%, hence drug metabolism is affected
2 Size of liver remains constant
3 ALP rises 3–4-fold owing to placental production
4 Other biochemistry remains the same

Liver disease in pregnancy

1 Any liver disease can occur in pregnancy
2 Hyperemesis gravidarum- can have abnormal LFTs and jaundice
3 Intrahepatic cholestasis of pregnancy – ↑ fetal mortality, third trimester, familial, cholestatic LFTs, resolves with delivery, common, treated with ursodeoxycholic acid
4 Acute fatty liver of pregnancy – third trimester, fulminant hepatitis, immediate delivery required, 20% mortality, rare
5 HELLP – haemolysis, elevated liver enzymes and low platelets, delivery required for treatment
6 Pre-eclampsia and eclampsia – may lead to fulminant hepatic failure; treatment is delivery

THE PANCREAS

Acute pancreatitis

Causes

   1 Gallstones
   2 Alcohol
   3 Trauma
   4 Post ERCP/surgery
   5 Viral: mumps, Coxsackie B, HIV
   6 Hyperlipidaemia
   7 Hypercalcaemia

8 Autoimmune – PAN
9 Hypothermia
10 Scorpion/snake venom
11 Drugs: azathioprine, steroids, frusemide, oral contraceptive pill, valproate, didanosine

Prognosis

Modified Glasgow prognostic score (validated for gallstones and alcohol) – worse prognosis if more than three of these present
1 WBC > 15
2 Glucose > 10
3 LDH > 600
4 AST > 200
5 Urea > 16
6 Calcium < 2
7 Albumin < 32
8 paO_2 < 8kPa

Complications

Early

1 ARDS
2 ARF
3 DIC
4 Jaundice
5 Anaemia
6 Hypocalcaemia
7 Hypoalbuminaemia
8 Hyperglycaemia
9 Metabolic acidosis

Late

1 Abscess
2 Pseudocyst
3 Chronic pancreatitis
4 Diabetes mellitus
5 Pancreatic ascites
6 Splenic vein thrombosis
7 Subcutaneous fat necrosis – Weber–Christian disease

Causes of hyperamylasaemia

1 Pancreatic
   (a) Acute pancreatitis
   (b) Pancreatic ascites
   (c) Pseudocyst
   (d) Pancreatic fistulae
   (e) Pancreatic carcinoma
   (f) ERCP
2 Other abdominal causes
   (a) Abdominal perforation
   (b) Mesenteric infarction
   (c) Cholecystitis/cholangitis
   (d) Salpingitis/ectopics
   (e) Acute and chronic hepatocellular disease
   (f) Ovarian neoplasm
3 Other non-abdominal causes
   (a) Salivary adenitis
   (b) End-stage renal disease
   (c) Anorexia
   (d) Burns
   (e) Metabolic disturbance

Essentials of chronic pancreatitis

1 Causes
   (a) Alcohol
   (b) Cystic fibrosis
   (c) Duct strictures
   (d) Hypercalcaemia
   (e) Hyperlipidaemia
   (f) Hereditary
   (g) Tropical pancreatitis
   (h) Idiopathic
2 Clinical features
   (a) Chronic severe pain
   (b) Weight loss
   (c) Diabetes
   (d) Malabsorption
3 Investigations
   (a) Calcification on AXR
   (b) ERCP/MRCP – dilated distorted duct with loss of side branches

(c) CT
(d) EUS
(e) Faecal elastase/pancreolauryl test
4 Treatment
   (a) Pancreatic enzyme supplements
   (b) Analgesia
   (c) Stop alcohol
   (d) Surgery

MISCELLANEOUS

Causes of calcification on the abdominal X-ray

1 Faecoliths
2 Phleboliths
3 Calcified lymph nodes
4 Calcified blood vessels
5 Calculi – renal, gallbladder, prostatic
6 Calcified pancreas, adrenal, liver, kidney, aorta, psoas muscle and costal cartilage
7 Calcified tumour – dermoid, fibroid, teratoma
8 Fetus
9 Calcification in the abdominal wall

Uncommon causes of abdominal pain

1 Gastric dilatation
2 Migraine
3 Epilepsy
4 Lead poisoning
5 Tabes dorsalis
6 Acute intermittent porphyria
7 Addison's disease
8 Haemochromatosis
9 Haemolytic crisis
10 Henoch–Schönlein Purpura
11 Hepatoma
12 Hyperparathyroidism
13 Uraemia
14 Intestinal parasites

Genetics

SINGLE GENE DISORDERS

Autosomal dominant inheritance

1. Alpha$_1$-antitrypsin deficiency (See page 404)
2. Acute intermittent porphyria (See page 276)
3. Adult polycystic kidney disease (See page 305)
4. Achondroplasia
5. Crigler–Najjar syndrome type 2 (See page 154)
6. Ehlers–Danlos syndrome
7. Facioscapulohumeral dystrophy
8. Familial adenomatous polyposis (FAP) (See page 150)
9. Gilbert's syndrome (See page 154)
10. Huntington's chorea (See page 359)
11. Hyperlipidaemia type II (familial hypercholesterolaemia) (See page 266)
12. Hereditary spherocytosis
13. Malignant hyperthermia
14. Marfan's syndrome (See page 177)
15. Myotonic dystrophy (See page 362)
16. Neurofibromatosis (type 1 and 2) (See below)
17. Noonan's syndrome (See page 177)
18. Osteogenesis imperfecta
19. Rotor syndrome (See page 154)
20. Retinoblastoma (See page 379)
21. Tuberous sclerosis (See page 176)
22. Von Willebrand's disease (See page 210)

Neurofibromatosis type I

1. Mutation or deletion of NF1 gene on chromosome 17
2. ↓ Neurofibromin (tumour suppressor)

3 Features
  (a) > 6 *café au lait* spots
  (b) Lisch nodules on iris
  (c) Peripheral neurofibromas
  (d) Axillary/inguinal freckling
  (e) Optic nerve gliomas
  (f) Scoliosis

Neurofibromatosis type 2 (central)

1 Mutation or deletion of NF2 gene on chromosome 22
2 ↓ Merlin (tumour suppressor)
3 Features
  (a) Bilateral acoustic neuromas
  (b) Other cranial and spinal tumours (meningioma, glioma, schwannoma)
  (c) Lens opacities/cataracts
  (d) Peripheral schwannomas
  (e) Few peripheral neurofibromas
  (f) < 6 *café au lait* spots

Tuberous sclerosis

1 Mutation of TSC1 (Ch 9) or TSC2 (Ch 16) genes
2 ↓ Hamartin (TSC1) or ↓ tuberin (TSC2) – both tumour suppressors
3 Features
  (a) Neurological
    (i) Low IQ (50%)
    (ii) Seizures
    (iii) Cortical tubers (cerebrum or cerebellum)
    (iv) Subependymal nodules
    (v) Subependymal giant cell astrocytomas
  (b) Skin
    (i) Ash-leaf macules
    (ii) Shagreen patches
    (iii) Adenoma sebacum
    (iv) Subungal fibromas
  (c) Others
  (d) Angiolipomata
  (e) Retinal hamartomas
  (f) Cardiac rhabdomyomas

Marfan's syndrome

1 Mutation of Fibrillin-1 gene (FBN-1) on chromosome 15
2 ↓ Fibrillin (constituent of connective tissue)
3 Features
    (a) Tall stature (armspan > height)
    (b) Arachnodactyly
    (c) Hyperextensile joints
    (d) Upward lens dislocation
    (e) High arched palate
    (f) Scoliosis
    (g) Aortic root dilatation (AR, aortic dissection)
    (h) MVP
    (i) Dural ectasia

Noonan syndrome

1 Features
    (a) Mental retardation (50%)
    (b) Short stature
    (c) Down-slanting eyes
    (d) Ptosis
    (e) Hypertelorism
    (f) Webbed neck
    (g) Congenital heart disease

Autosomal recessive inheritance

1 Albinism
2 Ataxia telangiectasia (See page 227)
3 Congenital adrenal hyperplasia (See page 109)
4 Crigler–Najjar syndrome type I (See page 154)
5 Cystinuria (See page 278)
6 Cystic fibrosis (See page 405)
7 Dubin–Johnson syndrome (See page 154)
8 Familial Mediterranean fever (See page 456)
9 Fanconi's anaemia
10 Friedreich's ataxia (See page 349)
11 Galactosaemia
12 Gaucher's disease
13 Glycogen storage diseases

14 Haemochromatosis (See page 273)
15 Homocystinuria (See page 278)
16 Hurler's syndrome
17 Limb girdle muscular dystrophy
18 Niemann–Pick disease
19 Phenylketonuria (See page 278)
20 Sickle cell disease (See page 189)
21 Thalassaemias (See page 189)
22 Wilson's disease (See page 272)

X-linked recessive inheritance

1 Agammaglobulinaemia (See page 225)
2 Becker's muscular dystrophy (See page 360)
3 Chronic granulomatous disease (See page 228)
4 Colour blindness
5 Complete testicular feminisation
6 Duchenne muscular dystrophy (See page 360)
7 Fabry's disease
8 Glucose-6-phosphate dehydrogenase (G6PD) deficiency (See page 58)
9 Haemophilia A (factor VIII) (See page 210)
10 Haemophilia B (factor IX) (See page 210)
11 Hunter's syndrome
12 Lesch–Nyhan syndrome (See page 429)
13 Nephrogenic diabetes insipidus (See page 282)
14 Retinitis pigmentosa (See page 378)
15 Wiskott–Aldrich syndrome (See page 227)

X-linked dominant inheritance

1 Vitamin D-resistant rickets

HLA disease associations

[See Table 29, opposite]

Table 29

Disease	Antigen
Idiopathic haemochromatosis	A3
Behçet's disease	B5
Ankylosing spondylitis	B27
Reiter's disease	B27
Subacute thyroiditis	B35
Narcolepsy	DR2
Goodpasture's disease	DR2
Multiple sclerosis	DR2
Dermatitis herpetiformis	DR3
Coeliac disease	DR3
Idiopathic membranous nephropathy	DR3
Sjögren's syndrome	DR3
SLE	DR3
Addison's disease	DR3
Graves' disease	DR3
IDDM	DR3
Myasthenia gravis	DR3
IDDM	DR4
Rheumatoid arthritis	DR4
Pernicious anaemia	DR5

CHROMOSOMAL ABNORMALITIES

Non-disjunction

Chromosomes fail to separate during meiosis and one zygote has three homologous chromosomes (eg trisomy 21 – Down's) or one chromosome (eg Turner's syndrome – XO)

Translocation

Part of one chromosome transferred to another non-homologous chromosome (eg part of chromosome 21 transferred to chromosome 15, leading to Down's syndrome)

Klinefelter's syndrome (47, XXY)

1 Male 1:600
2 Eunuchoid body
3 Tall stature

4 Gynaecomastia ($\uparrow$ risk of breast cancer)
5 Hypogonadism
6 Azoospermia
7 Low IQ
8 MVP (55%)
9 $\downarrow$ Testosterone $\uparrow$ FSH $\uparrow$ LH $\uparrow$ oestradiol

Turner's syndrome (45, XO)

1 1:2500 females
2 Short stature
3 Streak ovaries and hypogonadism
4 Webbed neck
5 Widely shaped nipples
6 $\uparrow$ Carrying angle of arms
7 Renal abnormalities (eg horseshoe kidney)
8 Coarctation of aorta (10–15%)
9 Bicuspid aortic valve
10 Diabetes and hypothyroidism common
11 Osteoporosis

Triple X syndrome (47, XXX)

1 Tall stature
2 Reduced intelligence
3 Mild developmental and behavioural difficulties

Down's syndrome (trisomy 21)

1 1:700 live births (more common as maternal age increases)
2 Features
   (a) Moderate mental retardation
   (b) Brachycephaly
   (c) Protruding tongue
   (d) Single palmer crease
   (e) Clinodactyly fifth finger
   (f) Upslanting palpebral fissures
   (g) Epicanthic folds prominent
   (h) Brushfield spots on iris
   (i) Increased incidence of:
      (i) Cardiovascular malformation

   (1) ASD
   (2) VSD
   (3) Fallot's tetralogy
   (4) PDA
  (ii) Haematological abnormalities:
   (1) ALL
   (2) AML
  (iii) GI abnormalities (eg Hirschsprung's disease)
  (iv) Hypothyroidism
  (v) Cataracts
  (vi) Early-onset Alzheimer's

Edward's syndrome (trisomy 18)

1 Mental retardation
2 Characteristic faces
3 Prominent occiput
4 Overlapping fingers
5 Rockerbottom feet
6 Congenital heart disease
7 Dislocated hips
8 Renal abnormalities

Patau's syndrome (trisomy 13)

1 Microcephaly
2 Cleft lip and palate
3 Polydactyly
4 CNS abnormalities
5 Congenital heart disease
6 Rectal abnormality

Cri-du-chat syndrome

1 Deletion of short arm of chromosome 5
2 Features
  (a) Mental retardation and behavioural problems
  (b) Growth retardation
  (c) Characteristic cry (laryngeal hypoplasia)
  (d) Congenital heart disease

Trinucleotide repeat disorders

1 Disorders where DNA contains multiple extra copies of trinucleotides, eg CAG = glutamine
2 Number of repeats varies and may enlarge in successive generations leading to increased severity and earlier onset of disease symptoms (anticipation)
3 Diseases
  (a) Huntington's disease (CAG) Huntingtin gene on chromosome 4
  (b) Spinocerebellar ataxia (CAG) multiple genes
  (c) Spinobulbar muscular atrophy (CAG) AR gene on X chromosome
  (d) Myotonic dystrophy (CTG) DMPK gene on chromosome 19
  (e) Friedreich's ataxia (GAA) frataxin gene on chromosome 9
  (f) Fragile X syndrome (CGG) FMR-1 gene on X chromosome

MITOCHONDRIAL DISORDERS

1 MELAS – **m**itochondrial **e**ncephalomyopathy, **l**actic **a**cidosis and **s**troke
2 MERRF – **m**yoclonic **e**pilepsy, **r**agged **r**ed **f**ibres
3 NARP – **n**europathy, **a**taxia, **r**etinitis **p**igmentosa
4 Leber's optic atrophy
5 Kearns–Sayre syndrome
6 Progressive external ophthalmoplegia

GENES ASSOCIATED WITH CANCER

Oncogene – genes associated with stimulation of cell division and predispose to cancer (dominant)
Tumour suppressor genes – mutation predisposes to cancer (recessive)

[See Table 30, opposite]

Table 30

Oncogene	Cancer
erb-B	Breast and brain
Ki-ras	Ovarian, pancreatic, lung, colon
N-ras	Leukaemia
BCR-ABL (Philadelphia chromosome)	CML
Bcl-1	Breast, head and neck
Bcl-2	Lymphoma
c-myc	Leukaemia, breast, stomach, lung
N-myc	Brain, nerve
L-myc	Lung
MEN2 (RET)	Medullary thyroid cancer, phaeochromocytoma

Tumour suppressor genes	Cancer
RB1	Retinoblastoma
WT1	Wilms' tumour
APC	FAP
p53	Wide range of tumours
VHL (Von Hippel–Lindau)	Renal cancers, haemangioblastomas, phaeochromocytoma, retinal angioma
MEN1	Parathyroid, pituitary adenomas, carcinoids, islet cell tumours
DPC4	Pancreatic
BRCA 1	Breast, ovarian
BRCA 2	Breast

Haematology

CAUSES OF ANAEMIA

1 Microcytic
   (a) Iron deficiency
   (b) Thalassaemia
   (c) Anaemia of chronic disease (some cases)
   (d) Sideroblastic anaemia
   (e) Lead poisoning
2 Normocytic, normochromic
   (a) Haemorrhage
   (b) Anaemia of chronic disease
   (c) Renal failure (reduced EPO)
   (d) Haemolytic anaemia
   (e) Bone marrow infiltration (carcinoma, leukaemia, myelofibrosis etc)
   (f) Polymyalgia rheumatica
   (g) Bone marrow failure (chemotherapy)
   (h) Aplastic anaemia
   (i) Some mixed deficiencies
3 Macrocytic
   (a) Megaloblastic (B_{12} or folate deficiency)
   (b) Reticulocytosis (some haemolytic anaemias)
   (c) Alcohol
   (d) Chronic liver disease
   (e) Hypothyroidism
   (f) Hypopituitarism
   (g) Myeloma
   (h) Myelodysplasia
   (i) Aplastic anaemia
   (j) Cytotoxic drugs

MICROCYTIC ANAEMIAS

Iron deficiency anaemia (IDA)

1 Features
  (a) Hypochromic microcytic cells
  (b) Pencil cells on blood film
  (c) Low ferritin
  (d) Low iron with normal/high TIBC
2 Causes
  (a) Chronic blood loss
    (i) Uterine
    (ii) GI tract
      (1) Peptic ulcer
      (2) GI malignancy
      (3) Colitis/Crohn's
      (4) Varices/portal hypertensive gastropathy
      (5) Hookworm infection (*Ankyostoma duodenale, Necator americanus*)
      (6) Angiodysplasia
      (7) Haemorrhoids
    (iii) Occasionally haemoglobinuria, haematuria, haemosiderosis, self-inflicted blood loss
  (b) Increased demands
    (i) Prematurity
    (ii) Growth
    (iii) Child-bearing
  (c) Malabsorption
    (i) Gastrectomy
    (ii) Coeliac disease
    (iii) Proximal small bowel disease
  (d) Nutritional deficiency

Sideroblastic anaemia

1 Anaemia with ring sideroblasts (normoblasts with iron around the nucleus)
2 Often dimorphic blood film (normal and microcytic cells)
3 Causes
  (a) Inherited (X linked)
  (b) Myelodysplasia

(c) AML
(d) Carcinoma
(e) Connective tissue disease
(f) Drugs
    (i) Isoniazid
    (ii) Chloramphenicol
    (iii) Alcohol
    (iv) Lead
4 Treatment
  (a) Pyridoxine may improve some cases
  (b) Iron chelation may be required

MACROCYTIC ANAEMIAS

Features of megaloblastic anaemia

1 Clinical
  (a) Yellow tinge to the skin
  (b) Glossitis
  (c) Mild splenomegaly
  (d) Low-grade pyrexia
  (e) Neurological signs (B_{12})
    (i) Optic atrophy
    (ii) Peripheral neuropathy
    (iii) Subacute combined degeneration of the cord
    (iv) Dementia
2 Blood film
  (a) Pancytopenia
  (b) Macrocytosis
  (c) Hypersegmented neutrophils
  (d) Occasionally megaloblasts in blood
  (e) Megaloblasts in bone marrow

Causes of low vitamin B_{12}

1 Nutritional (vegans)
2 Stomach disorders
  (a) Pernicious anaemia (autoantibodies to intrinsic factor or parietal cells)
  (b) Gastrectomy/partial gastrectomy

3 Chronic pancreatitis
4 Intestinal disorders
   (a) Terminal ileal disease
       (i)   Crohn's
       (ii) Ileal resection
       (iii) TB
       (iv) *Yersinia enterocolitica*
       (v)   Radiation enteritis
   (b) Bacterial overgrowth
   (c) Coeliac disease
   (d) Giardiasis
   (e) Whipple's disease
   (f) Tropical sprue
5 *Diphyllobothrium* infection (fish tapeworm)

Associations in pernicious anaemia

1 Female
2 Blue eyes
3 Early greying
4 North European
5 Familial
6 Blood group A
7 Vitiligo
8 Myxoedema
9 Hashimoto's disease
10 Thyrotoxicosis
11 Addison's disease
12 Hypoparathyroidism
13 Hypogammaglobulinaemia
14 Carcinoma of the stomach

Causes of folate deficiency

1 Dietary (alcoholics)
2 Increased demand
   (a) Pregnancy
   (b) Haemolytic anaemias
   (c) Malignancies (especially leukaemia, lymphoma and carcinoma)
   (d) Psoriasis or exfoliative dermatitis

3 Malabsorption
  (a) Coeliac disease
  (b) Crohn's disease
  (c) Pancreatic insufficiency
  (d) Partial gastrectomy
4 Drugs
  (a) Methotrexate
  (b) Sulfasalazine
  (c) Phenytoin

Macrocytosis with associated haematological diseases

1 Myeloma – ↑ ESR, leukoerythroblastic blood picture, paraproteins
2 Myelodysplasias – monocytosis, dysplastic morphology, cytopenias
3 Aplastic anaemia – pancytopenia, with hypoblastic bone marrow
4 Myeloproliferative disorders – polycythaemia rubra vera (PRV), essential thrombocythaemia, myelofibrosis, CML

HAEMOGLOBINOPATHIES

Thalassaemia

1 Genetic disorders leading to defective haemoglobinisation of the red cell
2 Haemoglobin normally is a tetramer of two α and two β chains
3 Four α haemoglobin genes and two β haemoglobin genes
4 Deletion of genes leads to varying degrees of thalassaemia
5 Common in Mediterranean populations

[See Table 31, overleaf]

Sickle cell disease

1 Due to production of abnormal β chain in haemoglobin
2 Valine replaces glutamic acid in position 6 of the β chain to form HbS
3 Common in black Africans
4 Heterozygotes HbAS = sickle cell trait
  (a) Mild, often asymptomatic. May get sickling under anoxic conditions

Table 31

	Clinical syndrome
α Genes chromosome 16	
4	Normal
3	Silent carrier – usually phenotypically normal
2	Thalassaemia minor – usually normal Hb with low MCV
1	HbH disease, Hb 8–9, low MCV hypersplenism
0	Hb Bart's – usually death in utero
β Genes chromosome 11	
2	Normal
1	Thalassaemia minor – usually asymptomatic $\uparrow$ HbA2, low MCV, Hb > 9
0	Thalassaemia major – severe anaemia Hb 2–3, splenomegaly, bone deformity due to bone marrow expansion (bossing of the skull) Need repeated transfusions, develop iron overload (see haemochromatosis) but this can be treated with desferrioxamine $\uparrow$ HbA2, $\uparrow$ HbF, absent HbA, reticulocytosis 4–10%

5 Homozygotes HbSS = sickle cell disease
  (a) Chronic haemolytic anaemia
  (b) Recurrent crises
6 Features of crisis
  (a) Pain – due to bone marrow infarction
  (b) Sickle dactylitis – infarction of small bones of hands and feet
  (c) Splenic sequestration crisis – occurs in children, rapid splenic enlargement and severe anaemia
  (d) Localised areas of splenic infarction – pleuritic pain
  (e) Thrombotic stroke – rare. Requires urgent exchange transfusion
  (f) Pulmonary infarction–chest syndrome – serious, again requiring exchange transfusion
  (g) Priapism – painful sustained erection. May require surgical intervention

(h) Other areas of sickle infarction
   (i) Retina
   (ii) Placenta
7 Other features
   (a) Avascular necrosis of neck of femur
   (b) Aplastic crisis – usually precipitated by parvovirus B_{19} infection
   (c) Leg ulcers
   (d) Renal failure
   (e) Chronic lung disease
   (f) Gallstones
   (g) Hyposplenism
   (h) Iron overload due to recurrent transfusion
8 Diagnosis
   (a) Haemoglobin electrophoresis
   (b) Blood film – anaemia, sickle cells, increased reticulocyte count, target cells
   (c) Positive sickling test

Aplastic anaemia

1 Pancytopenia with hypoplastic bone marrow
2 Causes
   (a) Idiopathic – probably autoimmune in most cases
   (b) Drugs
      (i) Gold
      (ii) Phenylbutazone
      (iii) Chloramphenicol
   (c) Infections (particularly hepatitis viruses)
   (d) Chemo-/radiotherapy
3 Treatment
   (a) Supportive
      (i) Antibiotics
      (ii) Transfusion blood and platelets
   (b) Specific
      (i) Growth factors (GCSF etc)
      (ii) Immunosuppression
      (iii) Bone marrow transplant

Haemolysis

1 Features
  (a) Destruction of RBCs (anaemia develops and the bone marrow cannot compensate)
  (b) Laboratory features suggestive of haemolysis
    (i) Elevated reticulocyte count (> 2%)
    (ii) ↑ LDH (released by RBC)
    (iii) ↓ Haptoglobins
    (iv) ↑ Unconjugated bilirubin
    (v) Blood film – spherocytes, fragmented red cells
2 Causes of haemolysis
  (a) Genetic
    (i) Membrane disorders
      (1) Hereditary spherocytosis
      (2) Hereditary elliptocytosis
    (ii) Haemoglobin
      (1) Sickling disorders (See page 189)
      (2) Thalassemia (See page 189)
    (iii) Enzyme defects
      (1) G6PD (See page 58)
      (2) Pyruvate kinase deficiency
  (b) Acquired
    (i) Immune
      (1) Isoimmune
        (a) Haemolytic disease of the newborn
        (b) Blood transfusion reaction
      (2) Autoimmune
        (a) Warm antibody mediated (See page 193)
        (b) Cold antibody mediated (See page 193)
        (c) Drug induced (See page 193)
    (ii) Non-immune
      (1) Trauma
        (a) Cardiac haemolysis
        (b) MAHA (See page 194)
      (2) Infection
        (a) Malaria
        (b) Toxoplasmosis
        (c) Septicaemia
      (3) Hypersplenism

(4) Membrane disorders
    (a) Paroxysmal nocturnal haemoglobinuria (See page 230)
    (b) Liver disease

Coombs' test – antiglobulin test

1 **Direct** Coombs' test detects antibody on a patient's red cells
  (a) The antibody may be
    (i) Opsonising the erythrocytes to attract phagocytes
    (ii) Complement fixing and causing a local enzymatic lysis in red cell membrane
    (iii) Agglutinating – clumping may be visible in the test tube
  (b) It detects acquired immune causes of haemolytic anaemia
2 **Indirect** Coombs' test detects antibody in the patient's serum
  (a) The patient's serum is incubated with test red cells bearing different antigen. This test is used frequently as part of the cross-matching process – the donor's cells are mixed with recipient's serum

Autoimmune haemolytic anaemia

1 Antibodies are present against red cell components, leading to haemolysis
2 Two types, 'warm' and 'cold'
3 Warm
  (a) Usually IgG antibody, which is most active at 37°C
  (b) Clinical features include haemolysis and features of the underlying disease
  (c) Causes
    (i) Idiopathic
    (ii) Secondary
      (1) SLE and other 'autoimmune diseases'
      (2) CLL
      (3) Lymphomas
      (4) Drugs
        (a) Methyldopa
        (b) Levodopa
        (c) Mefenamic acid
4 Cold
  (a) Usually IgM antibody that is most active at 4°C
  (b) Features include haemolysis and Raynaud's, and those of the underlying disease

5 Causes
  (a) Idiopathic
  (b) Secondary
     (i) Infections
        (1) *Mycoplasma pneumoniae*
        (2) Infectious mononucleosis
     (ii) Lymphoma
     (iii) Paroxysmal cold haemoglobinuria
     (iv) Syphilis (rare)

Microangiopathic haemolytic anaemia (MAHA)

1 Features
  (a) Anaemia
  (b) Helmet cells
  (c) Fragmented red cells
  (d) Polychromasia
  (e) Reticulocytosis
2 Causes (overlap between these conditions)
  (a) Disseminated intravascular coagulation (DIC) (See page 210)
  (b) Haemolytic uraemic syndrome (HUS)
     (i) Bloody diarrhoea
     (ii) Abdominal pain
     (iii) Fever
     (iv) Haemorrhage
     (v) MAHA
     (vi) Oliguria and ARF
     (vii) Associated with *Escherichia coli* 0157:H7
     (viii) Sporadic cases do occur
  (c) Thrombotic thrombocytopenic purpura (TTP)
     (i) Diarrhoea less marked
     (ii) Thrombocytopenia
     (iii) MAHA
     (iv) Fluctuating neurological signs
     (v) Renal impairment
  (d) Malignant hypertension
  (e) Severe pre-eclampsia

CAUSES OF ABNORMAL BLOOD CELL NUMBERS

Causes of reticulocytosis

1 Haemorrhage
2 Haemolysis
3 Infection
4 Polycythaemia
5 Myeloproliferative disorders
6 Recovery from chemo- or radiotherapy
7 Post EPO or iron therapy

Causes of a neutrophilia (>7.5 × 10^9/l)

1 Bacterial infections (generalised or localised)
2 Non-infectious inflammation
   (a) MI
   (b) Trauma
   (c) Vasculitis
   (d) Rheumatoid disorders
3 Metabolic disorders
   (a) Acidosis
   (b) Uraemia
   (c) Poisoning
   (d) Eclampsia
4 Corticosteroid therapy
5 Malignant neoplasms
6 Myeloproliferative disorders
7 Acute haemorrhage

Causes of a lymphocytosis (>3.5 × 10^9/l)

1 Acute viral infections
   (a) Influenza
   (b) EBV
   (c) CMV
   (d) Acute HIV (chronic HIV causes lymphopenia)
   (e) Mumps
   (f) Viral hepatitis
2 Chronic lymphocytic leukaemia
3 Thyrotoxicosis

4 Chronic infections
   (a) TB
   (b) *Brucella*
   (c) Syphilis
5 Other chronic leukaemias and lymphomas
6 Infancy

Causes of an eosinophilia (>0.5 × 10^9/l)

1 Allergy
   (a) Asthma
   (b) Hay fever
   (c) Drug hypersensitivity
2 Parasites (helminths)
   (a) Ankylosomiasis
   (b) Ascariasis
   (c) Toxocariasis
   (d) Schistosomiasis
3 Skin diseases
   (a) Eczema
   (b) Psoriasis
   (c) Dermatitis herpetiformis
4 Connective tissue disorders
   (a) RA
   (b) Polyarteritis nodosa and Churg–Strauss
   (c) Sarcoidosis
5 Neoplasms
   (a) Hodgkin's disease
   (b) Lymphoma
   (c) Paraneoplastic
   (d) Eosinophilic leukaemia
6 Tropical eosinophilia
7 Hypereosinophilic syndrome

Hypereosinophilic syndrome

1 Idiopathic disorder characterised by persistently elevated eosinophil count in the absence of a cause, that leads to end-organ damage
2 Clinical features
   (a) Weight loss
   (b) Rashes (urticarial or angio-oedema)

(c) Fever
(d) GI
  (i)   Splenomegaly
  (ii) Diarrhoea
(e) Respiratory
  (i)   Cough
  (ii) Pulmonary infiltrates
(f) Cardiac
  (i)   Pericarditis
  (ii) Cardiac mural thrombosis
  (iii) Chronic endocardial fibrosis
  (iv) CCF
(g) Peripheral neuropathy
(h) Stroke
(i) Arthropathy
3 Treatment
(a) Steroids

Causes of a monocytosis (>0.8 × 10⁹/l)

1 Recovery – especially after chemo-/radiotherapy
2 Chronic inflammatory disease
  (a) Sarcoidosis
  (b) Inflammatory bowel disease
  (c) RA
  (d) SLE
3 Infections
  (a) EBV
  (b) TB
  (c) Leishmaniasis
  (d) Trypanosomiasis
  (e) Malaria
  (f) *Brucella*
  (g) Syphilis
4 Hodgkin's disease
5 Myelodysplastic syndromes
6 Acute myelomonocytic leukaemias

Causes of neutropenia

1 Viral infections
2 Idiosyncratic drug reactions, e.g. carbimazole (See page 67)

3 Post chemo- or radiotherapy
4 Collagen vascular diseases
   (a) SLE
   (b) RA (Felty's syndrome)
   (c) Wegener's granulomatosis
5 Myelodysplasia
6 Marrow infiltration
7 B_{12} or folate deficiency
8 Autoimmune neutropenia
9 Hypersplenism
10 Glycogen storage diseases

Causes of thrombocytosis (platelets > 500 × 10^9/l)

1 Essential thrombocytosis
2 Secondary causes
   (a) Infection and inflammatory disorders
   (b) Post splenectomy or hyposplenism
   (c) Malignancy
   (d) Trauma
   (e) Bleeding
   (f) Iron deficiency anaemia
   (g) Infarction
   (h) Thrombosis

Causes of thrombocytopenia

1 Decreased production
   (a) Marrow failure (seen in leukaemias and MDS)
   (b) Megaloblastic anaemia
2 Excessive destruction
   (a) Immune thrombocytopenic purpura (ITP)
   (b) Viruses
   (c) Drugs, eg heparin
   (d) SLE
   (e) Lymphoma
   (f) Hypersplenism
   (g) Thrombotic thrombocytopenic purpura
   (h) Haemolytic uraemic syndrome
   (i) DIC
   (j) Platelet aggregation

Causes of a pancytopenia

1 Aplastic anaemia (including cytotoxic drug therapy)
2 Bone marrow failure
 (a) Leukaemia
 (b) Myelodysplasias
 (c) Myelofibrosis
 (d) Myeloma
 (e) Carcinoma
 (f) Lymphoma
3 Hypersplenism
4 Megaloblastic anaemia
5 Paroxysmal nocturnal haemoglobinuria – occasionally

Causes of a leukoerythroblastic blood picture

1 Invasion of marrow space
 (a) Tumour (metastatic carcinoma)
 (b) Myeloma
 (c) Lymphoma
 (d) Osteopetrosis
 (e) Storage disease
2 Severe illness
 (a) Severe haemolysis
 (b) Massive trauma
 (c) Septicaemia

ABNORMALITIES OF RED CELL MORPHOLOGY (SEEN ON BLOOD FILM)

[See Table 32, overleaf]

MORPHOLOGICAL ABNORMALITIES IN WHITE BLOOD CELLS

[See Table 33, overleaf]

Table 32

Tear drops	Myelofibrosis
Helmet cells and fragmented cell	Microangiopathic haemolysis
Pencil cells	IDA (with hypochromic microcytes)
Hereditary elliptocytosis	Elliptocytes
Sickle cells	Sickle cell diseases with target cells
Spherocytes	Hereditary spherocytosis
	Haemolysis (any cause)
Target cells	Liver disease
	Post splenectomy
	IDA
	Thalassaemias
	Sickle cell disease
Polychromasia	Reticulocytosis
Howell–Jolly bodies	Splenectomy
	Hyposplenism
	Megaloblastic anaemia
Heinz bodies	G6PD deficiency
	Splenectomy
Acanthocytes	Abetalipoproteinaemia
Burr cells	Uraemia
Basophilic stippling	Lead poisoning
	Thalassaemias

Table 33

Auer rods	AML
Atypical lymphocytes	EBV
	CMV
	Toxoplasmosis
	HIV
	Lymphoma
	Leukaemia
	Drug reactions
Left shifted – immature	Severe infections
	DKA
	CML
Hypersegmented nuclei (right shifted) – hypermature	Megaloblastic anaemia

LEUKAEMIAS

Acute lymphoblastic leukaemia (ALL)

1 Predominantly affects children
2 Presents with marrow failure
   (a) Fever (even in the absence of infection)
   (b) Anaemia
   (c) Bleeding
   (d) Infection
   (e) Hepatosplenomegaly
   (f) CNS signs
3 Diagnosis
   (a) Circulating blast cells
   (b) DIC (10%)
   (c) ↑ LDH
   (d) Bone marrow examination – morphology (L1–L3)/cytogenetics/ immunophenotype
4 Treatment
   (a) Chemotherapy (induction/consolidation/maintenance/CNS prophylaxis)
   (b) Bone marrow transplantation
   (c) 70–90% cure children (35% adults)
5 Prognostic indicators
   (a) Height of presenting WCC (blasts)
   (b) Age (<1 or >10 years of age do worse)
   (c) Sex (adult males do worse)
   (d) Cytogenetics
   (e) Immunophenotype

Acute myeloid leukaemia (AML)

1 Predominantly affects adults
2 Presents with marrow failure or leukaemic infiltration
   (a) Fever
   (b) Anaemia
   (c) Infection
   (d) Bleeding
   (e) DIC
   (f) Hepatosplenomegaly
   (g) Lymphadenopathy
   (h) Gum or orbital infiltration

3 Diagnosis
   (a) Auer rods on blood film
   (b) Bone marrow examination
   (c) Morphology (M0–M7), cytogenetics and immunophenotyping
4 Treatment
   (a) Chemotherapy (overall 30% cure rate)
   (b) Bone marrow transplantation
5 Prognostic indicators
   (a) Cytogenetics
   (b) Age (over 60 do worse)
   (c) Response to first chemotherapy

Acute promyelocytic leukaemia

1 M3 subtype of AML
2 Majority of cells are abnormal hypergranular promyelocytes
3 Auer rods are common
4 Strongly Sudan black/peroxidase positive
5 Characteristic chromosome abnormality t(15;17)
6 DIC very common with treatment

Chronic myeloid leukaemia (CML)

1 Disease of middle age
2 Clinical features
   (a) Often presents with tiredness, weight loss and sweating
   (b) Splenomegaly (90%) often massive
   (c) Anaemia
   (d) Bruising/bleeding
   (e) Complications associated with hyperleukocytosis may be found
   (f) All patients eventually develop blast crisis (1–10 years)
3 Diagnosis
   (a) High white cell counts
   (b) Anaemia
   (c) Platelets variable
   (d) High serum B_{12}
   (e) Low leukocyte ALP
   (f) Philadelphia chromosome (95%)
   (g) Marrow hyperplasia, sometimes with increased reticulin
4 Treatment
   (a) Hydroxyurea

(b) α-interferon
(c) Bone marrow transplantation
(d) Tyrosine kinase inhibitors (imatinib)

Chronic lymphoid leukaemia (CLL)

1 Most indolent of chronic leukaemias
2 Features
   (a) Many discovered as an incidental finding
   (b) Commonest cause of lymphocytosis in the elderly
   (c) Progression through lymphocytosis to lymphadenopathy to
        hepatosplenomegaly and marrow failure occurs (patients may
        skip stages)
3 95% of B-cell lineage
4 Mature-looking lymphocytes and smear cells seen on the film
5 Treatment
   (a) None
   (b) Chlorambucil
   (c) Fludrabine (nucleoside analogue)
   (d) Steroids if associated autoimmune phenomena
   (e) Radiotherapy

Philadelphia chromosome

1 A balanced translocation between chromosomes 9 and 22
   (a) 90% of CML
   (b) 5% of childhood ALL
   (c) 25% of adult ALL
   (d) 1% of AML

Leukocyte ALP

High in
1 Polycythaemia rubra vera
2 Essential thrombocythaemia
3 Myelofibrosis
4 Neutrophilia
5 Liver cirrhosis
6 Hodgkin's disease
7 Aplastic anaemia
8 Cushing's syndrome (and corticosteroids)

9 Pregnancy
10 Down's syndrome

Low in
1 Pernicious anaemia
2 AML
3 CML
4 Paroxysmal nocturnal haemoglobinuria

LYMPHOMA

Non-Hodgkin's lymphoma (NHL)

1 Progressive clonal expansion of B or T cells and/or natural killer (NK) cells
2 Tumours originating from lymphoid tissues, mainly of lymph nodes
3 85% B-cell origin
4 Low-grade lymphomas
   (a) Slowly progressive peripheral painless lymphadenopathy is most common presentation
   (b) Extranodal involvement and B symptoms (pyrexia, night sweats, weight loss) are common in patients with advanced or end-stage disease
   (c) Bone marrow is frequently involved and may be associated with cytopenia
   (d) Splenomegaly in 40%
   (e) Some have hepatomegaly
5 Intermediate and high-grade lymphomas
   (a) More varied clinical presentation
   (b) Most present with lymphadenopathy (rapidly growing and bulky)
   (c) More than one-third present with extranodal involvement, eg GI tract, skin, bone marrow, sinuses, genitourinary tract, thyroid and CNS
   (d) Splenomegaly
   (e) Hepatomegaly
   (f) Large abdominal mass
   (g) B symptoms are more common (30–40%)
6 Primary CNS lymphomas

(a) High-grade B-cell neoplasms
(b) 1% of all intracranial neoplasms
7 Causes
(a) Chromosomal translocations
(b) Viruses, eg HIV, EBV, HTLV1
(c) *Helicobacter pylori* causes GI MALToma
(d) Environmental factors
8 Investigations
(a) FBC results non-specific
(b) May be evidence of autoimmune haemolysis
(c) LDH (high levels suggest poor prognosis)
(d) β_2-Microglobulin (may be elevated, poor prognosis)
(e) Imaging to stage disease
(f) Biopsy lymph nodes
(g) Bone marrow examination
(h) Cytogenetics
9 Treatment
(a) Chemo-/radiotherapy depends on grade and stage

Hodgkin's lymphoma

1 Reed–Sternberg cells are characteristic
2 B-cell lymphoma
3 May present with
(a) Asymptomatic lymphadenopathy (above the diaphragm in 80%)
(b) B symptoms (eg unexplained weight loss, fever, night sweats) in 40%
(c) Chest pain, cough or SOB due to mediastinal mass
(d) Pruritus
(e) Alcohol-induced pain at sites of nodal disease is specific, but occurs in less than 10% of patients
(f) Pel–Ebstein fever (high fever for 1–2 weeks, followed by an afebrile period of 1–2 weeks) may occur
(g) Hepatosplenomegaly may occur
(h) Central nervous system (CNS) symptoms due to paraneoplastic syndromes may occur
4 Investigation
(a) Lymph node biopsy
(b) Bone marrow
(c) Imaging

5 Staging
  (a) Stage I – single lymph node area or single extranodal site
  (b) Stage II – 2 or more lymph node areas on the same side of the diaphragm
  (c) Stage III – lymph node areas on both sides of the diaphragm
  (d) Stage IV denotes disseminated or multiple involvement of extranodal organs
  (e) Presence or absence of B symptoms. One or more of
      (i)   Fever (temperature >38°C)
      (ii) Drenching night sweats
      (iii) Unexplained loss of more than 10% of body weight within the preceding 6 months
6 Treatment
  (a) Chemo-/radiotherapy depending on stage

Myeloma

1 Plasma cell neoplasm leads to production of a monoclonal paraprotein
2 Diffuse bone marrow infiltration and focal osteolytic deposits may occur
3 Peak age – 70 yrs
4 Paraproteins
  (a) IgG (55%)
  (b) IgA (25%)
  (c) Light chain disease (20%)
5 Symptoms
  (a) Bone pain (eg back, ribs, long bones, shoulder)
  (b) Renal failure – due to light chain deposition
  (c) Anaemia
  (d) Infection
  (e) Neuropathy
  (f) Amyloidosis
  (g) Bleeding
6 Diagnosis
  (a) Abundant plasma cells in marrow
  (b) Paraprotein on electrophoresis
  (c) Bence Jones protein in urine
  (d) Osteolytic bone lesions
  (e) Supported by ↑ ESR, ↑ Ca^{2+}, anaemia, 'pepper pot' skull

7 Treatment
   (a) Supportive (bone pain, transfusion, radiotherapy)
   (b) Chemotherapy +/– autologous bone marrow transplant
8 Prognosis
   (a) 50% alive at 2 years
   (b) Worse if Hb < 7.5 and urea >10 at presentation

Differentiation of myeloma from benign monoclonal gammopathy (MGUS)

Table 34

MGUS	Myeloma
Low level of paraprotein	High levels of paraproteinaemia
Paraproteinaemia remains low	Paraproteinaemia rises
Other immunoglobulins normal	Other immunoglobulins low
No clinical evidence of myeloma	Clinical evidence of myeloma

Myelodysplasias (MDS)

1 Healthy stem cells suppressed by abnormal clonal proliferation
2 Features
   (a) Cytopenias – ↓ Hb the most common, but also ↓ WCC and ↓ platelets or a combination
   (b) Dysplastic changes seen in blood and bone marrow
       (i)   Hypogranular neutrophils
       (ii) Abnormal neutrophil nuclear lobulation
       (iii) Changes in red cell precursors
       (iv) Mononuclear megakaryocytes
   (c) Propensity to transform into acute myeloid leukaemia (normally takes years)
   (d) Cytogenetic abnormalities as seen in AML
   (e) Mainstay of treatment is supportive – antibiotics, transfusion, platelet transfusion

Classification of myelodysplastic syndromes

[See Table 35, overleaf]

Table 35

MDS	Features
Refractory anaemia (RA)	Dysplastic morphological feature seen, but difficult to distinguish
Refractory anaemia with excess blasts (RAEB)	As above plus increased number of blast cells in marrow (5–20%)
Refractory anaemia with excess of blasts in transformation (RAEB-t)	As above but 20–30% blasts in marrow
Chronic myelomonocytic leukaemia (MCML)	Monocytosis in marrow and blood leukaemia
Primary acquired sideroblastic anaemia	Ring sideroblasts in marrow

Complications of bone marrow transplantation

1 Early
   (a) Infections – bacterial, fungal, CMV, HSV
   (b) Haemorrhage
   (c) Acute GVHD
   (d) Graft failure
   (e) Haemorrhagic cystitis
   (f) Interstitial pneumonitis
   (g) Veno-occlusive disease
2 Late
   (a) Infections – especially VZV
   (b) Chronic GVHD – hepatitis, malabsorption, scleroderma, serous effusions, arthritis
   (c) Chronic pulmonary disease
   (d) Cataracts
   (e) Infertility
   (f) Second malignancies

BLEEDING DISORDERS

1 Prothrombin time (PT)
   (a) Measures the extrinsic system and the final common pathway
   (b) Prolonged in
      (i)   Warfarin
      (ii) Liver disease

    (iii) Vitamin K deficiency
    (iv) Deficiency of factors I, II, V, VII and X
    (v) DIC
2 Activated partial thromboplastin time (APTT)
  (a) Measures intrinsic and final common pathway
  (b) Prolonged in
    (i) Heparin
    (ii) Modest increase with warfarin
    (iii) DIC
    (iv) Liver disease
    (v) Massive transfusion
    (vi) Haemophilia (A and B)
    (vii) Antiphospholipid antibody syndrome
3 Thrombin time (TT) – measures the final part of the common pathway
  (a) Prolonged in
    (i) DIC
    (ii) Heparin
4 Bleeding time
  (a) Measure of platelet function
  (b) Prolonged in
    (i) Low platelet count
    (ii) Von Willebrand's disease
    (iii) Aspirin and other antiplatelet agents
    (iv) Afibrinogenaemia
    (v) MDS

Table 36

Disease	PT	APTT	TT	BT	PL
Vitamin K deficiency (and warfarin)	↑↑	↑	N	N	N
Heparin	↑	↑↑	↑↑	N	N
Liver disease	↑	↑	N or ↑	N or ↓	N or ↓
Haemophilia	N	↑↑	N	N	N
Platelet defect	N	N	N	↑	N (↓ in ITP)
Von Willebrand's disease	N	↑↑	N	↑	N
DIC	↑↑	↑↑	↑↑	↑	↓

HAEMATOLOGY

Haemophilia A

1 Deficiency of factor VIII
2 X-linked recessive disorder
3 Presents often early in life after trauma/surgery, bleeds into joints, muscles
4 Diagnosis: ↑ APTT, low factor VIII
5 Management
   (a) Minor bleeds – desmopressin, pressure and elevation
   (b) Major bleeds – eg haemarthrosis, requires factor VIII

Haemophilia B

1 Also known as Christmas disease
2 Due to factor IX deficiency
3 Behaves clinically like haemophilia A

Von Willebrand's disease

1 Autosomal dominant condition (chromosome 12)
2 Commonest inherited coagulopathy in UK
3 Caused by a quantitive or a qualitative abnormality of vWF (von Willebrand Factor) production
4 vWF is made on endothelial cells. It is the glue that sticks platelets to the damaged subendothelium
5 Disease manifests as platelet-type bleeding disorder, with bruising, superficial purpura, menorrhagia, nose bleeds, bleeding from cuts and mucous membranes
6 Diagnosis is made by
   (a) Low factor VIIIc
   (b) Low vWF Ag
   (c) Prolonged bleeding time
   (d) Deficient ristocetin-induced platelet aggregation
7 Treatment is with DDAVP if mild and with vWF concentrate

Disseminated intravascular coagulation

1 Caused by release of procoagulant
2 Massive release of coagulation factors and platelets with laying down of fibrin
3 Fibrin immediately removed as the fibrinolytic system put into overdrive, worsening haemorrhagic tendency

4 Laboratory results
   (a) Prolongation of PT, APTT, TT and BT
   (b) ↑ fibrin degradation products/D-dimer
   (c) Thrombocytopenia
   (d) Microangiopathic blood film
5 Causes
   (a) Obstetric
       (i)   Retroplacental haemorrhage
       (ii) Retained dead fetus
       (iii) Amniotic fluid embolus
       (iv) Severe pre-eclampsia
   (b) Other causes
       (i)   Crush injury
       (ii) Septicaemia
       (iii) Haemolytic transfusion reaction
       (iv) Malignancy (leukaemia, carcinoma)
       (v)   Shock
       (vi) Liver failure
       (vii) Fat embolism
6 Treatment
   (a) Remove cause
   (b) Transfuse with blood, platelets, FFP or cryoprecipitate
   (c) Heparin if thrombotic phenomena prominent

THROMBOPHILIA

Causes of thrombophilia

1 Inherited
   (a) Antithrombin III deficiency
       (i) AD
       (ii) Inhibitors of factors Xa, XIa and XIIa
   (b) Protein C deficiency
       (i)   AD
       (ii) Vitamin K dependent
       (iii) Inhibits factors V and VIII
       (iv) Skin necrosis may occur in some cases with warfarin

(c) Protein S
  (i) AD
  (ii) Vitamin K dependent
  (iii) Inhibits factors V and VIII
(d) Factor V Leiden mutation (activated protein C resistance)
  (i) Most common inherited thrombophilia
  (ii) 5% of healthy individuals
  (iii) Point mutation in the factor V gene
  (iv) Tendency to venous thrombosis (lower risk than other thrombophilias)
(e) Prothrombin gene mutation
(f) Dysfibrinogenaemia
(g) Fibrinolytic defects
(h) Homocystinuria
2 Acquired
(a) Lupus anticoagulant/antiphospholipid syndrome
(b) OCP/oestrogens/tamoxifen
(c) Nephrotic syndrome
(d) Cancer
(e) IBD
(f) Behçet's syndrome
(g) Paroxysmal nocturnal haemoglobinuria

Clinical risk factors for DVT

1 All of the above
2 Increasing age
3 Obesity
4 Immobility
5 Varicose veins
6 Previous family history of thrombosis
7 Major abdominal surgery
8 Trauma to the lower limbs
9 Pregnancy and the puerperium
10 Increased blood viscosity
11 Post MI or stroke
12 Cigarette smoking
13 Diabetic hypermosmolar state

THE SPLEEN

Causes of splenomegaly

1 Myeloproliferative disorders
   (a) Myelofibrosis
   (b) CML
   (c) Polycythaemia rubra vera
   (d) Essential thrombocythaemia
2 Portal hypertension
3 Cirrhosis
4 Congestive cardiac failure
5 Chronic haemolytic anaemias
6 Autoimmune haemolytic anaemia
7 Hereditary spherocytosis
8 Haemoglobinopathies
9 Lymphoproliferative disorders
10 Most lymphomas
11 Chronic lymphocytic leukaemia
12 Hairy cell leukaemia
13 Infection
14 Bacterial
   (a) Typhoid
   (b) *Brucella*
   (c) TB
   (d) Endocarditis
15 Viral
   (a) EBV
   (b) CMV
16 Protozoal
   (a) Malaria
   (b) Leishmaniasis
   (c) Toxoplasmosis
17 Collagen diseases
   (a) RA
   (b) SLE
18 Storage diseases
   (a) Gaucher's syndrome

Indications for splenectomy

1 **Traumatic rupture** – although surgical repair of capsule preferable if possible
2 **Autoimmune destruction of blood cells** – ITP and warm autoimmune haemolytic anaemia after failure of steroids
3 **Haematological malignancies** – low-grade lymphoproliferative disorders with painful splenomegaly, hypersplenism and limited disease outside the spleen. Also sometimes indicated for myeloproliferative disorders, especially myelofibrosis
4 **Congenital haemolytic anaemias** – such as hereditary spherocytosis and elliptocytosis
5 **Staging in Hodgkin's disease and NHL** – done only where CT/MRI is unavailable

Haematological changes post splenectomy

1 Howell–Jolly bodies – nuclear remnants in red cells, normally removed by the spleen
2 Enhanced neutrophilia in response to infection
3 Target cells
4 ↑ Platelets
5 Spherocytes (occasionally)
6 Decreased IgM

Causes of hyposplenism

1 Splenectomy
2 Sickle cell disease
3 Coeliac disease
4 Myeloproliferative disorders
5 Congenital asplenism

Immunology

CELLS OF THE IMMUNE SYSTEM

Polymorphonuclear cells

Neutrophil

1 Multilobed nucleus
2 Half-life of 6 hrs in blood and 1–2 days in tissues
3 Active in bacterial and fungal infections
4 Stored in bone marrow and released in infection
5 Attracted to infected tissue by
   (a) Cytokines (IL-8, TNF-α, GM-CSF)
   (b) Bacterial proteins
   (c) Leukotrienes (LTB4)
   (d) Complement (C3b, C3a)
6 Adhesion molecules (integrins and ICAMs) on endothelium attach to neutrophils and allow them to migrate into the infected tissue
7 Neutrophils pass through endothelium by diapedesis
8 Kill microbes by phagocytosis
9 Oxygen-dependent killing – myeloperoxidase and hydrogen peroxide generate highly reactive oxygen species to kill microbes
10 Oxygen-independent killing involves lysozyme and lactoferrin
11 See page 195 for causes of neutrophilia

Eosinophils

1 Active against multicellular parasites
2 ↑ In allergic patients
3 Can bind IgE
4 Activated by C3b, C4b, C5a, LTB4, IL-3 and IL-5
5 Migrate like neutrophils
6 Phagocytose Ab–Ag complexes
7 See page 196 for causes of eosinophilia

Mast cells and basophils

1 Basophils circulate in blood
2 Mast cells are active in the tissues
3 Produce histamine, prostaglandins, leukotrienes and proteases
4 Involved in immune response to parasites
5 Immediate hypersensitivity (type 1) caused by interaction with Ag bound to IgE

Mononuclear phagocyte system

1 Monocytes present in blood
2 Macrophages active in tissue (Kupffer cells, alveolar macrophages and osteoclasts)
3 Functions
   (a) Cytotoxic (phagocytose opsonised micro-organisms, particularly intracellular parasites such as *Mycobacterium tuberculosis*)
   (b) Antigen-presenting cells
   (c) Produce cytokines
      (i)   IFN-α and -β
      (ii) IL-1
      (iii) IL-6
      (iv) IL-8
      (v) TNF-α
   (d) Involved in delayed hypersensitivity reactions (type 4)
   (e) May differentiate to multinucleate giant cells in granuloma

LYMPHOCYTES

B lymphocytes

1 Mature in bone marrow
2 Form 30% of lymphocytes
3 May differentiate into plasma cells
4 Express MHC 2 molecules on surface
5 Express highly specific monoclonal immunoglobulin on surface
6 Mainly activated by IL-4 (IL-2, -5, -6 also involved)
7 Activation requires both antigen and T-helper cells
8 When activated there is clonal expansion of the specific B cell, and production of plasma cells and memory cells

9 Plasma cells are non-circulating cells (present in lymphoid organs) that produce specific antibodies
10 Functions
   (a) Antibody production
   (b) Antigen presentation
   (c) Produce cytokines to activate T cells

T Lymphocytes

1 Arise from the thymus gland
2 Form 70% of lymphocyte population
3 Important in intracellular infections, tumour surveillance, and graft rejection
4 All T cells have CD3 receptors and T-cell receptors on their surface
5 Activated T cells also have
   (a) IL-2 receptors
   (b) Transferrin receptors
   (c) MHC 2 molecules
6 T-helper (Th) cells (66%)
   (a) Have CD4 receptors that interact with MHC 2 molecules
   (b) Th1 cells
      (i) Involved in cell-mediated immunity
      (ii) Activate macrophages
      (iii) Activate cytotoxic cells
      (iv) Antagonise Th2 cells
      (v) Produce and are activated /influenced by IFN-γ and IL-2
      (vi) Are suppressed by IL-10
      (vii) Produce type 4 hypersensitivity
   (c) Th2 cells
      (i) Involved in humoral immunity
      (ii) Activate and mature B cells
      (iii) Antagonise Th1 cells
      (iv) Produce IL-2, IL-4, IL-5, IL-6 and IL-10
      (v) Are suppressed by interferons
      (vi) Contribute to types 2 and 3 hypersensitivity
7 T-cytotoxic/suppressor cells (33%):
   (a) Have CD8 receptors that interacts with MHC 1 molecules
   (b) Are important in eliminating cells infected with viruses

8 General functions of T cells
   (a) Signalling for B-cell expansion and maturation
   (b) Recruitment and activation of
        (i)   Cells of the monocyte/phagocyte lineage
        (ii) Cytotoxic T cells
   (c) Secretion of cytokines
   (d) Regulation of immune reactions

NK cells

1 Resemble lymphocytes
2 Kill tumour cells or virally infected cells without prior activation
3 Produce IFN-γ
4 Activated by IFN-γ, IL-2, IL-12
5 Cause cell lysis with perforins

Antigen-presenting cells (APC)

1 Monocytes
2 Macrophages
3 Kupffer cells
4 Dendritic cells
5 Langerhans' cells in skin
6 B lymphocytes

IMMUNOGLOBULINS

1 Consist of two heavy and two light chains joined by disulphide
   bonds
2 C-region constant
3 V-region variable
4 Fab sites bind to antigen
5 Fc site receptor for immune cells

IgG

1 Monomer
2 Four subclasses (1 (65%), 2 (20%), 3 (10%), 4 (5%))
3 Most abundant in serum
4 Secondary immune response

5 Can cross the placenta
6 Activates complement via the classical pathway

IgA

1 Monomer (plasma) or dimer (mucosal surfaces and secretions)
2 Monomer > dimer
3 IgA1 and IgA2
4 Predominantly produced by MALT
5 Activates the alternative pathway
6 J chain joins two monomers, forming a dimer
7 Secretory piece facilitates secretion of dimer on to epithelial surfaces

IgM

1 Pentamer joined by J chain
2 Primary immune response
3 Very effective agglutinator
4 Opsonises bacteria
5 Includes blood group antibodies

IgD

1 Monomer
2 Present on B cells
3 Involved in B-cell activation

IgE

1 Involved in type 1 hypersensitivity reactions (anaphylaxis)
2 Present on mast cells and basophils
3 Rises in response to parasitic infections and atopy in patients

Immunoglobulin levels and age

1 At birth
 (a) IgG adult levels (active placental transport)
 (b) IgA absent (increased levels suggest acquired in utero infection)
 (c) IgM absent (increased levels suggest acquired in utero infection)
2 IgG levels fall at 3–6 months (prone to infection)

3 Adult levels
  (a) IgM 1 year
  (b) IgG 5–6 years
  (c) IgA puberty

COMPLEMENT

1 Positive feedback enzymatic cascade of > 40 proteins
2 Complement mainly made in the liver
3 Functions
  (a) Opsonisation and lysis of bacteria
  (b) Production of proinflammatory mediators
  (c) Solubilisation of antibody–antigen complexes
4 Critical step is activation of C3 to C3b
5 C3 is activated by the classical and alternative pathways
6 Classical pathway
  (a) Initiated by Ab–Ag complexes
  (b) Components involved: C1q, C1r, C1s, C2, C3, C4
  (c) C4b2a cleaves and activates C3
7 Alternative pathway
  (a) Activated by
    (i) Endotoxin
    (ii) Bacterial cell walls
    (iii) IgA
  (b) Components involved: C3, factor D, factor B and properdin
  (c) C3bBb activates C3
8 Membrane attack pathway
  (a) Final common pathway
  (b) Generates the more biologically active components, such as C5a and the membrane attack complex
  (c) C5, C6, C7, C8 and C9 involved
9 Some important components of the complement pathway
  (a) C3a
    (i) Mediates inflammation
    (ii) Anaphylatoxin
  (b) C3b
    (i) Cleaves C5
    (ii) Opsonises
    (iii) Activates alternative pathway

(c) C5a
   (i) Mediates inflammation
   (ii) Anaphylatoxin
   (iii) Chemotaxin
(d) Membrane attack complex
   (i) Structure that makes holes in cell membranes
   (ii) Causes lysis of cell membranes and cell death
10 Regulatory proteins
   (a) C1 inhibitor
      (i) Inhibits C1s and C1r irreversibly
   (b) C4 binding protein
      (i) Inhibits cleavage of C3
   (c) Factor H
      (i) Inhibits cleavage of C3
   (d) Decay accelerating factor (DAF)
      (i) Inhibits cleavage of C3
   (e) Complement receptor 1
      (i) Inhibits cleavage of C3

CYTOKINES

[See Table 37, overleaf]

HYPERSENSITIVITY

Type 1 (anaphylactic)

1 Immediate (< 30 min)
2 IgE mediated
3 Specific Ag + IgE + mast cell/basophil = vasoactive mediator release
4 Leads to
   (a) Smooth muscle contraction
   (b) Vasodilatation
   (c) Increased vascular permeability
   (d) Attraction of eosinophils
   (e) Oedema
   (f) Bronchial constriction
   (g) Wheals

Table 37

Cytokine	Major producer cells	Main action
IL-1α, IL-1β	Macrophages, endothelial cells	Acute-phase response, macrophage and neutrophil migration
IL-2	T cells	Proliferation of T cells, B cells and NK cells
IL-3	T cells	Early hematopoiesis
IL-4	T cells, mast cells	B-cell activation, IgE switch, inhibition of Th1 cells
IL-5	T cells, mast cells	Eosinophil growth and differentiation
IL-6	Macrophages, endothelial cells	T-cell and B-cell growth differentiation, induction of acute-phase proteins
IL-7	Bone marrow, thymic epithelium	Growth of pre-B and pre-T cells
IL-9	T cells	Stimulates mast cells and Th2 cells
IL-10	T cells, macrophages	Suppression of macrophage functions
IL-11	Stromal fibroblasts	Haematopoiesis
IL-12	Macrophages, dendritic cells	NK cell activation, Th1 cell differentiation
IL-13	T cells	B-cell growth and differentiation, inhibition of Th1 cells and macrophages
IL-15	Non-T cells	Growth of T cells and NK cells
IL-16	T cells, mast cells, eosinophils	Chemoattractant for CD4 T cells, monocytes and eosinophils
IL-17	CD4 memory cells	Cytokine production by epithelia, endothelia, and fibroblasts
IL-18	Macrophages	IFN-γ production by T cells and NK cells
IFN-γ	Leukocytes Fibroblasts	Macrophage activation, increase expression of MHC molecules, Ig class switching, inhibition of Th2 cells Antiviral, increases MHC class I expression

Table 37 (cont.)

Cytokine	Major producer cells	Main action
INF-α	Macrophages, NK cells, T cells	Induction of proinflammatory cytokines, endothelial cell activation, apoptosis
TNF-α	Macrophages T cells	Activates macrophages, increases MHC expression, increases neutrophil cytotoxicity, stimulates acute-phase response
TNF-β	T cells, B cells	Cell death, endothelial activation, lymphoid organ development
TGF-β	Monocytes, T cells	Anti-inflammatory, inhibits cell growth, induces IgA secretion
G-CSF	Fibroblasts and monocytes	Neutrophil development and differentiation
GM-CSF	Macrophages, T cells	Growth and differentiation of myelomonocytic lineage cells

5 Systemic reaction leads to anaphylaxis
6 Local reactions lead to atopy – asthma, hay fever, eczema, allergic rhinitis

Type 2 (cytotoxic)

1 IgG and IgM antibody mediated
2 Ig + tissue Ag = complement activation, lysis, opsonisation, phagocytosis and inflammation
3 Neutrophils attracted
4 Examples include
    (a) Transfusion reactions
    (b) Haemolytic disease of the newborn
    (c) ITP
    (d) Haemolytic anaemia
    (e) PA
    (f) Pemphigus
    (g) MG
    (h) Goodpasture's syndrome

(i)   Rheumatic fever
(j)   Drug-induced nephritis
(k) Hyperacute allograft rejection

Type 3 (immune complex)

1 Circulating antibody that reacts with free antigen, forming immune complexes
2 Ig–Ag deposits lead to complement, mast cell and neutrophil activation
3 Leads to
   (a) Vasculitis (deposited in vessels)
   (b) Nephritis (deposited in kidneys)
   (c) Extrinsic allergic alveolitis (deposited in lungs)
4 Examples include
   (a) Arthrus reaction
   (b) Serum sickness
   (c) SLE
   (d) RA
   (e) Glomerulonephritis
   (f) Vasculitis
   (g) SBE
   (h) Extrinsic allergic alveolitis
   (i) HSP

Type 4 (delayed hypersensitivity)

1 Involves cell-mediated cytotoxicity (CD4 T cells), mediator release and macrophage activation
2 Reaction after > 12 hrs
3 Leads to
   (a) Erythema
   (b) Granuloma formation
4 Examples include
   (a) TB
   (b) Mantoux test
   (c) Graft rejection
   (d) Graft versus host disease
   (e) Contact dermatitis

Type 5

1 Antibody reacts with a surface receptor to switch on a cell
2 Graves' disease due to thyroid-stimulating antibodies

IMMUNODEFICIENCY

Primary B cell and antibody deficiencies

X-linked infantile (Bruton's) agammaglobulinaemia

1 X linked (BTK gene)
2 Expressed at 5–6 months when maternal derived IgG ↓
3 Absent B cells
4 Pre-B cells present in bone marrow but cannot mature into plasma cells
5 Gene defect on X chromosome leading to absent Bruton's tyrosine kinase
6 Severe depression or absence of all immunoglobulins
7 Diagnosis by low CD19 lymphocytes with low IgG
8 Lymph nodes small and tonsils absent
9 Recurrent pyogenic bacterial infections (particularly encapsulated organisms)
10 Malabsorption syndrome due to *Giardia lamblia* infection
11 Many live 20–30 yrs
12 Often die of bronchiectasis
13 Treatment with iv γ-globulin and prophylactic antibiotics

Selective IgA deficiency

1 Recurrent sinus and respiratory infections
2 Chronic diarrhoeal diseases, eg *Giardia*
3 Increased incidence of coeliac disease
4 Associated with HLA B8 DR3 and autoimmune disease (below)
5 IgA antibodies in 30–40% – may lead to anaphylaxis during blood transfusion
6 20% have IgG subclass (2 and 4) deficiencies – more severe respiratory infections
7 Some patients develop increased IgM (hyper-IgM syndrome)
8 Symptomatic treatment
9 γ-Globulin only used if associated IgG subclass deficiency

T-cell disorders

Congenital thymic aplasia (Di George syndrome)

1 Thymus and parathyroids fail to develop (third and fourth pharyngeal pouches)
2 Defect on chromosome 22
3 Clinical features (NB CATCH 22)
   (a) **C**ongenital heart disease
   (b) **A**bnormalities of facial and ear structures
   (c) **T**hymic aplasia
   (d) **C**left palate
   (e) **H**ypoparathyroidism/hypocalcaemia/hypothyroidism
4 ↓ Cell-mediated immunity
   (a) Chronic rhinitis
   (b) Recurrent pneumonia
   (c) Candidiasis
   (d) Diarrhoea
5 Treatment
   (a) Symptomatic (calcium etc)
   (b) Surgery
   (c) Thymic transplantation

Combined B- and T-cell disorders

Severe combined immunodeficiency disease

1 X linked or AR
2 Failure of stem cells to differentiate into T and B cells
3 Some are caused by lack of adenosine deaminase (AR)
4 Infants have very few lymphocytes in blood or lymphoid tissue
5 Susceptible to all microbial infections, notably rotavirus, CMV, Candida, *Pneumocystis carinii*
6 Symptoms occur in early infancy and are fatal in the first year of life if untreated
7 Bone marrow transplant treatment of choice

Common variable immunodeficiency

1 AD/AR
2 Onset 15–35 years
3 Combined B-/T-cell defects

4 Impaired cell-mediated immunity
5 $\downarrow$ Immunoglobulins (< 3 g/l)
6 May follow EBV infection
7 Associated with IgA deficiency
8 Treatment with iv γ-globulin and prophylactic antibiotics
9 Clinical features
   (a) Recurrent pyogenic bacterial infections
   (b) Autoimmune diseases common (especially PA)
   (c) Increased incidence of *Giardia lamblia* and malabsorption
   (d) Lactose intolerance
   (e) Anaemia
   (f) Splenomegaly
   (g) Thrombocytopenia
   (h) Lymphoid malignancies
   (i) Arthritis
   (j) Leukopenia

Ataxia telangiectasia

1 AR (ATM gene chromosome 11)
2 Failure of DNA repair
3 Deficiencies of T cells, IgA, IgG2 and IgG4
4 Clinical features
   (a) Cerebellar ataxia (presents at 18 months)
   (b) Recurrent sinus/pulmonary infections
   (c) Oculocutaneous telangiectasia (age 6)
   (d) $\uparrow$ Malignancy
   (e) Endocrine abnormalities
      (i) Glucose intolerance
      (ii) Hypogonadism
      (iii) Abnormal liver enzymes
      (iv) $\uparrow$ AFP and CEA
5 Treatment
   (a) Antibiotics and sunscreens
   (b) Immunoglobulins reduce infective episodes

Wiskott–Aldrich syndrome

1 X-linked recessive
2 Defect in WASP gene – impaired intracellular signalling in T cells and failure of T cells to help B cells

3 Normal circulating lymphocyte numbers
4 IgG – normal
5 IgA – ↑
6 IgE – ↑
7 IgM – ↓
8 Clinical features
   (a) Thrombocytopenia (severe)
   (b) Multiple infections
   (c) Eczema
   (d) Lymphoid malignancies
   (e) Bleeding episodes
   (f) Autoimmune disease
9 Treated with bone marrow transplant

Primary phagocytic disorders

Chronic granulomatous disease

1 AR or X linked
2 Neutrophils lack NADPH oxidase, necessary to produce highly reactive oxygen species to kill micro-organisms
3 Normal numbers of neutrophils
4 Diagnosed by inability of phagocytes to reduce nitroblue tetrazolium dye
5 Leads to granuloma formation
6 Clinical features
   (a) Pneumonia
   (b) Lymphadenitis
   (c) Abscesses (skin, liver, other viscera)
7 Interferon-γ reduces infection rate

Leukocyte adhesion deficiency

1 AR
2 Defect in CD18
3 Leukocytes unable to adhere to vascular endothelium expressing ICAM-1, so cannot migrate
4 Blood shows dramatic leukocytosis
5 Cannot form pus efficiently
6 Present with severe bacterial infections
7 Can be treated with bone marrow transplant

Chediak–Higashi disease

1 AR (CHS-1 gene)
2 Defects in microtubules lead to inability of lysosomes to release their granules
3 Partial albinism and recurrent pyogenic infections
4 Poor prognosis, most dying in childhood
5 Diagnosed by giant granules in neutrophils
6 Treatment with bone marrow transplant and antibiotics

Job's syndrome

1 AD
2 Hyper-IgE
3 Neutrophils do not respond to chemotactic stimuli
4 Reduced production of interferon-γ
5 Recurrent cold staphylococcal abscesses (boils)
6 Chronic eczema
7 Otitis media

COMPLEMENT DEFICIENCY

Primary complement deficiencies

Table 38

Deficiency	Disorder
C1qrs, C2, C4	Immune complex disease
C1 esterase inhibitor	Hereditary angio-oedema
C3, factor H, factor I	Recurrent pyogenic infections
C5-8, properdin, factor D	Recurrent *Neisseria* infections
C9	Asymptomatic
CD59, DAF, HRF, proteins	Paroxysmal nocturnal haemoglobinuria

Hereditary angio-oedema

1 AD
2 85% due to deficiency of C1 esterase
3 15% due to defective C1 esterase
4 Clinical features
 (a) Recurrent oedema

      (i)   Subcutaneous (non-itchy, no erythema) – 91%
      (ii) Laryngeal (stridor) – 48%
      (iii) Intestinal (abdominal pain or obstruction)
  (b) Onset in 1–2 hrs
  (c) Resolves in 24–48 hrs
  (d) First attacks usually in childhood
  (e) Precipitating factors
      (i)   Intercurrent infection
      (ii) Stress
      (iii) Trauma
      (iv) Menstruation
      (v) Autoimmune disease
      (vi) ACEI
      (vii) OCP

5 Diagnosis
  (a) Decreased C2 and C4 during an attack
  (b) C3 normal
  (c) Decreased C1 esterase

6 Treatment
  (a) IV C1 esterase inhibitor/FFP
  (b) Prophylaxis with danazol or tranexamic acid

Paroxysmal nocturnal haemoglobinuria

1 Absence of inhibitors of complement activation (DAF/HRF/CD59)
2 Cells susceptible to complement induced lysis
3 Acquired clonal disorder
4 Leads to intravascular haemolysis
5 Predisposes to venous thromboembolism and infection
6 Can evolve into aplastic anaemia or acute leukaemia
7 Clinical features
  (a) Haemoglobinuria
  (b) Jaundice
  (c) Anaemia
  (d) Abdominal pain
8 Diagnosis by Ham's test
9 Treatment supportive with anticoagulation and antibiotics
10 Severe cases may need bone marrow transplant

Secondary complement deficiencies occur in

1 Post streptococcal nephritis
2 SLE
3 Chronic membranoproliferative GN
4 Serum sickness
5 Bacterial septicaemia with capsular micro-organism
6 Malaria
7 Liver disease

ACQUIRED IMMUNODEFICIENCY

Immunoglobulin deficiency

1 Drugs
  (a) Gold
  (b) Phenytoin
  (c) Penicillamine
  (d) Idiosyncratic reactions
2 Haematological malignancy
  (a) CLL
3 Protein loss
  (a) Nephrotic syndrome
  (b) Protein-losing enteropathy

Cell-mediated dysfunction

1 Drugs
  (a) Ciclosporin
  (b) Cyclophosphamide
  (c) Steroids
2 Haematological malignancy
  (a) Lymphoma
3 AIDS

MAJOR HISTOCOMPATIBILITY COMPLEX

1 Genes expressed on short arm of chromosome 6
2 Codes for human leukocyte antigens
3 HLA are molecules involved in antigen recognition by T lymphocytes

4 T lymphocytes will only recognise antigen that is presented by an HLA molecule
5 Class 1
(a) A, B, C
(b) Present on almost all cells
(c) Signals that carrier cell is 'infected' and suitable for destruction
(d) Only interacts with CD8 cytotoxic T cells
6 Class 2
(a) DP, DQ, DR
(b) Present on B cells, macrophages, dendritic cells and activated T cells
(c) Interacts with CD4 T-helper cells to protect against cytotoxic T cells
7 Class 3
(a) Codes for complement C4 and factor B

TRANSPLANTATION

Types of transplant

1 Autograft – transplant within one individual
2 Syngraft – transplant between genetically identical individuals
3 Allograft – transplant between non-identical individuals
4 Xenograft – transplant between species

Rejection

Table 39

Type	Time	Pathophysiology
Hyperacute	Minutes	Due to preformed antibodies, ie ABO mismatch, antibodies to HLA class 1 molecules from previous transfusion or transplant
Acute	< 10 days	Mediated by CD8 cytotoxic T cells
Chronic	Years	Unclear. Could be due to immune complex deposition and complement activation

Graft versus host disease

1 Immunocompetent T cells from the graft recognise alloantigens from the recipient and cause an immune response
2 Relatively common after bone marrow transplant
3 Clinical features:
   (a) Dermatitis (mild to severe necrolytic)
   (b) Diarrhoea (mild to severe)
   (c) Cholestatic liver disease
   (d) Destruction of red blood cells
   (e) Can be fatal
4 Chances reduced by close HLA matching and selective destruction in the T lymphocytes using monoclonal antibodies
5 Treatment with ciclosporin, methylprednisolone and antithyrocyte globulin

VACCINES

Live attenuated

1 Measles
2 Mumps
3 Rubella
4 Polio (Sabin)
5 Varicella zoster
6 BCG (TB)
7 Yellow fever

Inactivated (killed)

1 Polio (Salk)
2 Influenza
3 Rabies
4 Cholera
5 Typhoid
6 Pertussis
7 Hepatitis A
8 Japanese encephalitis

IMMUNOLOGY

Subunit vaccines

1 Hepatitis B
2 Influenza
3 *Streptococcus pneumoniae*
4 *Neisseria meningitidis* types A and C
5 *Haemophilus influenzae* type b

Preformed antibody vaccines

1 Tetanus
2 Hepatitis B
3 Botulism
4 Rabies
5 Varicella
6 Diphtheria
7 CMV

Current immunisation guidelines

2, 3 and 4 months

1 Triple vaccine (diphtheria, tetanus, pertussis)
2 Hib
3 Meningococcal C
4 Polio
5 (BCG in high risk children)

12–15 months

1 MMR

4–5 years

1 Polio booster
2 Diphtheria and tetanus booster
3 MMR booster

10–14 years

1 BCG

15–18 years

1 Diphtheria and tetanus booster
2 Polio booster

Adulthood

1 Rubella in women seronegative for rubella
2 Tetanus 10-yearly

High-risk groups

1 Hepatitis A
2 Hepatitis B
3 Influenza
4 Pneumococcal
5 Rabies
6 Anthrax

Travellers to high-risk areas

1 Yellow fever
2 Typhoid
3 Cholera
4 Hepatitis A
5 Japanese encephalitis

MISCELLANEOUS

Indications for iv immunoglobulin

Primary immunodeficiency

1 X-linked hypogammaglobulinaemia
2 Common variable immunodeficiency

Secondary immunodeficiency

1 CLL
2 Bone marrow transplantation
3 Paediatric AIDS
4 Myeloma

Inflammatory conditions

1 Kawasaki's disease
2 ITP
3 Guillain–Barré syndrome

The acute-phase response

1 Normocytic anaemia
2 ↑ Immunoglobulins
3 CRP
4 Serum amyloid P
5 Mannose-binding protein
6 Ferritin
7 ↑ Fibrinogen leads to ↑ ESR
8 ALP
9 ↓ Albumin
10 ↑ Platelets
11 ↑ Complement
12 ↑ Caeruloplasmin
13 ↑ Alpha$_1$-antitrypsin
14 ↑ Angiotensin
15 ↑ Haptoglobin
16 ↑ Fibronectin

CRP

1 Useful in monitoring inflammation
2 Acute-phase reactant
3 Rises within hours
4 Falls in 2–3 days
5 Marked elevation
   (a) Bacterial infection
   (b) Abscess
   (c) Crohn's disease
   (d) Connective tissue diseases (except SLE)
   (e) Neoplasia
   (f) Trauma
   (g) Necrosis
6 Normal or slight elevation
   (a) Viral infection

(b) Steroids/oestrogens
(c) UC
(d) SLE

Autoantibodies in autoimmune disease

Table 40

Disease	Antigen
Hashimoto's thyroiditis	Thyroglobulin
	Thyroid peroxidase
Graves' disease	TSH receptor
PA	Intrinsic factor
	Parietal cell
Addison's disease	Adrenal cortex cells (17/21 hydroxylase)
IDDM	Cytoplasm of islet cell
	Insulin
	Glutamic acid decarboxylase (GAD) – also in stiff man syndrome
Myasthenia gravis	ACh receptor
Lambert Eaton syndrome	Calcium channels on nerve endings
Guillain–Barré syndrome	Peripheral nerve myelin components
Paraneoplastic polyneuropathies	CNS proteins – Hu, Yo, Ri.
Goodpasture's syndrome	Glomerular and lung basement membrane
Pemphigoid	Skin basement membrane
Pemphigus	Desmosomes between prickle cells in epidermis
Autoimmune haemolytic anaemia	Erythrocytes
ITP	Platelets
PBC	Mitochondria
Autoimmune hepatitis	ANA
	Smooth muscle
	Liver/kidney/microsomal
Some male infertility	Spermatozoa

Autoantibodies in rheumatological disorders (See Rheumatology, page 450)

Autoimmune polyglandular syndromes

Type 1

1 Mucocutaneous candidiasis
2 Adrenal failure
3 Hypoparathyroidism
4 Gonadal failure
5 Alopecia
6 Malabsorption
7 Autoimmune hepatitis

Type 2

1 Adrenal failure
2 Thyroid disease
3 Type 1 diabetes
4 Gonadal failure
5 Vitiligo
6 Coeliac disease
7 Myasthenia gravis

EICOSANOIDS

Prostaglandins

1 Produced by cyclo-oxygenase from arachidonic acid
2 PGI_2
   (a) Prostacyclin
   (b) Produced in vascular endothelium
   (c) Causes vasodilatation
   (d) Inhibits platelet aggregation
3 PGD_2
   (a) Mainly produced in mast cells
   (b) Produces vasodilatation and oedema
4 PGE_2
   (a) Causes vasodilatation and oedema
   (b) ↑ Pain
   (c) ↑ Fever

5 $PGF_{2\alpha}$
   (a) Causes vasodilatation and oedema
6 Thromboxane A2
   (a) Produced in platelets
   (b) Causes platelet aggregation
   (c) Vasoconstrictor

Leukotrienes

1 Produced by lipo-oxygenase from arachidonic acid in neutrophils
2 LTB4
   (a) Potent chemotactic factor
   (b) Aggregates neutrophils
3 LTC4, D4, E4
   (a) Vasoconstrict
   (b) Cause bronchospasm
   (c) Increase vascular permeability

Infectious Disease

MODES OF TRANSMISSION

1 Airborne – eg measles, diphtheria, tonsillitis, whooping cough, tuberculosis
2 Intestinal – eg enterovirus, viral hepatitis, poliomyelitis, salmonellosis, Q fever
3 Direct contact – eg impetigo, scabies
4 Venereal route – eg gonorrhoea, syphilis
5 Insect or animal bite – eg malaria, leishmaniasis, trypanosomiasis, rabies
6 Bloodborne – eg hepatitis B, C, HIV
7 Congenital transmission

FACTORS AFFECTING VULNERABILITY TO DISEASE

1 Immunological
   (a) Genetic deficiency – immunoglobulin/complement/T-cell deficiency
   (b) Prior immunity – natural or vaccine
   (c) Acquired deficiency – HIV, malignant disease, transplant patients
   (d) Miscellaneous – eg diabetes, pregnancy, splenectomy
2 Other
   (a) Psychological status
   (b) Nutritional status
   (c) Foreign bodies
   (d) Behavioural factors (smoking, alcoholics)
   (e) Previous antibiotics (eg *Clostridium difficile*, MRSA)

241

NOTIFIABLE DISEASES

Table 41

Acute encephalitis	Opthalmia neonatorum
Acute poliomyelitis	Paratyphoid fever
Anthrax	Plague
Cholera	Rabies
Ebola	Food poisoning
Leprosy	Relapsing fever
Leptospirosis	Scarlet fever
Malaria	Small pox
Measles	Tetanus
Meningitis	Tuberculosis
Meningococcal septicaemia	Typhoid fever
Mumps	Yellow fever
Viral hepatitis	Viral haemorrhagic fever
Whooping cough	Dysentery (amoebic or bacillary)

ANTIBIOTICS

Choice of antibiotic

1 Blind
   (a) Clinical diagnosis
   (b) Geographical location
   (c) Awaiting microbiological sensitivities
2 Spectrum of activity
   (a) Narrow as possible, although blind treatment is usually broad spectrum
   (b) Bactericidal vs bacteriostatic (no firm evidence except bactericidal in bacterial endocarditis)
3 Patient factors
   (a) Site of infection
   (b) Renal/hepatic impairment
   (c) Allergies

Types of antibiotic

1 Inhibitors of cell wall synthesis
   (a) Beta-lactams

    (i)   Penicillins – eg benzylpenicillin, ampicillin, piperacillin
    (ii) Cephalosporins – eg cephalexin, cefotaxime
    (iii) Monobactams – eg aztneonem
    (iv) Carbopentems – eg imipenem
  (b) Glycopeptides – vancomycin, teicoplanin
2 Inhibitors of protein synthesis
  (a) Macrolides – erythromycin, azithromycin, clarithromycin
  (b) Aminoglycosides – gentamicin, tobramycin, amikacin
  (c) Tetracycyline
3 Miscellaneous
  (a) Chloramphenicol
  (b) Clindamycin
  (c) Fusidic acid
4 Inhibitors of DNA replication
  (a) Quinolones (DNA gyrase)
  (b) Metronidazole
5 Inhibitors of folate synthesis
  (a) Co-trimoxazole

Bactericidal antibiotics

1 Penicillins
2 Cephalosporins
3 Aminoglycosides

Antituberculous drugs

1 Rifampicin – inhibits DNA-dependent RNA polymerase
2 Isoniazid – inhibits cell wall synthesis
3 Pyrazinamide – poorly understood, probably works inside phagosomes
4 Ethambutol – inhibits bacterial RNA synthesis
5 Streptomycin – inhibits bacterial protein synthesis

Antiviral drugs (non-HIV)

1 Aciclovir – active against HSV and VZV
2 Ganciclovir – CMV, HSV and VZV
3 Ribavirin – RSV (aerosol), HCV and Lassa (has to be early)

Antihelmintic drugs

1 Benzimidazoles (eg albendazole, thiabendazole, mebendazole)
   (a) *Trichuris*
   (b) Hookworms
   (c) *Enterobius*
   (d) *Ascaris*
   (e) *Taenia*
   (f) *Echinococcus*
2 Piperazines (eg diethylcarbamazine – DEC)
   (a) *Ascaris* and *Enterobius*
   (b) Microfilarial disease – *Onchocerca volvulus, Wuchereria bancrofti, Brugia malayi*
3 Praziquantel
   (a) *Schistosoma*
   (b) *Taenia*

PYREXIA OF UNKNOWN ORIGIN (PUO)

1 Infection (35%)
   (a) TB
   (b) Hidden abscesses
   (c) Subacute bacterial endocarditis
   (d) Infectious mononucleosis
   (e) CMV
   (f) Brucellosis
   (g) Chronic prostatitis
2 Neoplasia (25%)
   (a) Hodgkin's disease and other lymphomas
   (b) Leukaemias
   (c) Solid tumours – eg renal, pancreatic, hepatocellular
   (d) Metastatic carcinoma
3 Connective tissue disease (20%)
   (a) Rheumatoid
   (b) SLE
   (c) PAN
4 Miscellaneous (15%)
   (a) Sarcoid
   (b) Multiple pulmonary emboli

(c) Crohn's disease
(d) Familial Mediterranean fever
(e) Drugs
5 Undiagnosed (5–10%)

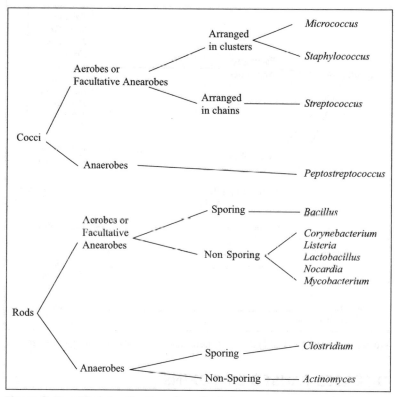

Figure 2 Simplified classification of medically important gram-positive bacteria

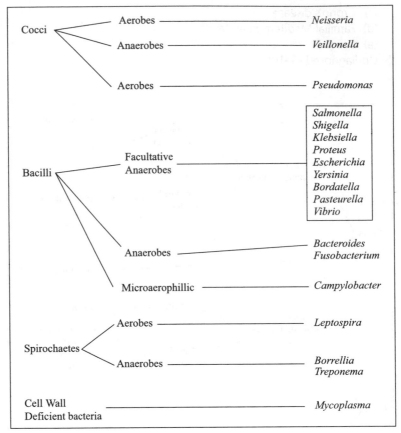

Figure 3 Simplified classification of medically important gram-negative bacteria

DISEASES CAUSED BY TOXINS

1 Diphtheria
  (a) *Corynebacterium diphtheriae* is the causative Gram-positive organism
  (b) Clinical features
      (i)   Incubation 2–5 days
      (ii) Upper respiratory tract illness
      (iii) Sore throat
      (iv) Low-grade fever
      (v)   An adherent membrane of the tonsil(s), pharynx and/or nose

(c) Complications
  (i) Cardiotoxic (heart failure)
  (ii) Neurotoxic (cranial and peripheral nerve paralysis)
  (iii) Death from suffocation caused by obstruction of airways by membrane
(d) Diagnosis
  (i) Throat swab
  (ii) Culture on Loeffler or tellurite media
(e) Treatment/prevention
  (i) Antitoxin
  (ii) Antibiotics (penicillin or erythromycin)
  (iii) Tracheotomy – to relieve laryngeal obstruction
  (iv) Vaccine

2 Tetanus
(a) Causative organism is *Clostridium tetani*
(b) Affects the nervous system and causes painful, uncontrolled muscle spasms
(c) Spores enter the body through an open wound and produce a powerful neurotoxin
(d) Spores are found throughout the environment, usually in soil, dust and animal waste
(e) Preventable through immunisation
(f) Because of widespread use of tetanus vaccine, the condition is now rare
(g) Recent outbreaks amongst intravenous drug users

3 Botulism
(a) Causative organism is *Clostridium botulinum*
(b) Human botulism is a serious but relatively rare disease
(c) Disease results from intoxication by extremely potent toxins in preformed foods
(d) No person-to-person transmission
(e) Clinical features
  (i) Marked fatigue
  (ii) Weakness and vertigo, followed by blurred vision, dry mouth, and difficulty in swallowing and speaking
  (iii) Vomiting, diarrhoea, constipation and abdominal swelling may occur
  (iv) Can progress to weakness in the neck and arms and the respiratory muscles
(f) Prevention of botulism is based on good food preparation (particularly preservation) practices and hygiene

(g) Antitoxin administration is indicated as soon as possible after clinical diagnosis has been made

4 Toxic shock syndrome
  (a) Mediated by toxin TSST-1, produced by *Staphylococcus aureus*
  (b) Rare, life-threatening
  (c) Associated with the use of superabsorbent tampons and occasionally with the use of contraceptive sponges

ZOONOSES

1 An infectious disease that can be transmitted from animals to humans
2 The list is long and encompasses many different species
  (a) Anthrax (cattle/sheep)
  (b) Brucellosis (cattle, goats, sheep)
  (c) Cat scratch disease and related *Bartonella* spp infections (cats)
  (d) Chagas' disease (trypanosomiasis) (dogs and various wild animal species, including raccoons, armadillos and opossums)
  (e) Dermatophytosis (ringworm), dermatophilosis, sporotrichosis, erysipelas (horses, cattle and dogs)
  (f) *Escherichia coli* O157 (deer, pigs, cows)
  (g) Gastroenteritis agents
    (i) *Campylobacter*
    (i) *Salmonella*
    (iii) *Yersinia*
    (iv) *Giardia*
    (v) *Cryptosporidium*
  (h) Japanese encephalitis virus (shore birds, such as herons and egrets, and pigs)
  (i) Larva migrans and *Echinococcus* hydatidosis (dogs and livestock)
    (i) Cutaneous, visceral and ocular larva migrans; *Cuterebra* myiasis; screw worm myiasis; human infection with canine whipworm
    (ii) *Strongyloides stercoralis* larva migrans
    (iii) *Echinococcus* hydatidosis
  (j) Leptospirosis (rats, dogs, pigs, cattle)
  (k) Listeriosis (many different species)
  (l) Lyme disease (dogs) – see below
  (m) Orf and milkers' nodules (cows, goats)

(n) Plague (rats)
(o) Q fever (sheep, cattle and goats)
(p) Rocky Mountain spotted fever (dogs)
(q) Systemic mycoses (dogs and cats)
  (i) Blastomycosis
  (ii) Histoplasmosis
  (iii) Coccidioidomycosis
  (iv) Cryptococcosis
(r) Toxoplasmosis (cats)
(s) Tuberculosis/*Mycobacterium* infections
(t) Tularaemia (rabbits, squirrels, voles, muskrats, beavers and other species)
(u) Visceral leishmaniasis (dogs and small mammals)
(v) West Nile virus (birds)

Lyme disease

1 Tickborne disease – most common in USA
2 Aetiologic agent is *Borrelia burgdorferi*
3 Transmitted from animals to humans by harbouring infected ticks
4 First diagnosed among a group of children in Lyme, USA, in 1975
5 Typically divided into three clinical phases
  (a) Early local disease (previously called stage 1)
    (i) Fever, malaise
    (ii) Arthralgia (joint pain)
    (iii) Myalgia (muscle pain)
    (iv) Headaches
    (v) Erythema migrans – target lesions at site of tick bite
  (b) Early disseminated disease (previously called stage 2)
    (i) Occurs weeks to months after initial infection
    (ii) Neurological disease (especially meningitis and Bell's (facial nerve) palsy)
    (iii) Myocarditis
    (iv) Arthropathy without joint effusion
  (c) Late disseminated disease (previously called stage 3)
    (i) Occurs months to years after initial infection
    (ii) Typified by chronic arthritis and/or encephalopathy (sleep disturbances, fatigue, personality changes)
6 Controlled by regular examination of dogs for ticks
7 A recombinant vaccine containing only the ospA (outer-surface protein) from *B. burgdorferi* is available for dogs

RESPIRATORY TRACT INFECTIONS

Viral causes of upper respiratory tract infections (URTI)

1 Rhinoviruses
2 Coronaviruses
3 Adenoviruses
4 Parainfluenza viruses
5 Coxsackie groups A and B
6 Respiratory syncytial virus
7 Epstein–Barr virus

Epstein–Barr virus (infectious mononucleosis/glandular fever)

1 Member of the herpesvirus family and one of the most common human viruses
2 95% of adults between 35 and 40 years of age have been infected
3 Symptoms of infectious mononucleosis
    (a) Fever
    (b) Sore throat
    (c) Swollen lymph glands
    (d) Hepatosplenomegaly
    (e) Cardiac or CNS involvement occurs only rarely
4 No known associations between active EBV infection and problems during pregnancy, such as miscarriage or birth defects
5 Transmission of EBV requires intimate contact with the saliva (found in the mouth) of an infected person ('kissing' fever)
6 Clinical diagnosis of infectious mononucleosis is suggested on the basis of the symptoms
7 Positive reaction to a 'monospot' test

Bacteria responsible for URTI

1 Beta-haemolytic group A streptococcus
2 *Haemophilus influenzae*
3 *Neisseria menigitidis* and *N. gonorrhoea* (mostly asymptomatic)
4 *Moraxella catarrhalis*
5 *Mycoplasma pneumoniae*

Organisms responsible for lower respiratory tract infections (LRTI)

Common

1 *Streptococcus pneumoniae*
2 *Haemophilus influenzae*
3 *Streptococcus pyogenes*
4 *Legionella pneumophila*
5 *Staphylococcus aureus*
6 *Mycoplasma pneumoniae*
7 *Klebsiella pneumoniae*

Uncommon

1 *Chlamydia* spp.
2 *Coxiella burnetii*
3 *Leptospira icterohaemorrhagiae*
4 *Fusobacterium necrophorum*
5 *Salmonella typhi*
6 *Francisella tularensis*
7 *Yersinia pestis*

Immunocompromised

1 *Pseudomonas* spp.
2 *Pneumocystis*
3 *Aspergillus*
4 CMV

Viral

1 RSV
2 Influenza
3 Parainfluenza

GASTROINTESTINAL INFECTIONS

1 Majority of gut infections cause diarrhoea
2 Small bowel infections are usually toxin mediated and cause watery diarrhoea with no blood

3 Large bowel infections typically cause bloody diarrhoea with mucus and sometimes pus – 'dysentery'

Small bowel, toxin-mediated 'secretory' infective agents

1 *Salmonella* spp. – from eggs and chickens (incubation 12–48 hours)
2 Some *Campylobacter* spp. – account for most acute gastroenteritis in UK (2–5 days)
3 Enterotoxigenic *E. coli* (ETEC) – main cause of traveller's diarrhoea (12–72 hours)
4 Rotavirus (1–7 days)
5 *Staphylococcus aureus* (2–6 hours)
6 *Clostridium perfringens* (8–22 hours)
7 *Clostridium botulinum* – canned or bottled food (18–36 hours)
8 *Vibrio cholerae*
9 *Bacillus cereus/subtilis* – contaminated rice (1–5 hours emetic, 12–24 hours diarrhoeal)
10 *Yersinia enterocolitica* (24–36 hours)
11 *Giardia lamblia* (1–4 weeks)
12 Small round structured viruses
13 *Aeromonas* spp.

Large bowel (bloody diarrhoea) invasive agents

1 *Campylobacter* spp.
2 *Shigella* spp. (incubation 2–3 days)
3 *Yersinia enterocolitica*
4 Enteroinvasive *E. coli* (EIEC)
5 *Entamoeba histolytica* – steroids are lethal in amoebiasis, but presents similarly to ulcerative colitis

Large bowel, toxin-mediated infective agents

1 *Clostridium difficile* (toxin A and B)
2 Enterohaemorrhagic *E. coli* (EHEC) – typically serotype O157, responsible for epidemic form of haemolytic–uraemic syndrome – eg Lanarkshire outbreak, 1999

URINARY TRACT INFECTIONS

Causal organisms

1 *Escherichia coli* – 60–90%
2 *Proteus mirabilis* – 10%
3 *Staphylococcus saprophyticus* – an important cause in sexually active women
4 *Klebsiella* spp.
5 *Streptococcus faecalis*
6 'Fastidious' Gram-positive bacteria – lactobacillus, streptococci, corynebacteria
7 Organisms after catheterisation – eg *Pseudomonas aeruginosa*, *Staphylococcus aureus*
8 *Mycobacterium tuberculosis*

Suitable oral antibiotics

All excreted in urine

1 Trimethoprim
2 Co-trimoxazole
3 Amoxicillin
4 Co-amoxiclav
5 Nitofurantoin
6 Nalidixic acid
7 Cephalexin

SEXUALLY TRANSMITTED INFECTIONS

Gonorrhoea

1 *Neisseria gonorrhoeae*
2 Transmission by oral/vaginal/anal intercourse
3 Large asymptomatic population
4 Symptoms include pus-like discharge, PU, itch, pain
5 In UK predominantly sensitive to penicillin, ciprofloxacin, cephalosporin or tetracycline
6 Untreated may cause urethral strictures, PID (women), prostatitis/epididymitis (men)
7 Responsible for ophthalmia neonatorum

Chlamydia

1 *Chlamydia trachomatis*
2 Responsible for >50% of cases of non-specific urethritis (NSU)
3 Cause of PID in women and infertility
4 Can cause conjunctivitis and a diffuse pneumonia in neonates
5 Sensitive to doxycycline and erythromycin

Trichomoniasis

1 Caused by *Trichomonas vaginalis* – flagellated protozoan
2 Cause of foul-smelling greeny/yellow discharge PV and vaginitis
3 Treated with metronidazole

Herpes simplex virus (HSV)

1 Types 1 and 2
2 Can be dormant for very long periods
3 Leads to painful genital ulceration
4 Aciclovir helps reduce time lesions are present
5 Can recur after initial infection, but normally less aggressively

Anogenital warts

1 Caused by human papilloma virus (HPV) – up to 60 different types
2 Benign tumours of the skin
3 Can cause large lesion around anus, glans, labia or vagina
4 Treated with cryotherapy and podophyllin
5 Often recur
6 Types 16 and 18 associated with carcinoma of cervix

Syphilis

1 Aetiological agent is *Treponema pallidum*
2 Transmission mainly sexual. Incubation 2–4 weeks
3 Four clinical stages
   (a) Primary
      (i)   Painless genital ulceration – the classic chancre
      (ii) Heals in 3–8 weeks
   (b) Secondary

     (i) Presents with generalised maculopapular rash 6–8 weeks later
     (ii) Generalised lymphadenopathy
     (iii) Rare manifestations include periostitis, arthritis, hepatitis, glomerulonephritis
(c) Tertiary
     (i) 3–10 years after the primary lesion
     (ii) Gummata (granulomatous nodules) form in skin, mucous membranes or bones
     (iii) Gummata can break down to form shallow punched-out ulcers
(d) Late or quaternary
(e) 10–20 years after primary syphilis
     (i) Two main forms
         (1) Cardiovascular
             (a) Aortitis and aneurysm
             (b) Aortic incompetence
             (c) Coronary ostial stenosis
         (2) Neurological
             (a) Tabes dorsalis
             (b) General paralysis of the insane (dementia, tremor, spastic paralysis)
             (c) Meningovascular syphilis (headache, cranial nerve palsies, pupillary loss of reaction to light (Argyll Robertson pupils)
4 Diagnosis is by direct demonstration of the spirochaete in the fluid of a chancre or ulcerated secondary lesion
5 Treated with penicillin

[See Table 42, overleaf]

HELMINTH INFECTIONS

Cestodes – tapeworms

1 *Taenia saginatum* (beef) – cause of cystericosis
2 *Taenia solium* (pork) – as above
3 *Diphyllobothrium latum* (fish)
4 *Echinococcus granulosus* (dog) – cause of cystic hydatid disease

Table 42

Stage of disease	VD Reference Laboratory (VDRL)	*Treponema pallidum* haemagglutination (TPHA)	Fluorescent Treponema antibody absorbed (FTA)
Primary	+ or –	–	+
Late primary	+	+ or –	+
Secondary and tertiary	+	+	+
Late – quarternary	+	+	+
Latent	+	+	+
Treated syphilis	–	+	+
Congenital syphilis	+	+	+

Nematodes – roundworms

1 *Necator americanus* and *Ancylostoma duodenale* – hookworms. Larvae enter feet and migrate to the gut and cause IDA
2 *Strongyloides stercoralis* causes IDA; larvae penetrate feet
3 *Ascaris lumbricoides* – looks like earthworm, can cause GI obstruction
4 *Trichenella spiralis* – transmitted by uncooked pork, migrates to muscle
5 *Enterobius vermicularis* – threadworm/pinworm. Causes pruritus ani. Commonest in UK
6 *Toxocara canis/cati* (dog/cat roundworm) causes visceral larva
7 *Ancylostoma braziliense/canium* (non-human hookworm) – causes cutaneous larva migricans
8 *Dracunculus medinensis* (guinea worm) – very long worm which appears at skin
9 Filariasis – very common
   (a) *Onchocerca volvulus* – causes blindness
   (b) *Wuchereria bancroftii* and *Brugia malayi* – cause lymphadanitis, elephantiasis and tropical pulmonary eosinophilia syndrome
   (c) Loa Loa – may migrate across the conjunctiva

Trematodes – flukes

1 Schistosomiasis (bilharzias) – caused by *Schistosoma haematobuim* (vesical veins) and *Schistosoma mansoni* and *japonicum* (mesenteric veins)

2 *Fasciola hepatica* – liver fluke
3 *Paragonimus westermani* – lung fluke

TROPICAL INFECTIOUS DISEASE AND TRAVEL MEDICINE

[See Table 43, overleaf]

Yellow fever

1 A viral haemorrhagic fever
2 Belongs to the flavivirus group
3 Occurs only in Africa and South America
4 In South America sporadic infections occur almost exclusively in forestry and agricultural workers from occupational exposure in or near forests
5 Transmitted between humans by a mosquito
6 Very rare cause of illness in travellers
7 General precautions are to avoid mosquito bites
8 Yellow fever vaccine is a live virus vaccine
9 The virus remains silent in the body during an incubation period of 3–6 days
10 There are then two disease phases
  (a) 'acute'
    (i) Fever, paradoxically associated with a slow pulse
    (ii) Muscle pain (with prominent backache)
    (iii) Headache
    (iv) Shivers
    (v) Loss of appetite
    (vi) Nausea and/or vomiting
  (b) 15% enter a 'toxic' phase within 24 hours
    (i) Jaundice
    (ii) Abdominal pain with vomiting
    (iii) Bleeding can occur from the mouth, nose, eyes and/or GI tract
    (iv) Renal impairment
    (v) Half of the patients in the toxic phase die within 10–14 days. The remainder recover without significant organ damage

Table 43

Disease	Parasite	Vector
Bilharzia/schistosomiasis	*S. mansoni*	Freshwater snails:
	S. japonicum	*Biomalphalaria*
	S. haematobium	*Oncomelania*
Guinea worm	*Dracunculus mediensis*	Water flea – Cyclops
Blinding worm/onchocerciasis	*Onchocerca volvulus*	Buffalo fly – *Simulium damnosum*
Eye worm	*Loa loa*	Fly – Chrysops
Lung fluke	*Paragonimus westermani*	Crustacean
Visceral leishmaniasis – Kala azar	*L. donovani*	Sandfly
Cutaneous leishmaiasis	*L. infantum*	
Mucocutaneous leishmaniasis –	*L. tropica*	
Espundia	*L. major*	
	L. braziliensis	
	L. mexicana	
African trypanosomiasis –	*T. brucei rhodesiense*	Tsetse fly – *Glossina* sp.
sleeping sickness	*T. brucei gambiense*	
South American trypanosomiasis –	*T. cruzi*	Riduvid bug, cone bug – *Triatoma* sp.
Chagas' disease		
Malaria	*P. falciparum*	Mosquito
	P. vivax	
	P. ovale	
	P. malariae	

11 Differential diagnoses include
  (a) Malaria
  (b) Typhoid
  (c) Rickettsial diseases
  (d) Haemorrhagic viral fevers (eg Lassa)
  (e) Arboviral infections (eg dengue)
  (f) Leptospirosis
  (g) Viral hepatitis
  (h) Poisoning (eg carbon tetrachloride)

Typhoid fever

1 Caused by the bacterium *Salmonella typhi*
2 Still common in the developing world, where it affects about 12.5 million persons each year
3 *Salmonella typhi* lives only in humans
4 Transmission is as a result of poor hygiene/sewage systems. Infected individuals become carriers
5 Clinical features include
  (a) Sustained fever as high as 39–40°C
  (b) Lethargy/anorexia
  (c) Abdominal pains
  (d) Headache
  (e) Rash – 'rose spots'
6 Diagnosis made by culture of *S. Typhi* in stool or blood
7 Vaccine available
8 Ampicillin, trimethoprim–sulfamethoxazole and ciprofloxacin are all used to treat infections

PROTOZOAL INFECTIONS

1 Gastrointestinal
  (a) *Cryptosporidium parvum*
  (b) *Giardia intestinalis (lamblia)*
  (c) Amoeba
  (d) *Entamoeba histolytica*
  (e) *Entamoeba coli*
  (f) *Endolimax nana*

2 Blood and tissue
   (a) Malaria
   (b) Leishmaniasis
   (c) Trypanosomiasis
   (d) Toxoplasmosis
   (e) Babeosis

Malaria

1 A life-threatening parasitic (protozoal) disease
2 Transmitted from person to person through the bite of a female *Anopheles* mosquito
3 40% of the world's population is at risk of malaria
4 90% of deaths due to malaria occur in Africa, mostly among young children
5 There are four types of human malaria
   (a) *Plasmodium vivax*
   (b) *P. malariae*
   (c) *P. ovale*
   (d) *P. falciparum*
6 *P. vivax* and *P. falciparum* are the most common species
7 *P. falciparum* the most serious type of malaria infection
8 In the human host the parasite undergoes a series of changes as part of its complex lifecycle
9 Its various stages allow plasmodia to evade the immune system, infect the liver and erythrocytes, and finally develop into a form that is able to infect a mosquito again when it bites an infected person
10 Inside the mosquito, the parasite matures until it reaches the sexual stage, where it can again infect a human host when the mosquito takes her next blood meal, 10–14 or more days later
11 Resistance to chloroquine is common throughout Africa

Leishmaniasis

1 A globally widespread group of parasitic diseases
2 Transmitted by the bite of the infected female phlebotomine sandfly (about 30 species of sandfly can become infected when taking a blood meal from a reservoir host)
3 Sandfly vector is usually infected with one species of flagellate protozoan belonging to the genus *Leishmania*
4 Most leishmaniases are zoonotic

5 Leishmaniasis presents itself in humans in four different forms, with a broad range of clinical manifestations
  (a) Visceral leishmaniasis (VL) (*Kala azar*)
      (i) Most severe form of the disease
      (ii) Untreated, has a mortality rate of almost 100%
      (iii) Characterized by
          (1) Irregular bouts of fever
          (2) Substantial weight loss
          (3) Hepatosplenomegaly
          (4) Anaemia
  (b) Mucocutaneous leishmaniasis (MCL) (*Espundia*)
      (i) Lesions that can lead to extensive and disfiguring destruction of mucous membranes of the nose, mouth and throat cavities
  (c) Cutaneous leishmaniasis (CL)
      (i) Skin ulcers – as many as 200 in some cases – on the exposed parts of the body, such as the face, arms and legs, causing serious disability and leaving the patient permanently scarred
      (ii) Diffuse cutaneous leishmaniasis (DCL) never heals spontaneously and tends to relapse after treatment
      (iii) Cutaneous forms of leishmaniasis are the most common and represent 50–75% of all new cases

RICKETTSIAL INFECTIONS

1 Most notorious is 'typhus'
2 Transmitted by arthropod vectors, often the reservoirs of the infection
3 Incubation tends to be 1–2 wks
4 Signs/symptoms – acute febrile illness with rash, headache, malaise, haemorrhage and petechiae are common in spotted fevers
5 Rash – maculopapular
6 Eschar – skin ulcer with blackened centre
7 Fatality – varies. With untreated typhus may be as high as 10–15%. In untreated Rocky Mountain fever from 15–20%
8 Treatment is with tetracycline

[See Table 44, overleaf]

Table 44

Disease	Causal organism	Reservoir	Vector	Geographical distribution
Typhus group				
Typhus	*R. prowazeki*	Man	Louse	America, Africa Asia
Murine	*R. typhi*	Rats, mice	Flea	Worldwide
Scrub typhus	*R. tsutsugamushi*	Mites	Mites	Far East
Spotted fever group				
Rocky Mountain spotted fever	*R. rickettsii*	Ticks	Ticks	Americas
Boutonneuse fever	*R. conorii*	Ticks	Ticks	Mediterranean, Africa
Queensland tick typhus	*R. australis*	Ticks	Ticks	Australia
North Asian tick fever	*R. siberica*	Ticks	Ticks	Eastern Russia, China, Mongolia
Rickettsial pox	*R. akari*	Mice	Mites	USA, Russia

FUNGAL INFECTIONS

1 Aerobic
2 Grow readily on simple media
3 Ubiquitous
4 Often a problem in immunocompromised
5 Types
   (a) Yeasts
   (b) Filamentous fungi
   (c) Dimorphic fungi

Yeasts

1 *Candida* – mucous membranes (thrush), chronic mucocutaneous candidosis. Can involve lower respiratory and urinary tract, eye, meninges, kidney and bone
2 *Cryptococcus* – lung granuloma normally primary focus, haematogenous spread ‡ subacute or chronic meningoencephalitis

Filamentous fungi

1 Dermatophytes – ringworm/tinea. Affects nails, skin, hair
2 *Aspergillus* (see below)
3 Zygomycosis
4 *Penicillium*

Dimorphic fungi

1 Coccoidomycosis
2 Histoplasmosis
3 Blastomycosis

Aspergillus fumigatus (See page 402)

Invasive aspergillosis

1 Acute (<1 month course)
2 Subacute/chronic necrotising (1–3 months)

Chronic aspergillosis (>3 months)

1 Chronic cavitary pulmonary
2 Aspergilloma of lung

3 Chronic fibrosing pulmonary
4 Chronic invasive sinusitis
5 Maxillary (sinus) aspergilloma

Allergic

1 Allergic bronchopulmonary (ABPA)
2 Extrinsic allergic (broncho)alveolitis (EAA)
3 Asthma with fungal sensitisation
4 Allergic aspergillus sinusitis (eosinophilic fungal rhinosinusitis)

Metabolic Medicine

LIPIDS

Lipoproteins

1 Very low-density lipoprotein (VLDL)
  (a) Synthesised continuously by liver
  (b) Carries 60% triglycerides and some cholesterol
  (c) Enzymic degradation to intermediate density lipoprotein (IDL) and then LDL
2 Low-density lipoprotein (LDL)
  (a) Formed from IDL by hepatic lipase
  (b) Major carrier of cholesterol
  (c) Binds to, and levels regulated by feedback on to, hepatic LDL receptor
3 High-density lipoprotein (HDL)
  (a) Synthesised in gut wall and liver
  (b) Carries cholesterol from periphery to liver
  (c) Inverse association with ischaemic heart disease
4 Chylomicrons
  (a) Carry dietary lipid from gut to liver
  (b) Broken down by lipoprotein lipase in portal vessels to free fatty acids

Hyperlipidaemias

1 Can be primary or secondary
2 Atherosclerotic disease associated with high total cholesterol and LDL
3 HDL protective

Primary disorders

1 Familial hypercholesterolaemia
  (a) Autosomal dominant
     (i) Heterozygotes ≈ 1:500
     (ii) Homozygotes very rare
  (b) Around 400+ defects in LDL receptor known
  (c) Defect in the receptor means half-life of LDL in plasma is prolonged, leading to increased serum levels
  (d) Heterozygotes
     (i) Total cholesterol 9–15 mmol/l
     (ii) 6–8 times increased risk of IHD (MI at young age)
     (iii) Xanthelasma and tendon xanthoma
  (e) Homozygotes
     (i) Xanthomas in early childhood
     (ii) MI as child
  (f) Treat with diet and statins
2 Familial triglyceridaemia
  (a) AD
  (b) Plasma turbid
  (c) Associated with eruptive xanthomata, pancreatitis, retinal vein thrombosis, hepatosplenomegaly, lipaemia retinalis
  (d) Treat with diet and fibrates
3 Lipoprotein lipase deficiency
  (a) Rare
  (b) AR
  (c) Failure to break down chylomicrons
  (d) Raised triglycerides
4 Familial combined hyperlipidaemia
  (a) Elevated cholesterol and triglycerides
  (b) Prevalence 1:200
  (c) Main feature is atherosclerosis

Causes of secondary hyperlipidaemia

1 Mainly raised cholesterol
  (a) Hypothyroidism
  (b) Cholestasis
  (c) Nephrotic syndrome
  (d) Renal transplant

2 Mainly raised triglycerides
  (a) Obesity
  (b) Chronic alcohol excess
  (c) Insulin resistance and diabetes
  (d) Chronic liver disease
  (e) Thiazide diuretics
  (f) High-dose oestrogens

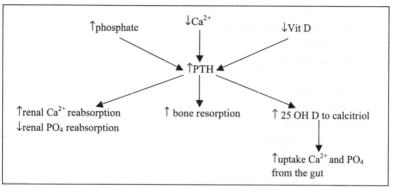

Figure 4 Bones and minerals

VITAMIN D

1 Mostly made in skin by action of UV light
2 25-hydroxylated in liver
3 Hydroxylated again to 1,25-OH D (calcitriol) in kidney

Hypercalcaemia

1 Causes
  (a) Primary hyperparathyroidism (adenoma of parathyroid gland)
  (b) Malignancy – PTH-related protein and bone metastases, commonly breast, kidney, thyroid, squamous cell tumours
  (c) Calcium intake (and milk-alkali syndrome)
  (d) Vitamin D
  (e) Tertiary hyperparathyroidism
  (f) Hyperthyroidism
  (g) Sarcoid – macrophages in lesions produce 1,25 vitamin D_3
  (h) Thiazides
  (i) Lithium

   (j)   Addison's
   (k) Theophylline toxicity
   (l)   Phaeochromocytoma
  (m) Familial hypocalciuric hypercalcaemia

2 Features
   (a) As underlying condition, plus
   (b) Lethargy, malaise and depression
   (c) Polyuria and polydipsia
   (d) Weakness
   (e) Confusion and psychosis
   (f) Constipation
   (g) Peptic ulceration
   (h) Nausea
   (i) Renal stones
   (j) Nephrocalcinosis
   (k) Pseudogout
   (l)   Proximal myopathy
  (m) Diabetes insipidus
   (n) Pancreatitis

3 Treatment
   (a) Aggressive rehydration
   (b) Bisphosphonate (pamidronate)
   (c) Frusemide
   (d) Steroids

Hyperparathyroidism

1 Primary
   (a) Single adenoma in > 80%
   (b) Multiple in around 5%
   (c) Commonest in women aged 40–60
   (d) Carcinoma very rare
   (e) Results in ↑ PTH, ↑ serum and urinary calcium, ↑ alkaline
      phosphatase and ↓ serum phosphate
   (f) Causes increased osteoblasts and osteoclasts with woven
      osteoid and osteatitis fibrosa cystica

2 Secondary
   (a) Due to hypertrophy of glands in response to chronic
      hypocalcaemia (eg in renal failure)

3 Tertiary
   (a) Consequence of long-standing secondary hyperparathyroidism.
      Further gland hyperplasia raises calcium levels. Treatment is
      parathyroidectomy

Hypocalcaemia

1 Causes
   (a) Hypoparathyroidism (including pseudohypoparathyroidism)
   (b) Chronic renal failure
   (c) Low levels of vitamin D_3
   (d) Hyperphosphataemia
   (e) Hypomagnesaemia
   (f) Sepsis
   (g) Respiratory alkalosis
   (h) Calcium deposition (eg acute pancreatitis)
   (i) Carcinoma of prostate
2 Features
   (a) Muscle weakness
   (b) Neuromuscular excitability
   (c) Confusion, seizures
   (d) Tetany
   (e) Alopecia
   (f) Brittle nails
   (g) Cataracts
   (h) Dental hypoplasia
3 Treatment
   (a) Supplementation of calcium, vitamin D_3

Hypoparathyroidism

1 Causes
   (a) Parathyroidectomy (intentional and accidental)
   (b) Autoimmune
   (c) Receptor defect (pseudohyperparathyroidism)
   (d) Di George syndrome
2 Diagnosis (hypoparathyroidism)
   (a) ↓ Calcium, ↓ PTH

Pseudohypoparathyroidism

1 Receptor defect leading to resistance of target tissues to PTH
2 X-linked dominant
3 ↓ Calcium, ↑ PTH
4 Clinical features
    (a) Short stature
    (b) Round face
    (c) Short neck
    (d) Shortening of the metacarpals and metatarsals

Causes of hyperphosphataemia

1 Renal failure
2 Hypoparathyroidism
3 Acromegaly
4 Vitamin D excess
5 Overintake of phosphate
6 Tumour lysis syndrome

Causes of hypophosphataemia

1 Intravenous glucose
2 Deficiency during parenteral feeding
3 Recovery phase of DKA
4 Primary hyperparathyroidism
5 Renal tubular disease
6 Vitamin D deficiency
7 Alcohol withdrawal

Osteomalacia/rickets

Decreased mineralisation of osteoid
1 Causes
    (a) Calciopenic
        (i) Vitamin D deficiency
        (ii) Impaired calcium metabolism
    (b) Phosphopenic
        (i) Proximal renal tubular disease
2 Clinical features
    (a) Pain
    (b) Deformity

(c) Fractures
(d) Proximal myopathy
(e) Raised alkaline phosphatase

Paget's disease

1 Increased bone turnover with abnormal new bone turnover
2 Causes pain, deformity, arthritis, nerve compression, fractures, sarcoma
3 ↑↑ ALP
4 Calcium only raised with immobility
5 Diagnosis – clinical, typical X rays or bone scan
6 Treatment: analgesia and bisphosphonates

MAGNESIUM

Hypomagnesaemia

1 Usually associated with low Ca^{2+} and low K^+
2 Associated with ventricular arrhythmias, fits, tetany and paraesthesiae

Causes

1 Renal loss
   (a) Loop/thiazide diuretics
   (b) Alcohol
   (c) DKA
   (d) Volume expansion
   (e) Hypercalcaemia
2 Loop of Henle disorder
   (a) Acute tubular necrosis
   (b) Post obstruction diuresis
   (c) Renal transplant
3 Nephrotoxic drugs
   (a) Aminoglycosides
   (b) Cisplatin
   (c) Ciclosporin
   (d) Amphotericin
4 GI loss
   (a) High-volume diarrhoea
   (b) Malabsorption

(c) Other small bowel disease
(d) Acute pancreatitis
5 Primary renal magnesium wasting
(a) Rare familial condition

Hypermagnesaemia

1 Causes
(a) Magnesium infusion
(b) Magnesium enema
(c) Oral magnesium overdose
(d) Renal failure
(e) Adrenal insufficiency
(f) Milk-alkali syndrome
(g) Theophylline toxicity
(h) Lithium
2 Treat with iv calcium if symptomatic

COPPER

1 50% of amount ingested is absorbed
2 Transported to liver by albumin
3 Binds with globulin to form caeruloplasmin

Wilson's disease

1 Autosomal recessive
2 Gene on chromosome 13
3 Abnormality of caeruloplasmin formation, hence accumulation of
   copper in body
4 Features: acute/chronic hepatitis, cirrhosis, Kayser–Fleischer rings,
   CNS symptoms, arthropathy, RTA
5 Diagnosis: low caeruloplasmin, high urinary copper, liver biopsy, KF
   rings
6 Treatment: penicillamine (copper chelator), liver transplant

IRON

1 4 g in normal human body, two-thirds in haemoglobin
2 20 mg/day in normal diet; only 10% absorbed
3 Fe^{2+} more readily absorbed than Fe^{3+}

4 Transferrin one-third saturated normal
5 Ferritin increased in iron overload (NB: acute-phase protein), decreased in deficiency
6 Plasma iron varies ++

Haemochromatosis

1 Autosomal recessive
2 Commoner, more severe in men
3 Gene on chromosome 6
4 Features: micronodular cirrhosis chondrocalcinosis, pseudogout, skin bronzing, diabetes, cardiomyopathy, arrhythmias
5 Diagnosis: raised serum iron and ferritin. Transferrin > 45% saturated. Liver biopsy
6 Treatment: venesection, desferrioxamine

Causes of secondary iron overload

1 Multiple transfusions
2 Alcoholic cirrhosis
3 Chronic hepatitis B/C
4 Beta-thalassaemia
5 Aplastic anaemia
6 Sideroblastic anaemia

ACID–BASE HOMOEOSTASIS

Table 45

	pH	pCO_2	HCO_3
Metabolic acidosis	N or ↓	↓	↓↓
Metabolic alkalosis	N or ↑	Slight ↑	↑↑
Respiratory acidosis	N or ↓	↑↑	↑
Respiratory alkalosis	N or ↑	↓↓	Slight ↓

$H^+ + HCO_3 \leftrightarrow H_2O + CO_2$
Anion gap $= \{[Na^+] + [K^+]\} - \{[CL^-]+[HCO_3^-]\} = 10–18$ mmol/l

Metabolic acidosis

1 Normal anion gap
  (a) Direct loss of bicarbonate (↑ chloride)

      (i) Diarrhoea
      (ii) Pancreatic fistulae
      (iii) Ureterosigmoidostomy
      (iv) RTA (See page 310)
      (v) Acetazolamide
   (b) Ingestion of acidifying agents
      (i) Ammonium chloride
2 High anion gap
   (a) DKA
   (b) Lactic acidosis
   (c) Renal failure
   (d) Salicylate poisoning
   (e) Methanol poisoning
   (f) Ethylene glycol poisoning

Respiratory acidosis

1 Hypoventilation leading to increased CO_2 and acidosis
2 Causes
   (a) COPD
   (b) Severe asthma
   (c) Obesity
   (d) Neuromuscular disorders leading to hypoventilation
      (i) Guillain–Barré
      (ii) MND
      (iii) Myasthenia gravis
      (iv) Muscular dystrophy
      (v) Flail chest
      (vi) Severe kyphoscoliosis
   (e) Muscle relaxants

Respiratory alkalosis

1 Hyperventilation leading to low CO_2 levels and alkalosis
2 Causes
   (a) Psychogenic
   (b) Pulmonary disease
   (c) Altitude
   (d) Right to left shunt
   (e) CO poisoning
   (f) Salicylates
   (g) Acute liver failure

Metabolic alkalosis

1 Vomiting
2 Potassium depletion
3 Hyperaldosteronism
4 Rapid diuresis
5 Fulminant hepatic failure
6 Milk-alkali syndrome
7 Forced alkaline diuresis

Lactic acidosis

1 Type A
  (a) Poor tissue perfusion with or without hypoxia
    (i)   Exercise
    (ii) Post epileptic seizure
    (iii) Shock
    (iv) Severe hypoxia
2 Type B
  (a) Administration of drugs or metabolic disturbance leading to increased production of lactate
    (i)   Metformin
    (ii) Alcohol
    (iii) Recovery from DKA
    (iv) Liver failure
    (v)   Paracetamol poisoning
    (vi) Thiamine deficiency

Osmolar gap

1 Normally gap between serum osmolality and calculated osmolality is < 10
2 If the value is greater then this suggests another osmotically active substance in the blood
3 Calculated with formula
  (a) $2(Na^+ + K^+) + urea + glucose$
4 Causes of raised osmolar gap
  (a) Methanol
  (b) Ethylene glycol
  (c) Diethylene glycol
  (d) Ethanol

PORPHYRIAS

1 Hereditary defects of enzymes involved in haem synthesis pathway
2 Overproduction of intermediates – porphyrins
3 Several different types; most important are
4 Acute intermittent porphyria
   (a) Autosomal dominant
   (b) Rare, commoner in females
   (c) Due to low levels of porphobilinogen deaminase in liver
   (d) Presents in youth
   (e) Increased urinary porphobilinogen in attack; urine turns dark red after standing
   (f) Clinical features
      (i) Severe abdominal pain
      (ii) Neuropsychiatric symptoms
      (iii) Vomiting
      (iv) Hypertension
      (v) Tachycardia
      (vi) Motor polyneuropathy
   (g) Commonly precipitated by hepatic enzyme-inducing drugs, eg alcohol, phenytoin, oral contraceptives, sulphonamides, rifampicin, benzodiazepines
   (h) Treatment of attacks
      (i) High-carbohydrate diet
      (ii) Haematin
      (iii) Opiate analgesia
      (iv) Fluid restriction for hyponatraemia
      (v) Conservative management of seizures, as antiepileptics can precipitate attacks
5 Porphyria cutanea tarda
   (a) Chronic hepatic condition
   (b) Many patients drink excessive alcohol
   (c) Autosomal dominant and acquired
   (d) Reduced hepatic uroporphyrinogen decarboxylase
   (e) Accumulation of uroporphyrinogen (raised in urine)
   (f) Many have evidence of iron overload and require venesection
   (g) Photosensitive bullous rash main feature

Amino acid metabolism disorders

[See Table 46, overleaf]

DEFICIENCIES

Protein–energy malnutrition

1 Undernutrition
 (a) Weight 60–80% of standard for age, no oedema
2 Marasmus
 (a) Deficient in protein and calories
 (b) Weight < 60% of standard, no oedema
3 Kwashiorkor
 (a) Solely due to protein deficiency
 (b) Weight 60–80% of standard, oedema present
 (c) Fatty liver often seen

Vitamin deficiencies

[See Table 47, overleaf]

DISORDERS OF SODIUM AND WATER HOMOEOSTASIS

Sodium is regulated by volume receptors. In health, water is adjusted to maintain a normal osmolarity and, in the absence of abnormal osmotically active solutes, a normal sodium. Therefore, disturbances of sodium concentration are caused by disturbances of water balance.

Causes of hyponatraemia – with normal extracellular water

1 Pseudohyponatraemia
 (a) Hyperlipidaemia
 (b) Hyperproteinaemia
2 Abnormal ADH release
 (a) Hypothyroidism
 (b) Severe potassium depletion

Table 46

Condition	Genetics	Clinical features	Diagnosis	Management
Cystinosis	Autosomal recessive; short arm of 17	Lymphadenopathy, growth retardation, Fanconi syndrome, renal failure	Measure cystine content of neutrophils	Dialysis, renal transplant Death usual
Cystinuria	AR	Renal stones	Urinary cystine/stone analysis	Fluids, penicillamine, alkalisation of urine
Homocystinuria	AR	Osteoporosis, arterial thrombosis, downward dislocation of lens, mental retardation	Cyanide-nitroprusside test – raised urinary homocysteine	Methionine restriction Supplements of cystine and pyridoxine
Alkaptonuria	AR	Arthritis, disc calcification, pigmentation of ears	Clinical; urine darkens on standing	Symptomatic for arthritis
Phenylketonuria	AR	Mental retardation, irritability, eczema, decreased pigmentation	Guthrie screening test perinatally	Dietary restriction of phenylalanine, tyrosine supplements
Oxalosis	AR	Renal stones/calcification, bone, cardiac and arterial disease	Urinary oxalate increased; may need liver biopsy	Pyridoxine, treat renal failure, fluids

Table 47

Vitamin	Cause of deficiency	Consequence of deficiency
A	Protein–energy malnutrition	Night blindness, dry corneas, keratomalacia
B_1 (thiamine)	Alcoholism, dietary restriction	Dry beri beri: Wernicke–Korsakoff, polyneuropathy
		Wet beri-beri: high output cardiac failure
B_2 (riboflavin)	Protein–energy malnutrition	Glossitis, angular stomatitis
Niacin	Alcoholism, isoniazid, carcinoid syndrome	Pellagra – **dermatitis**, **diarrhoea**, **dementia** and **death**
B_6 (pyridoxine)	Hydralazine, isoniazid	Peripheral neuropathy, glossitis
B_{12} (cyanocobalamin)	Pernicious anaemia, gastrectomy, ileal disease, vegans	Macrocytic anaemia, subacute combined degeneration of the cord
C	Dietary deficiency	Scurvy: gingivitis, bleeding, joint swelling
D	Renal failure, dietary	Osteomalacia, rickets
E	Fat malabsorption, abetalipoproteinaemia	Spinocerebellar degeneration
K	Biliary obstruction, antibiotic therapy	Bleeding diathesis

METABOLIC MEDICINE

3 ADH-like substances
   (a) Oxytocin
   (b) DDAVP
4 Unmeasured osmotically active substances stimulating osmotic ADH
   release
   (a) Glucose
   (b) Alcohol
   (c) Mannitol
5 Syndrome of inappropriate ADH secretion (SIADH)
6 Stress
   (a) Surgery
   (b) Nausea

Causes of hyponatraemia – with decreased extracellular volume

1 Kidney
   (a) Osmotic diuresis (hyperglycaemia, severe uraemia)
   (b) Diuretics
   (c) Adrenocortical insufficiency
   (d) Tubulointerstitial disease
   (e) Unilateral renal artery stenosis
   (f) Recovery post ATN
2 Gastrointestinal
   (a) Vomiting
   (b) Diarrhoea
   (c) Haemorrhage
   (d) Fistula
   (e) Obstruction

Causes of hyponatraemia – with increased extracellular volume

1 Oliguric renal failure
2 Heart failure
3 Liver failure
4 Hypoalbuminaemia

Causes of hypernatraemia

1 Dehydration
2 Iatrogenic (administration of hypertonic sodium solution)

3 Diabetes insipidus
4 Osmotic diuresis
   (a) Total parenteral nutrition
   (b) Hyperosmolar diabetic coma

Causes of SIADH

1 Malignancy
   (a) Bronchus, bladder, prostate, pancreas
   (b) Lymphoma
   (c) Ewing's sarcoma
   (d) Mesothelioma
   (e) Thymoma
2 Pulmonary disorders
   (a) Pneumonia
   (b) Abscess
   (c) TB
   (d) PEEP
   (e) Asthma
3 Central nervous system
   (a) Encephalitis
   (b) Meningitis
   (c) Trauma
   (d) Subarachnoid haemorrhage
   (e) Guillain-Barré syndrome
   (f) Hydrocephalus
   (g) Acute psychosis
   (h) Acute intermittent porphyria
4 Drugs
   (a) Opiates
   (b) Carbamazepine
   (c) Oxytocin
   (d) Chlorpropamide
   (e) Phenothiazines
   (f) TCAs
   (g) Cytotoxics (vincristine, cyclophosphamide)
   (h) Rifampicin
   (i) Porphyria (drug induced)

Causes of diabetes insipidus

1 Cranial (reduced secretion of ADH)
   (a) Idiopathic
   (b) Familial (eg DIDMOAD syndrome)
   (c) Craniopharyngioma
   (d) Infiltrative processes of hypothalamus
       (i) Sarcoidosis
       (ii) Histiocytosis X
   (e) Trauma
   (f) Pituitary surgery
   (g) Lymphocytic hypophysitis
   (h) Dysgerminomas
2 Nephrogenic (reduced action of ADH)
   (a) Primary
       (i)   Childhood onset
       (ii) X-linked/dominant
       (iii) Tubular receptor abnormality
   (b) Secondary
       (i)   Hypercalcaemia
       (ii)   Hypokalaemia
       (iii) Renal disease
       (iv)   Chronic pyelonephritis
       (v)   APKD
       (vi)   Post obstruction
       (vii) Sarcoidosis
       (viii) Drugs
             (1) Lithium
             (2) Demeclocycline (used to treat SIADH)
             (3) Amphotericin
             (4) Glibenclamide

Causes of polyuria

1 Excessive intake
   (a) Beer drinking
   (b) Primary polydipsia (lesion of hypothalamus)
   (c) Psychogenic polydipsia
2 Osmotic diuresis
   (a) Diabetes mellitus
   (b) CRF

3 ARF (diuretic phase)
4 Diuretics
5 Diabetes insipidus (cranial and nephrogenic)
6 Hypokalaemia
7 Hypercalcaemia
8 Obstructive uropathy
9 Tubulointerstitial disease

Investigation of polyuria

1 Record fluid intake
2 Record urine volume (if < 3l/24 hrs and normal biochemistry excludes significant abnormality)
3 Blood glucose, U&E, calcium
4 Urinalysis
5 Early morning urine osmolality
6 Water deprivation test
   (a) To identify the cause of polyuria and/or polydipsia
   (b) Hourly urine and plasma osmolality measured until 3% of bodyweight lost
   (c) Injection of DDAVP (synthetic ADH)

Interpretation of water deprivation test

Table 48

	Initial plasma osmolality	Final urine osmolality (mmol/kg)	Urine osmolality post DDAVP (mmol/kg)	Final plasma ADH
Normal	Normal	> 600	> 600	High
Cranial DI	High	< 300	> 600	Low
Nephrogenic DI	High	< 300	< 300	High
Primary polydipsia	Low	300–400 (approx.)	400 (approx.)	Moderate
Partial cranial DI	High	300–400	400–600	Relatively low

POTASSIUM

Potassium is the major intracellular ion. Excretion of potassium is increased by aldosterone.

Causes of hypokalaemia

1 Decreased intake
   (a) Oral (uncommon except in starvation)
   (b) Parenteral
1 Redistribution into cells
   (a) Metabolic alkalosis
   (b) Insulin
   (c) Alpha-adrenergic antagonists
   (d) Beta-adrenergic agonists
   (e) Vitamin B_{12} or folic acid when correcting megaloblastic anaemia
   (f) Total parenteral nutrition (TPN)
   (g) Hypokalaemic periodic paralysis
   (h) Pseudohypokalaemia
   (i) Hypothermia
2 Increased excretion
   (a) Gastrointestinal
      (i) Purgative abuse
      (ii) Vomiting
      (iii) Villous adenoma
      (iv) Severe diarrhoea
      (v) Ileostomy/uterosigmoidostomy
      (vi) Fistulae
   (j) Renal
      (i) Thiazides
      (ii) Loop diuretics
      (iii) Renal tubular damage
      (iv) Mineralocorticoid excess
         (1) Primary hyperaldosteronism (Conn's)
         (2) Secondary hyperaldosteronism
         (3) Apparent mineralocorticoid excess
            (a) Liquorice
            (b) Carbenoxolone
         (4) Cushing's syndrome
      (v) Bartter's syndrome
      (vi) Renal tubular acidosis type 1 and 2

Hyperkalaemia

1 Causes
   (a) Spurious
      (i) Haemolysis
      (ii) Delayed separation of serum
      (iii) Contamination
      (iv) Excessive intake (parenteral, oral)
   (b) Decreased excretion
      (i) Acute oliguric renal failure
      (ii) Chronic renal failure
      (iii) Mineralocorticoid deficiency (Addison's disease)
      (iv) Hypoaldosteronism
      (v) Drugs
         (1) Spironolactone
         (2) Amiloride
         (3) Triamterene
         (4) ACE inhibitors
         (5) NSAIDs
         (6) Ciclosporin
   (c) Redistribution
      (i) Acidosis
      (ii) Rhabdomyolysis
      (iii) Tumour lysis syndrome
      (iv) Digoxin poisoning
2 ECG changes
   (a) Tenting of T waves
   (b) Reduction in size of P waves
   (c) Increase in PR interval
   (d) Widening QRS complexes
   (e) Disappearance of P waves
   (f) Further QRS widening
   (g) Sinusoidal waveform
3 Treatment
   (a) IV calcium gluconate (stabilises cardiac membranes)
   (b) IV insulin and dextrose
   (a) Calcium resonium
   (b) Frusemide
   (c) Salbutamol nebulisers
   (d) Dialysis

Nephrology

PHYSIOLOGY

Glomerular filtration rate (GFR)

1 Passive process
2 Reduces with age (peak age 20–30, reduces by 1 ml/min per year after this)
3 Normal
   (a) 130 ml/min/1.73 m male
   (b) 120 ml/min/1.73 m female
4 Calculating GFR
   (a) 24 hour urine collection for creatinine clearance
   (b) Cockcroft and Gault equation
      (i)
      $$GFR = \frac{(140 - \text{age in yrs}) \times \text{wt (kg)} \times 1.23 \text{ (male) or } 1.04 \text{ (female)}}{\text{Serum creatinine (μmol/l)}}$$
   (c) Inulin clearance
   (d) Radioisotope studies (^{51}Cr EDTA, ^{125}I isothalamate, ^{99m}Tc DTPA)

The renal tubule

1 Proximal tubule
   (a) 50% sodium reabsorbed
   (b) 90% bicarbonate reabsorbed
   (c) Phosphate reabsorption (PTH)
   (d) Drug secretion into urine – trimethoprim, cimetidine, most diuretics
   (e) Creatinine and urate secretion
2 Loop of Henle
   (a) Medullary concentration gradient
   (b) 40% sodium reabsorption
   (c) Loop diuretic action, eg frusemide

3 Distal tubule
  (a) 5% sodium reabsorption
  (b) Thiazide diuretic action
  (c) Aldosterone receptors
4 Collecting duct
  (a) 2% sodium reabsorption
  (b) Spironolactone acts on aldosterone receptors
  (c) Hydrogen ion secretion (acidifying urine)
  (d) Antidiuretic hormone action

Hormone effects on the kidney

1 Aldosterone – increases tubular reabsorption of Na^+, increases H^+ and K^+ secretion
2 Atrial natriuretic peptide – increases Na^+/H_2O excretion
3 Catecholamines – increase renin secretion
4 1,25-dihydroxyvitamin D – increase tubular calcium reabsorption
5 Erythropoietin – produced by kidney
6 Prostaglandins – autoregulation of renal blood flow, increases renin
7 PTH – increases excretion of phosphate and bicarbonate; increases calcium reabsorption; increases synthesis of 1, 25-dihydroxyvitamin D
8 Renin – autoregulation of renal blood flow
9 Vasopressin – increase antidiuresis

INVESTIGATIONS

Urea and creatinine

1 Raised creatinine
  (a) Large muscle bulk
  (b) Rhabdomyolysis
  (c) Decreased tubular secretion
      (i)   Trimethoprim
      (ii) Potassium-sparing diuretics
      (iii) Cimetidine
2 Reduced creatinine
  (a) Small muscle mass
  (b) Pregnancy
  (c) SIADH

3 Raised urea
  (a) Reduced GFR, eg dehydration
  (b) Diuretics
  (c) GI bleeding
  (d) Corticosteroids/tetracycline
  (e) High-protein diet
  (f) Increased catabolism
4 Reduced urea
  (a) Chronic liver disease
  (b) Starvation/anabolic state
  (c) Alcohol abuse
  (d) SIADH
  (e) Pregnancy

Urinalysis

1 Protein
  (a) Normally excrete < 150 mg/day
  (b) Dipstix sensitive for albumin
  (c) False positive with alkaline urine
  (d) 24 hr urine required for quantification
2 Blood
  (a) Dipstix sensitive for blood
  (b) Should be confirmed by microscopy
3 Glucose
  (a) Not quantitative
4 pH
  (a) Normal 4–8
  (b) If > 8 may indicate false positive for protein
5 Nitrite
  (a) Most Gram-negative organisms reduce nitrates to nitrites (30% false negative)
6 Leukocytes
  (a) Good correlation with quantitative microscopy

Urine microscopy

1 White cells
  (a) UTI
  (b) TB
  (c) Calculi of renal tract

   (d) Chemical cystitis
   (e) Glomerulonephritis
   (f) Analgesic nephropathy
   (g) Urethral/vaginal infection
2 Bacteria
   (a) UTI
   (b) Asymptomatic bacteriuria (without pyuria)
   (c) Contamination
3 Red cells (See Causes of haematuria, below)
4 Hyaline casts
   (a) Tamm–Horsfall protein
   (b) Can be present in concentrated urine or after exercise
   (c) Febrile illness
   (d) Diuretics
5 Granular casts
   (a) Dense granular casts are pathological
   (b) Chronic proliferative or membranous GN
   (c) Diabetic nephropathy
   (d) Amyloidosis
6 Red cell casts
   (a) Glomerular bleeding
   (b) Glomerular inflammation, eg GN
7 White cell casts
   (a) Pyelonephritis
8 Epithelial cell casts
   (a) ATN
   (b) Acute GN

Causes of haematuria

  1 Urinary tract malignancy
  2 Urinary infections
  3 Renal calculi
  4 Acute GN
  5 IgA nephropathy
  6 Interstitial nephritis
  7 Polycystic disease
  8 Renal papillary necrosis
  9 Prostatic hypertrophy
10 Hypertension
11 Endometriosis

12 AV malformations
13 Trauma
14 Fictitious

Causes of coloured urine

1 Haematuria
2 Haemoglobinuria
3 Myoglobinuria
4 Obstructive jaundice
5 Drugs, eg rifampicin
6 Beetroot
7 Porphyria
8 Alkaptonuria

Causes of proteinuria

1 Mild (< 500 mg/day)
   (a) Fever
   (b) Obstructive nephropathy
   (c) Hypertension
   (d) Prerenal failure
   (e) Chronic pyelonephritis
   (f) Renal tumour
   (g) Tubulointerstitial disease
   (h) Orthostatic proteinuria
2 Moderate (< 3 g/day)
   (a) UTI
   (b) Chronic pyelonephritis
   (c) ATN
   (d) Acute GN
   (e) Chronic GN
   (f) Obstructive nephropathy
   (g) Hypertension
   (h) Orthostatic proteinuria
3 Heavy (> 3 g/day)
   (a) Acute GN
   (b) Chronic GN
   (c) Myeloma
   (d) Pre-eclampsia
   (e) Nephrotic syndrome

ACUTE RENAL FAILURE

Causes

1 Prerenal
  (a) Appropriate renal response to poor renal perfusion
  (b) Drugs, eg ACEIs
2 Renal
  (a) Acute tubular necrosis (ATN)
    (i)   Circulatory compromise (hypovolaemia, cardiogenic shock)
    (ii) Sepsis
    (iii) Nephrotoxic (eg drugs)
    (iv) Often multiple causes
  (b) Vascular causes
    (i)   Acute cortical necrosis
    (ii) Large vessel occlusion
      (1) Embolus
      (2) Thrombosis
      (3) Renal artery stenosis
      (4) Dissection
    (iii) Small vessel disease
      (1) Accelerated hypertension
      (2) Scleroderma
    (iv) Renal vein thrombosis
  (c) Glomerulonephritis
  (d) Interstitial nephritis
  (e) Vasculitis
  (f) Haematological
    (i)   Myeloma
    (ii) Haemolytic uraemic syndrome/TTP/DIC
  (g) Others
    (i)   Rhabdomyolysis
    (ii) Hepatorenal syndrome
    (iii) Acute cortical necrosis
3 Postrenal
  (i)   Urinary obstruction (stone, neoplasia, bladder outflow
      obstruction)

Investigation of acute renal failure

1 Full history and examination
  (a) ?Systemic cause
  (b) Drug history – penicillin or NSAIDs
  (c) Family history
2 Ultrasound scan
  (a) Rule out obstruction
  (b) Kidney size (if small, then acute on chronic)
3 Urine
  (a) Microscopy of urine (See page 289)
  (b) Protein
  (c) Haematuria
  (d) Casts
4 IVU (intravenous urogram) or CT to look for nephrolithiasis
5 Isotope renography
  (a) Static, eg DMSA
  (b) Dynamic, eg MAG3, DTPA
  (c) Captopril renogram to look for renovascular disease
6 Blood tests
  (a) Specific

(i)	Anti-GBM antibodies	Goodpasture's disease
(ii)	ANCA	Systemic vasculitis
(iii)	Anti-dsDNA and Anti-Sm	SLE
(iv)	C3 nephritic factor	MCGN type 2
(v)	ASOT and Anti-DNAase	Post streptococcal GN
(vi)	Blood cultures	Infection, especially endocarditis

  (b) Less specific

(i)	Complement	High in vasculitis Low in SLE, MCGN type1 & type 2, mixed essential cryoglobulinaemia, post infectious
(ii)	Immunoglobulins	Polyclonal increase in SLE, vasculitis, post infectious and sarcoid Monoclonal increase in myeloma Raised IgE in Churg–Strauss Raised IgA in Henoch–Schönlein purpura and IgA nephropathy

(iii)	Cryoglobulins	Cryoglobulinaemia
		Also in SLE and post infectious
(iv)	CRP	Increased in most cases but not usually in SLE
(v)	Neutrophilia	Systemic vasculitis
(vi)	Thrombocytosis	Systemic vasculitis
(vii)	Eosinophilia	Drug-induced interstitial nephritis
		Churg–Strauss syndrome
(viii)	Lymphopenia	SLE
(ix)	Thrombocytopenia	Drug-induced interstitial nephritis SLE

Acute tubular necrosis (ATN)

1 Ischaemic damage
2 Renal hypoperfusion
3 Reversible in time, but time taken varies (may need dialysis until recovery occurs)

Prerenal produces low-volume concentrated urine
ATN gives low- or high-volume, dilute, 'poor quality' urine

Symptoms of uraemia

1 Cardiovascular
   (a) Pericarditis (can be haemorrhagic leading to tamponade)
   (b) Poor LV function
   (c) IHD
2 Respiratory
   (a) Pleurisy
   (b) Dyspnoea
   (c) Kussmaul breathing (acidosis)
3 Gastrointestinal
   (a) N+V
   (b) GI bleeding (peptic ulcer, angiodysplasia)
   (c) Constipation
   (d) Diarrhoea
4 Haematological
   (a) Bleeding (poor platelet function)
   (b) Anaemia

(i) Reduced erythropoietin
(ii) Bone marrow suppression
(iii) Shortened red cell survival
(iv) Increased blood loss
5 Dermatological
  (a) Pruritus
  (b) Purpura
  (c) Pallor
  (d) Pigmentation
6 CNS
  (a) Fatigue
  (b) Encephalopathy (toxins)
  (c) Depression
  (d) Involuntary movements
  (e) Seizures
  (f) Paraesthesiae
  (g) Neuropathy
  (h) Coma

Rhabdomyolysis

1 Muscle damage
2 Myoglobin release
3 ARF
4 Raised potassium and phosphate
5 Creatinine kinase massively raised
6 Creatinine raised disproportionately to urea
7 Causes
  (a) Trauma/compression injury
  (b) Uncontrolled fitting
  (c) Statins
  (d) Burns
  (e) Infectious mononucleosis
  (f) Viral necrotising myositis
  (g) Barbiturate, alcohol or heroin overdose
  (h) Severe exercise
  (i) Heat stroke
  (j) Polymyositis
  (k) Malignant hyperpyrexia

Criteria for urgent renal replacement therapy

1 Severe hyperkalaemia
2 Fluid overload leading to pulmonary oedema
3 Acidosis resulting in circulatory compromise
   (a) Uraemia giving encephalopathy
   (b) Pericarditis
   (c) Bleeding

CHRONIC RENAL FAILURE

1 Causes (in the UK)
   (a) Diabetes mellitus 20%
   (b) Chronic GN 20%
   (c) Renovascular 15%
   (d) Chronic reflux nephropathy 15%
   (e) Polycystic kidney disease 10%
   (f) Post obstructive 10%
   (g) Myeloma 3%
   (h) Amyloidosis 3%
   (i) Others
       (i) Chronic interstitial nephritis
       (ii) Analgesic nephropathy
       (iii) Renal calculi
       (iv) Post ARF
       (v) Other hereditary disorders
2 Management of chronic renal disease
   (a) Blood pressure control
       (i) ACE inhibitors
       (ii) Other antihypertensives
       (iii) Diuretics
   (b) Reduction in proteinuria
       (i) ACE inhibitors
   (c) Treat acidosis
   (d) Treatment of anaemia
       (i) IV iron
       (ii) Erythropoietin
   (e) Diet
       (i) Low salt intake

    (ii) Low potassium intake
    (iii) High calorie intake
  (f) Treatment of hyperphosphataemia and hypocalcaemia
    (i) Phosphate binders
    (ii) Oral calcium
    (iii) Alphacalcidol
  (g) Glucose control in diabetics
  (h) Lipid control
  (i) Volume status
  (j) Avoid nephrotoxic drugs and radiocontrast

Anaemia of CRF

1 GFR < 35 ml/min
2 Due to lack of erythropoietin (normally produced by the kidneys)
3 Other contributing factors
  (a) Reduced iron intake
  (b) Impaired iron absorption
  (c) Toxic effect of uraemia in bone marrow
  (d) Capillary fragility
  (e) Reduced RBC survival
4 Management
  (a) Subcutaneous erythropoietin (EPO) injections
  (b) If ferritin < 100 then iv iron
  (c) Resistance to EPO therapy
    (i) Iron deficiency
    (ii) Sepsis or chronic inflammation
    (iii) GI blood loss
    (iv) Hyperparathyroidism
    (v) Aluminium toxicity (rare now)

Renal osteodystrophy

1 Pathophysiology
  (a) Low plasma ionised calcium
    (i) Reduced 1,25-dihydroxy vitamin D
    (ii) Malnutrition
    (iii) Hyperphosphataemia
  (b) Increased parathyroid hormone release
    (i) Secondary hyperparathyroidism response to
      (1) Hypocalcaemia

NEPHROLOGY

(2) Hyperphosphataemia
(3) Low 1,25(OH)$_2$ vitamin D
(c) Low vitamin D levels
(d) Acidosis
2 Treatment
(a) Phosphate binders (eg calcium acetate) to lower phosphate
(b) Bicarbonate
(c) Vitamin D (1-alphacalcidol)
(d) Parathyroidectomy

Conditions when haemodialysis preferred to peritoneal dialysis

1 Recent abdominal surgery or irremediable hernias
2 Recurrent or persistent peritonitis (eg *Pseudomonas* or fungal infection)
3 Peritoneal membrane failure
4 Severe malnutrition – protein loss during dialysis
5 Intercurrent severe illness with hypercatabolism
6 Chronic severe respiratory disease
7 Age and general frailty – physical or mental reason why unable to do dialysis
8 Loss of residual renal function

Complications of dialysis

1 Peritoneal dialysis
   (a) Infection
   (b) Catheter malfunction
   (c) Hernias
   (d) Peritoneal membrane failure
2 Acute complications of haemodialysis
   (a) Bleeding
   (b) Hypotension
   (c) Air embolus
   (d) Hypo/hypernatraemia
   (e) Haemolysis
   (f) Haemorrhage
3 Long term (all)
   (a) Loss of vascular access
   (b) Anaemia

(c) Vascular disease
(d) Hypertension
(e) Abnormal bleeding
(f) Dialysis amyloid (β_2-microglobulin)
(g) Renal osteodystrophy
(h) Acquired cystic disease
(i) Aluminium toxicity (rare)
(j) Malignancy
(k) Malnutrition

Renal transplantation

1 In UK 2000 patients per year
2 Graft survival 90% at 1 year, 70% at 5 years
3 Live donors – 10–15% of transplants
4 Contraindications to live donation
    (a) Pre-existing renal disease
    (b) Disease of unknown aetiology (eg MS or sarcoid)
    (c) Overt ischaemic heart disease
5 Matching
    (a) Donors must be ABO compatible (rhesus not important)
    (b) HLA typing
       (i) Antigens on chromosome 6
       (ii) Importance of HLA matching: DR > B > A > C
       (iii) Acceptable: 1 DR or 1B mismatch
       (iv) Good match: 0 DR with 0 or 1 B mismatch
6 Nephrectomy prior to transplant if
    (a) Uncontrollable hypertension
    (b) Infection in urinary tract
    (c) Massive kidneys (eg polycystic)
    (d) Renal or urothelial malignancy
7 Post-transplant complications
    (a) Acute and chronic rejection (See page 232)
    (b) Infections
    (c) Surgery-related complications
       (i) Vascular occlusion
       (ii) Ureteric occlusion
    (d) Increased risk of
       (i) Malignancy – NHL, cervical cancer (especially ciclosporin)
       (ii) Skin cancer (especially azathioprine)

      (iii) Cardiovascular – IHD 10–20 times more prevalent
      (iv) Hypertension
      (v) Opportunistic infections, eg PCP, CMV, VZV etc.
   (e) Drug toxicity, especially ciclosporin

8 Immunosuppression
   (a) Triple therapy with
      (i)   Tacrolimus or ciclosporin
      (ii) Azathioprine or mycophenolate
      (iii) Low-dose prednisolone

9 Diseases that recur in the transplanted kidney
   (a) Alport's syndrome – anti-GBM disease
   (b) Mesangiocapillary GN (universal recurrence)
   (c) IgA nephropathy (universal recurrence)
   (d) FSGS
   (e) Membranous GN
   (f) Vasculitis (monitor autoantibody level)
   (g) All GN can recur

RENAL SYNDROMES

1 Renal disorders commonly present as one of the renal syndromes
2 Definitions of common renal syndromes
   (a) Asymptomatic proteinuria
      (i)   < 3 g/day
   (b) Nephrotic syndrome
      (i)   > 3 g/day
      (ii) Oedema
      (iii) Serum albumin < 25 g/l
      (iv) Increased cholesterol
   (c) Nephritic syndrome
      (i)   Hypertension
      (ii) Haematuria
      (iii) Oedema
      (iv) Oliguria
   (d) Haematuria
      (i)   Microscopic or macroscopic
3 Glomerulonephritis is an inflammatory condition affecting the renal glomeruli

4 Interstitial nephritis is an inflammatory disorder affecting the renal interstitium
5 Screening tests
   (a) Dipstick urine
       (i) Proteinuria
       (ii) Haematuria
   (b) Quantify proteinuria with 24-hr urine collection
   (c) Urine microscopy for red cells and casts

Nephrotic syndrome

1 Causes
   (a) Primary glomerular disease
       (i)   Minimal change GN
       (ii)   Membranous GN
       (iii) Focal segmental GN
       (iv)   Mesangiocapillary GN
   (b) Secondary glomerular disease
       (i)   Diabetes mellitus
       (ii)   Infection (malaria, leprosy, hepatitis B)
       (iii) Pre-eclampsia
       (iv)   Accelerated hypertension
       (v)   Myeloma
       (vi)   Carcinoma
       (vii) Amyloidosis
       (viii) SLE
       (ix)   RA
   (c) Drugs
       (i)   Gold
       (ii)   Penicillamine
       (iii) Captopril
       (iv)   NSAIDs
       (v)   Mercury
2 Complications of nephrotic syndrome
   (a) Susceptibility to infection
   (b) Thromboses
   (c) Hyperlipidaemia
   (d) ARF
   (e) Protein malnutrition
   (f) Oedema/ascites/effusions

Acute nephritic syndrome

1 Bacterial
 (a) *Streptococcus*
 (b) Bacterial endocarditis
 (c) Shunt nephritis
 (d) *Meningococcus*
2 Viral
 (a) CMV
 (b) EBV
 (c) Hepatitis viruses
3 Parasitic
 (a) *Plasmodium falciparum*
4 Systemic disease
 (a) Wegener's granulomatosis
 (b) Goodpasture's disease
 (c) SLE
 (d) HUS
 (e) HSP
 (f) Vasculitis
 (g) Acute tubulointerstitial nephritis

GLOMERULONEPHRITIS

1 Inflammatory condition affecting the renal glomeruli that leads to structural and functional change
2 Structural changes are cellular proliferation, leukocyte proliferation, basement membrane thickening, hyalinisation and electron-dense deposits in characteristic patterns
3 Functional changes are proteinuria, haematuria and reduced GFR

Minimal change GN

1 Presents with nephrotic syndrome
2 Renal function usually normal
3 May be secondary to Hodgkin's disease, carcinoma or NSAIDs
4 More common in children
5 Selective proteinuria
6 Electron microscopy shows fusion of the epithelial foot processes
7 Treat with steroids (90% respond)
8 Excellent prognosis

Membranous GN

1 Presents with either
  (a) Nephrotic syndrome
  (b) Proteinuria
  (c) Chronic renal failure
2 Thickening of the glomerular basement membrane with subepithelial deposits of IgG or complement
3 Causes
  (a) Idiopathic
  (b) Malignancy – bronchus, stomach, lymphoma, colon, CLL
  (c) Chronic infection – hepatitis B, malaria, syphilis
  (d) Drugs – gold, penicillamine, captopril
  (e) Connective tissue diseases – SLE, rheumatoid arthritis, MCTD, Sjögren's syndrome
  (f) Others – sarcoidosis, Guillain–Barré syndrome, primary biliary cirrhosis
4 Prognosis – Rule of Thirds
  (a) 1/3 progress CRF to ESRF
  (b) 1/3 respond to immunosuppressive therapy
  (c) 1/3 remit spontaneously

Focal segmental glomerulosclerosis (FSGS)

1 Presents with proteinuria, nephrotic syndrome or hypertension
2 Associated with HIV/AIDS
3 Focal segmental sclerotic lesions of the glomeruli with IgM or C3 deposits
4 Poor response to steroids
5 25% progress to ESRF

Mesangioproliferative GN (IgA nephropathy or Berger's disease)

1 Mainly young adults
2 Presents with recurrent haematuria (micro- or macroscopic)
3 Mesangial proliferation with IgA deposits
4 Associated with URTI
5 Increased incidence in Far East
6 50% have increased serum IgA
7 Most have a benign course
8 25% progress to ESRF after 20 years

Mesangiocapillary GN

1 Presents with nephrotic or nephritic syndrome, proteinuria or hypertension
2 Two types
   (a) Type 1
      (i) Associations
         (1) SLE
         (2) Post streptococcal
         (3) Endocarditis
         (4) Abscess
         (5) Shunt nephritis
         (6) Hepatitis B and C
         (7) Cryoglobulinaemia
         (8) Sickle cell disease
         (9) $Alpha_1$-antitrypsin deficiency
   (b) Type 2
      (i) Often familial and associated partial lipodystrophy
3 Most type 2 have low C3 and 60% have C3 nephritic factor
4 Double contour on basement membrane (immune deposition)
5 Poor prognosis – 50% to ESRF

Diffuse proliferative GN

1 Nephritic or ARF
2 Post streptococcal
3 Preceded by sore throat or skin disease (impetigo)
4 Children or young adults
5 Low C3 and positive ASOT
6 Treatment with antibiotics and supportive care
7 Prognosis variable

Rapidly progressive GN (crescentic)

1 ARF with systemic disease or nephritic syndrome
2 Most severe GN
3 Necrotising GN with crescent formation
4 Main causes
   (a) Goodpasture's (anti-GBM antibodies) (See page 305)
   (b) Systemic vasculitis (ANCA positive or negative)
   (c) SLE

5 Management
   (a) Immunosuppressant +/- plasma exchange
   (b) Mortality > 20%

Causes of GN with hypocomplementaemia

1 SLE
2 Shunt nephritis – coagulase-negative staphylococcal infection of shunts
3 Primary complement deficiency
4 Endocarditis
5 Post streptococcal GN
6 Mesangiocapillary GN
7 Cryoglobulinaemia type 2

ESSENTIAL INHERITED RENAL DISEASES

Polycystic kidney disease

1 Autosomal dominant
2 PKD1 chromosome 16 (86%)
3 PKD2 chromosome 4 (10%)
4 Cysts develop in teenage years
5 Presentation varies
   (a) Haematuria
   (b) Hypertension
   (c) Loin pain
   (d) Infections or CRF
6 Associations
   (a) Liver cysts
   (b) Berry aneurysms
   (c) Malignant change
   (d) Pancreatic cysts
   (e) MV prolapse or AR
   (f) Hepatic fibrosis
   (g) Diverticular disease

Alport's syndrome

1 85% X-linked dominant
2 Defect in α5 chain of type 4 collagen (type 4 collagen major constituent of GBM)
3 Variable thickness and splitting of GBM
4 Presentation
   (a) Deafness
   (b) Microscopic haematuria
   (c) Proteinuria
   (d) CRF
   (e) Anterior lenticonus (eye)
   (f) 'Dot and fleck' retinopathy
5 Nephrotic syndrome in one-third
6 Males – all develop renal failure
7 Females – minor abnormalities only

TUBULOINTERSTITIAL NEPHRITIS

Acute

1 Inflammatory disorder affecting structures other than the glomeruli in the kidney
2 Presents with
   (a) Nephritic syndrome
   (b) Mild renal impairment
   (c) Hypertension
   (d) Microscopic haematuria or sterile pyuria
   (e) May develop eosinophiluria or eosinophilia
   (f) Interstitial oedema on biopsy with acute tubular necrosis
3 Causes
   (a) Most commonly hypersensitivity reaction to drugs
       (i) NSAIDs
       (ii) Rifampicin
       (iii) Frusemide
       (iv) Cephalosporins
       (v) Penicillins
       (vi) Sulphonamides
       (vii) Allopurinol

(viii) Thiazides
(ix) Cimetidine
(b) Others
  (i) Infections
    (1) CMV
    (2) HIV
    (3) Hantavirus
    (4) HBV
    (5) Bacterial infection secondary to obstruction
    (6) Leptospirosis
    (7) Mycobacterial
  (ii) SLE
  (iii) Goodpasture's
  (iv) Lymphoma
  (v) Leukaemia
  (vi) Sarcoidosis
4 Treatment
  (a) Stop cause, eg drug
  (b) Some require small dose of steroids
  (c) Most have complete recovery

Chronic

1 Chronic inflammatory condition of the renal interstitium
2 Presents with
  (a) CRF
  (b) ESRF
  (c) RTA type 1
  (d) Nephrogenic diabetes insipidus
  (e) Salt-wasting states
3 Biopsy – chronic inflammation, scarring, tubule loss
4 Causes
  (a) Drugs
    (i) Analgesics
    (ii) Ciclosporin
    (iii) Cisplatin
    (iv) Lithium
    (v) Iron
  (b) Atherosclerotic
  (c) Obstructive uropathy and reflux nephropathy

(d) Chronic transplant rejection
(e) Metabolic
    (i) Hypercalcaemia
    (ii) Hypokalaemia
    (iii) Hyperuricaemia
(f) Heavy metals
    (i) Lead
    (ii) Cadmium
(g) Haematological
    (i) Myeloma
    (ii) Light chain nephropathy
    (iii) Sickle cell disease
(h) Autoimmune
    (i) SLE
    (ii) Rheumatoid arthritis
    (iii) Wegener's granulomatosis
(i) Others
    (i) Irradiation
    (ii) Tuberculosis
    (iii) Sarcoidosis
    (iv) Alport's syndrome
    (v) Balkan nephropathy
5 Treatment
    (a) Remove causative factor
    (b) Supportive care
    (c) Steroids may be beneficial

ANALGESIC NEPHROPATHY

1 Chronic analgesic usage (phenacetin, paracetamol, NSAIDs)
2 Leads to papillary necrosis (haematuria, loin pain, obstruction and infection)
3 Chronic interstitial nephritis
4 Cup and spill calyces on IVU
5 CT may reveal microcalcification at the papillary tips
6 Increased risk of TCC
7 Treatment is supportive

NSAIDS AND THE KIDNEY

1 Renal failure secondary to reduced GFR (reduced prostaglandins)
2 Acute interstitial nephritis
3 Minimal change GN
4 Chronic interstitial nephritis
5 Tubular necrosis
6 Papillary necrosis

RENAL CALCULI

1 Prevalence in UK 3%
2 Calcium-containing most common (85%)
3 Predisposition
  (a) Metabolism
    (i) Hypercalciuria
    (ii) Primary hypercalcaemia
    (iii) Renal tubular acidosis
    (iv) Uric aciduria
    (v) Hyperoxaluria
    (vi) Increased oxalate intake
    (vii) Cystinuria
  (b) Structural
    (i) Polycystic kidney disease
    (ii) Reflux nephropathy
    (iii) Nephrocalcinosis
    (iv) Medullary sponge kidney
  (c) Others
    (i) Dehydration
    (ii) Cadmium
    (iii) Beryllium
    (iv) Triamterene
4 Presents with
  (a) Renal colic
  (b) Infection
  (c) Haematuria
  (d) Can be asymptomatic (staghorn calculi)

5 Investigation
  (a) KUB (85% sensitive)
  (b) Ultrasound (may not detect stones < 5 mm)
  (c) IVU
  (d) CT (currently thought to be the best investigation)
6 Treatment
  (a) Increase fluid intake
  (b) Decrease protein in diet
  (c) Treat underlying cause
  (d) Thiazide diuretic (reduces calciuria)
  (e) Stone removal and/or lithotripsy

UTI

1 Causes
  (a) *E. coli*
  (b) Enterococci
  (c) *Proteus*
  (d) *Enterobacter*
  (e) *Pseudomonas*
  (f) *Klebsiella*
  (g) TB
2 Predisposing factors
  (a) Female
  (b) Bladder outflow obstruction
  (c) Anatomical disorders of bladder (diverticula, tumours)
  (d) Vesicoureteric reflux
  (e) Renal stones
  (f) Pregnancy
  (g) Diabetes
  (h) Immunosuppression (HIV)
  (i) Foreign body (including catheters)

RENAL TUBULAR ACIDOSIS

Metabolic acidosis caused by a disorder of renal tubules (different from uraemic acidosis).

[See Table 49, opposite]

Table 49

	Type 1 (distal)	Type 2 (proximal)	Type 4
Defect	Reduced H+ secretion Impaired acidification of urine	Defect in reabsorption of bicarbonate (bicarb loss)	Hypoaldosteronism or failure of aldosterone action Reduced H+ and K+ secretion
Diagnosis	Urine pH > 5.5 (never acidified) Metabolic acidosis Normal anion gap Hyperchloraemia Normal or near normal urea and creatinine Ammonium chloride load fails to acidify urine	Urine pH < 5.4 Rarely isolated defect Usually other proximal tubular defects, eg glycosuria, hyperphosphaturia etc. Metabolic acidosis Normal anion gap Hyperchloraemia Normal or near normal urea and creatinine Often polyuria Fractional bicarbonate rises after iv load of bicarbonate	Urine pH < 5.4 Hyperkalaemia Metabolic acidosis Normal anion gap Hyperchloraemia GFR usually reduced, so may have increased urea and creatinine

NEPHROLOGY

continued

Table 49 (cont.)

	Type 1 (distal)	Type 2 (proximal)	Type 4
Plasma bicarbonate	< 12 mmol/l	Plasma 14–20 mmol/l	14–20 mmol/l
Plasma K	Low	Normal or low	High
Complications	Nephrocalcinosis	Osteomalacia	Hyperkalaemia
	Severe hypokalaemia	Rickets	
	Calculi	Fanconi syndrome	
	Growth failure		
	UTIs		
Treatment	Replace potassium, then	High doses of bicarbonate	Mineralocorticoid
	iv bicarbonate	Thiazides	Fludrocortisone
	Long-term oral bicarbonate	Potassium	

Causes of type 1 RTA

1 Hereditary (AD)
2 Autoimmune
   (a) SLE
   (b) Sjögren's syndrome
   (c) Autoimmune hepatitis
3 Renal disorders
   (a) Chronic pyelonephritis
   (b) Chronic interstitial nephritis
   (c) Obstructive nephropathy
   (d) Transplant rejection
   (e) Medullary sponge kidney
4 Others
   (a) Hypercalcaemia
   (b) Lithium
   (c) Amphotericin
   (d) Idiopathic

Causes of type 2 RTA

1 Hereditary (AD)
2 Wilson's disease
3 Sjögren's syndrome
4 Interstitial nephritis
5 Amyloidosis
6 Myeloma
7 Vitamin D deficiency
8 Drugs
   (a) Tetracycline
   (b) Sulphonamides
   (c) Acetazolamide
9 Lead
10 Mercury
11 Cystinosis
12 Fructose intolerance

Causes of type 4 RTA

1 Hypoadrenalism
2 Hyporeninaemic hypoaldosteronism

3 Diabetic nephropathy
4 Gout nephropathy
5 Urinary obstruction
6 NSAIDs
7 Potassium-sparing diuretics

FANCONI SYNDROME

1 Tubular dysfunction leading to abnormal excretion of amino acids, phosphate, bicarbonate, glucose and small proteins
2 Often have type 2 RTA and metabolic bone disease
3 Causes
  (a) Primary inherited
  (b) Secondary inherited
      (i)   Cystinosis
      (ii)   Wilson's disease
      (iii) Galactosaemia
      (iv)   Fructose intolerance
  (c) Acquired
      (i)   ATN
      (ii)   Hypokalaemic nephropathy
      (iii) Myeloma
      (iv)   Sjögren's syndrome
      (v)   Transplant rejection
      (vi)   Hyperparathyroidism
      (vii) Heavy metals
      (viii) Tetracycline
      (ix)   6-Mercaptopurine
4 Treatment
  (a) Treat underlying cause
  (b) Bicarbonate
  (c) Potassium
  (d) Oral phosphate
  (e) Calcitriol

SYSTEMIC DISORDERS AND THE KIDNEY

Amyloidosis

1 Chronic infiltrative disorders
2 Deposition of extracellular fibrillar material (ie amyloid)
3 20 types of proteins isolated
4 Can get systemic or localised forms
5 Some examples
   (a) Primary amyloid – (AL) light chains
   (b) Secondary amyloid – (AA) inflammatory associated
   (c) Senile amyloid (Alzheimer's) – β-protein precursor
   (d) Dialysis amyloid – β_2-microglobulin
   (e) Cardiac amyloid – transthyretin
   (f) CJD – prion protein
6 Presentation
   (a) Proteinuria (asymptomatic to nephrotic)
   (b) Chronic renal failure
7 Clinical features of systemic amyloidosis
   (a) Hepatosplenomegaly
   (b) Nephrotic syndrome
   (c) Renal failure
   (d) Macroglossia
   (e) GI bleeding
   (f) Malabsorption
   (g) Restrictive cardiomyopathy
   (h) Skin deposition
   (i) Neuropathy
   (j) Bleeding disorder
8 Associations of secondary amyloidosis
   (a) Myeloma
   (b) Rheumatoid conditions
      (i) Rheumatoid arthritis
      (ii) Psoriatic arthritis
      (iii) Ankylosing spondylitis
      (iv) Behçet's syndrome
      (v) Reiter's syndrome
      (vi) Juvenile arthritis
      (vii) Polymyositis
      (viii) Scleroderma

    (c) GI conditions
       (i) Whipple's disease
       (ii) Inflammatory bowel disease
    (d) Infections
       (i) Tuberculosis
       (ii) Osteomyelitis
       (iii) Leprosy
       (iv) Syphilis
       (v) Bronchiectasis
    (e) Familial Mediterranean fever
9 Diagnosis
    (a) Biopsy
       (i) Rectal biopsy
       (ii) Subcutaneous fat aspiration
       (iii) Organ biopsy
    (b) Histology: Congo red stain on biopsy
    (c) SAP scan
10 Treatment
    (a) Remove or treat underlying cause
    (b) Cytotoxic therapy
    (c) Bone marrow transplant
    (d) Prognosis
       (i) 44% 5-year survival on dialysis
       (ii) Worse if on dialysis: faster speed of onset and multisystem involvement

Renovascular disease

1 Associated with general vascular disease
2 Risk factors (See page 24)
3 Presentation
    (a) Hypertension
    (b) Flash pulmonary oedema
    (c) End-stage renal failure
    (d) Chronic renal failure
    (e) Acute renal failure following ACE inhibitor or angiotensin 2 antagonist
4 Investigations
    (a) Asymmetrical kidneys on ultrasound scan
    (b) Captopril renogram

(c) CT/MR angiogram
(d) Conventional angiography
5 Treatment
  (a) Angioplasty +/- stenting to prevent deterioration in renal function or to salvage renal function
  (b) Aspirin
  (c) Antihypertensives
  (d) Lipid-lowering treatment

Connective tissue disorders

1 Renal disease associated with
  (a) Rheumatoid arthritis
  (b) Mixed connective tissue disease
  (c) Sjögren's syndrome
  (d) Systemic sclerosis
  (e) SLE

SLE nephritis

1 40% have clinical renal involvement (near 100% histologically)
2 Women:men = 10:1
3 Any renal presentation possible
4 Histology variable (Table 50)

Table 50

Type	Histological appearance
1	Normal
2a	Mesangial deposits
2b	Mesangial hypercellularity
3	Focal segmental nephritis
4	Diffuse proliferative nephritis
5	Membranous nephritis

5 Wire loop characteristic
6 Treatment
  (a) ARF and SLE – aggressive immunosuppressant therapy with pulsed methylprednisolone and iv cyclophosphamide, then high-dose oral prednisolone
  (b) Maintenance with oral steroids and azathioprine
  (c) Plasma exchange – if severe or pulmonary haemorrhage

Systemic sclerosis

1 Present in one-third of patients (almost all with diffuse disease)
2 Presents with
   (a) Slowly progressive renal failure with hypertension
   (b) Accelerated hypertension
   (c) Microangiopathic haemolytic anaemia (MAHA)
   (d) Acute renal failure
3 Histology
   (a) 'Onion skin' appearance of interlobular arteries
   (b) Glomeruli show appearances of ischaemia
4 Treatment
   (a) ACE inhibitor
   (b) Aggressive BP control
   (c) Dialysis
   (d) Transplantation
5 Prognosis
   (a) Many progress to end-stage renal failure
   (b) Poor, owing to other organs being affected

Diabetes mellitus (DM)

1 Most common cause of ESRF in UK
2 49% type 1 20–40 years from diagnosis
3 Presentation
   (a) Microalbuminuria (30–250 mg/day)
   (b) Proteinuria (> 0.5 g/day)
   (c) Hypertension
   (d) Nephrotic syndrome
   (e) Chronic renal failure
4 Biopsy
   (a) Diffuse glomerular sclerosis
   (b) Kimmelstiel–Wilson nodules are characteristic
   (c) Mesangial expansion
5 Treatment
   (a) ACE inhibitors and angiotensin blockers
   (b) Tight glycaemic control
   (c) Tight blood pressure control (target < 130/75)
6 Outcome
   (a) Established nephropathy to ESRF
   (b) Poor prognosis due to other comorbidity, eg cardiovascular

Hypertension and the kidney

1 Significant renal dysfunction in uncomplicated essential hypertension is rare, so other causes such as primary renal disease should be sought
2 Hypertension is more likely to lead to progressive renal dysfunction in Afro-Caribbeans
3 Renal blood flow is reduced in hypertension but GFR is preserved, and this leads to hyalinisation in the afferent arterioles
4 Ageing leads to a gradual decline in renal function, with hypertension, atherosclerosis and glomerulosclerosis
5 Uncontrolled hypertension in CRF accelerates loss of renal function
6 Biopsy findings in hypertension
  (a) Arterial fibrinoid necrosis (accelerated hypertension)
  (b) Severe tubular and glomerular ischaemia (ARF)
  (c) Interstitial fibrosis and glomerulosclerosis (CRF)

Myeloma

1 Acute renal failure
  (a) Light chain nephropathy
  (b) Hypercalcaemia
  (c) Hyperuricaemia
  (d) Dehydration
  (e) Contrast nephropathy
2 Chronic renal failure
  (a) Amyloidosis
  (b) Glomerulonephritis
  (c) Chronic interstitial nephritis
  (d) Papillary necrosis (hyperviscosity)
  (e) Plasma cell infiltration
  (f) Usually progress to end-stage renal failure
3 Light chain nephropathy
  (a) Kappa and lamda chains deposited
  (b) Direct toxicity
  (c) Cast formation
  (d) Acute tubular necrosis
  (e) Tubular atrophy

NEPHROLOGY

Goodpasture's syndrome

1 Autoimmune disorder (anti-GBM antibody)
2 Autoantibody to type 4 collagen in glomerular and alveolar basement membrane
3 Pathology
   (a) Crescentic GN
   (b) Pulmonary haemorrhage
4 Presents with
   (a) Haemoptysis
   (b) Haematuria
   (c) Breathlessness
   (d) Massive pulmonary haemorrhage
5 Management
   (a) Steroids
   (b) Cyclophosphamide
   (c) Plasma exchange
6 Prognosis
   (a) Depends on renal function at presentation
   (b) Poor if ITU necessary

Risk factors for radiocontrast nephropathy

1 Hypovolaemia
2 Diabetes mellitus
3 Pre-existing CRF
4 Hypercalcaemia
5 Hyperuricaemia
6 Age
7 Myeloma
8 High contrast dose
9 Contrast increased iodine content

TUMOURS OF THE RENAL TRACT

1 Benign
   (a) Adenoma
   (b) Hamartoma
   (c) Renin-secreting (juxtaglomerular cell)

2 Malignant
  (a) Renal cell carcinoma
    (i)   From tubular epithelium
    (ii) Some cases hereditary
      (1) von-Hippel–Lindau
        (a) 40% have renal cell carcinoma
        (b) Phaeochromocytoma
        (c) Pancreatic cysts and islet cell tumors
        (d) Retinal angiomas
        (e) Central nervous system haemangioblastomas
        (f) Endolymphatic sac tumours
        (g) Epididymal cystadenomas
      (2) Hereditary papillary renal carcinoma (HPRC)
      (3) Familial renal oncocytoma (FRO) associated with Birt–Hogg–Dube syndrome (BHDS)
      (4) Hereditary renal carcinoma (HRC)
    (iii) Risk factors
      (1) Smoking
      (2) Obesity
      (3) Hypertension
      (4) Exposure to solvents or heavy metals
      (5) Renal transplantation
      (6) Analgesic abuse
      (7) Dialysis
    (iv) Local and haematogenous spread
    (v)   30% metastatic disease at presentation
    (vi) Clinical features
      (1) Haematuria
      (2) Loin pain
      (3) Abdominal masses
      (4) Renal vein invasion
      (5) Pulmonary emboli
      (6) Pyrexia of unknown origin
      (7) Left testicular vein occlusion leads to varicocoele on left
      (8) Polycythaemia – excess erythropoietin production
      (9) Hypercalcaemia – PTH-like substance
      (10) Hypertension – renin secretion
      (11) Cushing's – ACTH production
    (vii) Diagnosis
      (1) USS
      (2) CT

      (viii) Treatment
          (1) Surgical excision
          (2) Some respond to interferon or IL-2
      (ix) Prognosis
          (1) 50% 5-year survival rate
  (b) Wilms' tumour
      (i) Present in children
      (ii) Embryonic renal tissue
      (iii) Hypertension common
      (iv) Early metastasis
      (v) Treatment
          (1) Nephrectomy and actinomycin D
      (vi) 65% 3-year survival
  (c) Urothelial tumours
      (i) Transitional cell origin
      (ii) Clinical features
          (1) Presents with haematuria, renal pain or obstruction
      (iii) Often multiple lesions
      (iv) Risk factors
          (1) Smoking
          (2) Analgesic nephropathy
          (3) Rubber and aniline dye exposure
          (4) Renal calculi
          (5) Cystic kidney disease
          (6) Chronic cystitis
          (7) Schistosomiasis infection
          (8) Cyclophosphamide
      (v) Diagnosis
          (1) IVU
          (2) CT
      (vi) Treatment
          (1) Renal pelvis or ureter
              (a) Nephroureterectomy
          (2) Bladder
              (a) Intravesical chemotherapy
              (b) TURBT
              (c) Cystectomy
              (d) Radiotherapy
      (vii) 50% 5-year survival

Neurology

INTERPRETING CEREBRAL LESIONS

The cerebral cortex

Motor – precentral gyrus (frontal lobe)
Somatosensory – postcentral gyrus
1 Auditory – superior temporal lobe
2 Visual – occipital cortex
3 Olfactory – frontal lobe
4 Broca's area – dominant frontal lobe, speech output
5 Wernicke's area – dominant posterior superior temporal gyrus, word comprehension.

Frontal lobe lesions may cause

1 Personality change – apathetic or disinhibited
2 Broca's aphasia (expressive)
3 Abnormal affective reactions
4 Difficulty planning or maintaining motivation
5 Primitive reflexes (eg grasp, rooting, pout)
6 Perseveration

Parietal lobe lesions may cause

1 Dominant hemisphere
   (a) Apraxia (inability to perform purposeful tasks)
   (b) Acalculia (inability to perform calculations)
   (c) Alexia (inability to read)
   (d) Agraphia (inability to write)
   (e) Drawing apraxia (inability to draw)
   (f) Gerstmann's syndrome
      (i) Alexia
      (ii) Agraphia
      (iii) Right/left confusion
      (iv) Finger agnosia (inability to name fingers)

2 Non-dominant
   (a) Dressing apraxia (inability to get dressed)
   (b) Ideomotor apraxia (inability to imitate gestures)
   (c) Visuospatial neglect or extinction
3 Both
   (a) Homonymous inferior quadrantanopia (upper loop of optic radiation)
   (b) Constructional apraxia (inability to build or arrange objects)
   (c) Astereognosis (inability to recognise objects by feel)

Occipital lesions may result in

1 Cortical blindness
2 Homonymous hemianopia
3 Visual agnosia (inability to comprehend memory of objects)

Temporal lobe lesions may result in

1 Wernicke's aphasia (receptive)
2 Cortical deafness (auditory cortex – bilateral)
3 Reduced language comprehension
4 Memory impairment
5 Impaired musical perception
6 Emotional disturbance – limbic cortex damage
7 Homonymous superior quadrantanopia (lower loop optic radiation)

Cerebellum

1 Signs of cerebellar pathology
   (a) Ataxia (wide-based gait)
   (b) Nystagmus
   (c) Dysarthria (scanning speech)
   (d) Dysdiadochokinesia
   (e) Past pointing
   (f) Intention tremor
2 Causes of cerebellar pathology
   (a) Alcoholism
   (b) Demyelination (MS)
   (c) Vascular
   (d) Drugs (phenytoin, barbiturates)
   (e) Neoplastic lesions of the posterior fossa

(f) Congenital syndromes (Freidreich's ataxia, ataxia–telangiectasia)
(g) Paraneoplastic degeneration
(h) Hypothyroidism (very rare)

CEREBROVASCULAR DISEASE

1 TIAs
   (a) Focal CNS disturbance that develops in minutes with full recovery within 24 hrs of onset
   (b) Embolic
2 Stroke (cerebrovascular accident)
   (a) Clinically as for TIA, but deficit persists
   (b) Embolic
   (c) Thrombotic
   (d) Haemorrhagic
3 Clinical presentation
   (a) Anterior circulation
       (i)   Motor or sensory dysfunction of the contralateral extremities and/or face
       (ii) Loss of vision in the ipsilateral eye (amaurosis fugax)
       (iii) Homonymous hemianopia
       (iv) Aphasia (dominant hemisphere)
       (v)   Dysarthria
   (b) Posterior circulation
       (i)   Motor or sensory dysfunction of the ipsilateral face and/or contralateral extremities
       (ii) Loss of vision in one or both of the homonymous visual fields
       (iii) Ataxia
       (iv) Vertigo
       (v)   Dysphagia
       (vi) Diplopia
   (c) Lacunar infarctions
       (i)   Small subcortical infarction due to occlusion of penetrating end artery
       (ii) Pure motor hemiparesis – posterior internal capsule
       (iii) Pure sensory stroke – thalamus
       (iv) Clumsy hand, dysarthria – pons

NEUROLOGY

    (v) No higher cortical functions affected

    (vi) Associated with better prognosis

4 Diagnosis

  (a) Clinical

  (b) CT/MRI brain

  (c) Risk factor investigation (See page 24)

    (i)   BP

    (ii)   ECG ?AF

    (iii) Cholesterol

    (iv) Glucose

    (v)   ESR/CRP ?vasculitis

    (vi) Thrombophilia screen if < 45 years

    (vii) Carotid Doppler to look for internal carotid stenosis

    (viii) Echocardiogram/TOE ?cardiac source of embolus or PFO

5 Treatment/secondary prevention

  (a) Treat on stroke unit

  (b) IV fluids to keep hydrated

  (c) Assess swallowing (if poor NBM)

  (d) Treat hyperglycaemia with insulin

  (e) Treat fever with paracetamol

  (f) DVT prophylaxis

  (g) Physiotherapy, speech therapy, occupational therapy

  (h) Infarct

    (i)   Aspirin (reduces risk of further infarct)

    (ii)   Dipyridamole (second line for those who infarct while on aspirin)

    (iii) Clopidogrel (if intolerant of aspirin)

    (iv) Thrombolysis (in some centres) within 3 hrs of onset

    (v)   Treat hypertension (2 weeks after CVA, immediately if TIA)

    (vi) Stop smoking

    (vii) Statin (reduces risk of further CVA)

    (viii) Anticoagulation if AF, mitral stenosis or mural thrombus (2 weeks after infarct, immediate if TIA)

    (ix) Carotid endarterectomy if carotid artery stenosis (> 80%)

  (i) Haemorrhage

    (i)   Neurosurgery if indicated

    (ii)   Treat hypertension

6 Prognosis

  (a) 20–30% mortality

  (b) 25–30% remains significantly disabled

Lateral medullary syndrome (Wallenberg's)

1 Infarction of lateral medulla and inferior olivary nucleus
2 Vertebral artery or posterior inferior cerebellar artery occlusion
3 Features
  (a) Ipsilateral pain and temperature loss on face (CN V)
  (b) Ipsilateral paralysis of palate, pharynx, vocal cords (CN IX, X)
  (c) Ipsilateral ataxia (cerebellar)
  (d) Contralateral pain and temp loss on body (spirothalamic tract)
  (e) Ipsilateral Horner's syndrome (descending sympathetic outflow)
  (f) Vertigo, nausea and vomiting, nystagmus (vestibular nuclei)

Subarachnoid haemorrhage (SAH)

1 Causes
  (a) Rupture of aneurysm – 80% anterior circulation (mainly ant. communicating artery)
  (b) Arteriovenous malformation
  (c) Trauma
  (d) Cocaine or amphetamine abuse
  (e) Hypertension
2 Symptoms
  (a) Headache (sudden onset and severe)
  (b) Vomiting
  (c) Coma
3 Diagnosis
  (a) CT scan (90% diagnostic yield)
  (b) Lumbar puncture:
    (i) Xanthochromia (> 4 hrs post episode, clears after 2 weeks)
    (ii) ↑ Blood cell count on microscopy (unreliable, as 20% of taps are traumatic)
  (c) CT angiography/MR angiography/cerebral angiography to find aneurysms
4 Treatment
  (a) Nimodipine – reduces vasospasm
  (b) Neurosurgical clipping of aneurysm
  (c) Endovascular embolisation of aneurysm
5 Prognosis
  (a) 30% mortality from first episode
6 Complications
  (a) Vasospasm – ischaemic injury

(b) 30% rebleed
(c) Hydrocephalus
(d) Hyponatraemia and SIADH
(e) Fever
(f) 30% recover to be independent
7 Conditions associated with SAH
(a) Polycystic kidney disease
(b) Ehlers–Danlos syndrome
(c) Marfan's syndrome
(d) Neurofibromatosis type 1
(e) Medium vessels vasculitis (eg PAN)
(f) Coarctation of aorta
(g) Fibromuscular dysplasia causing renal artery stenosis

MIGRAINE

1 Symptoms
(a) Unilateral throbbing headache
(b) Usually preceded by visual aura
(c) Nausea
(d) Photophobia
(e) Paraesthesiae
(f) Rarely reversible neurological signs
2 Pathophysiology unclear, but thought to be vascular in origin
3 Treatment
(a) Acute
(i) Paracetamol
(ii) NSAIDs
(iii) $5HT_1$ agonists, eg sumatriptan
(iv) Dopamine antagonists
(v) Ergotamine
(b) Prophylactic (two or more disabling attacks per month)
(i) Propranolol
(ii) Pizotifen
(iii) Amitryptiline
(iv) Valproate
(v) Calcium channel blockers
(vi) Methysergide

BENIGN INTRACRANIAL HYPERTENSION

1 Raised intracranial pressure in the absence of mass lesion or hydrocephalus
2 Symptoms
   (a) Headache
   (b) Most commonly overweight females
3 Examination
   (a) Papilloedema
   (b) Sixth cranial nerve palsy
   (c) Scotomas (optic nerve damage)
4 Investigation
   (a) Brain scan normal
   (b) CSF pressure increased (> 200 mm)
5 Treatment
   (a) Weight loss
   (b) Sequential lumbar puncture
   (c) Acetazolamide
   (d) Ventriculoperitoneal shunt
6 Causes
   (a) Obesity (90%)
   (b) OCPs
   (c) Vitamin A (excess or deficiency) also vitamin A derivatives, eg retinoids
   (d) Nalidixic acid
   (e) Nitrofurantoin
   (f) Tetracycline

DEMENTIA

1 Acquired, global impairment of intellect, memory and personality
2 Causes
   (a) Potentially treatable
       (i) B_{12} deficiency
       (ii) Folate deficiency
       (iii) Hypothyroidism
       (iv) Syphilis
       (v)   Wilson's disease

    (vi)   Normal-pressure hydrocephalus
    (vii) HIV associated
    (viii) Chronic subdural haematoma
  (b) Usually progressive
    (i)   Alzheimer's
    (ii)   Multi-infarct dementia
    (iii) Pick's disease
    (iv) Huntington's disease
    (v)   Parkinson's disease
    (vi) Lewy body dementia
    (vii) Chronic head injury
    (viii) Chronic alcoholism or drug intoxication
    (ix) CJD
    (x)   Progressive multifocal leukoencephalopathy (PML)
    (xi) Primary and secondary tumours

Alzheimer's disease

1 Progressive memory loss and cognitive impairment
2 Deterioration of language, disorientation and personality change
3 Pathology
  (a) Senile plaques (β-amyloid) – neurotoxic
  (b) Neurofibrillary tangles (τ protein)
  (c) Hippocampus particularly affected
  (d) Loss of cholinergic neurones and reduced choline
     acetyltransferase activity
2 Genes implicated
  (a) Amyloid precursor protein APP gene, chromosome 21
  (b) Presenilin 1 (PS1) gene, chromosome 14
  (c) Presenilin 2 (PS2) gene, chromosome 1
  (d) Apolipoprotein E4
3 Treatment
  (a) Will only lead to modest improvement in cognition
  (b) Cholinesterase inhibitors (reduce acetylcholine depletion)
    (i)   Donepezil
    (ii) Rivastigmine
  (c) NMDA antagonist (improves function of hippocampal neurones)
    (i)   Memantine

Pick's disease

1 Focal lobar atrophy affecting frontal and temporal lobes
2 Severe atrophy, neuronal loss and gliosis
3 Pick bodies in cellular cytoplasm
4 Severe progressive dementia with prominent frontal lobe features language disturbance

Lewy body dementia

1 Lewy bodies are a pathological feature of Parkinson's disease (in substantia nigra)
2 Diffuse Lewy bodies leads to dementia

Normal-pressure hydrocephalus

1 Defect CSF absorption – basal meningeal thickening leads to intermittent rise in CSF pressure
2 Triad of
   (a) Dementia
   (b) Gait abnormality ('glued to the floor' sign)
   (c) Urinary incontinence (frontal lobe)
3 Causes
   (a) Meningitis
   (b) Head injury
   (c) Subarachnoid haemorrhage
   (d) Idiopathic
4 Radiology
   (a) Cortical atrophy
   (b) Dilated ventricles
   (c) Hydrocephalus
5 Treatment
   (a) Ventriculoperitoneal shunt

Creutzfeldt–Jakob disease (CJD)

1 Prion disease
2 Accumulation of prion protein in CNS leads to disease
3 Three forms
   (a) Familial
      (i) Autosomal dominant
      (ii) PRNP gene

       (iii) Variable symptoms
          (1) Ataxia
          (2) Dementia
          (3) Sleep abnormality
    (b) Infectious/iatrogenic (Kuru, variant CJD)
       (i)   Causes
          (1) Following neurosurgery
          (2) Corneal transplants
          (3) GH therapy
       (ii) Incubation 2–10 years
       (iii) Variant CJD
          (1) Younger-age onset (median age at death 29 years)
          (2) Behavioural disturbance
          (3) Psychiatric disturbance
          (4) Cerebellar syndrome
          (5) Myoclonus
          (6) Later severe cognitive impairment
          (7) EEG features absent
          (8) Spongiform change and neuronal loss
          (9) Astrogliosis of basal ganglia and thalamus
  (c) Sporadic
       (i)   85% of all cases
       (ii) Incidence 1 in 2 million worldwide
       (iii) Mean age 65 years
       (iv) Severe dementia
       (v) Myoclonus
       (vi) Cerebellar syndrome
  (g) EEG – periodic synchronous discharge

NEUROLOGICAL INFECTIONS

Causes of meningitis

1 Acute bacterial causes
  (a) Adults
       (i)   *Meningococcus*
       (ii) *Pneumococcus*
  (b) Neonates
       (i)   Group B streptococcus
       (ii) *E. coli*

   (c) Rarities (lymphocytic CSF)
     (i) *Listeria monocytogenes*
     (ii) Leptospirosis
     (iii) Syphilis
     (iv) Lyme disease
   (d) Rarities (polymorphs in CSF)
     (i) *Mycobacterium tuberculosis*
     (ii) *Staphylococcus aureus*
     (iii) *Listeria*
     (iv) *Pseudomonas*
   (e) Chronic bacterial cause
     (i) *Mycobacterium tuberculosis*
2 Chronic fungal causes
   (a) Cryptococcosis
3 Acute viral causes
   (a) Mumps
   (b) Enteroviruses (especially polio)
   (c) HSV
4 Amoebic meningitis

Encephalitis

1 Features
   (a) Headache
   (b) Fever
   (c) Confusion
   (d) Altered conscious level
   (e) Seizures
   (f) Focal neurology.
2 Viral causes
   (a) HSV (mainly type 1)
   (b) Enteroviruses eg Coxsackie
   (c) Arboviruses (eg Japanese encephalitis)
   (d) VZV
   (e) HIV
   (f) Rabies

Herpes simplex encephalitis

1 Anterior temporal lobe pathology
2 Gross cerebral oedema

3 Investigation
  (a) CSF
    (i) Lymphocytosis
    (ii) Mildly raised protein
    (iii) Usually normal glucose
    (iv) HSV PCR
  (b) EEG – focal temporal lobe involvement
  (c) MRI – temporal lobe lesions
4 Treatment
  (a) IV aciclovir
  (b) Phenytoin for seizures

EPILEPSY

1 Disorder characterised by two or more seizures
2 Paroxysmal discharge of neurones owing to imbalance of inhibitory and excitatory neurones
3 Prevalence 0.7% constant at all ages
4 Incidence greater in young and elderly
5 Partial seizures
  (a) Simple partial seizures
    (i) Seizure with preservation of consciousness
    (ii) Many types exist, including sensory, motor, autonomic, and psychic experiences
    (iii) Last a few seconds to a few minutes
    (iv) EEG – local discharge in corresponding area
    (v) May progress
  (b) Complex partial seizures
    (i) Consciousness impaired
    (ii) A typical complex partial seizure lasts about 60–90 sec and is followed by brief postictal confusion
    (iii) Preceded by aura – *déjà vu*, strong smell, or rising sensation in abdomen
    (iv) Automatisms
  (c) Secondary generalised seizures
    (i) Begin with an aura and evolves into a complex partial seizure, and then into a generalised tonic–clonic seizure
6 Generalised seizures
  (a) Absence seizures

    (i) Episodes of impairment of consciousness with no aura or postictal confusion
    (ii) Typically last less than 20 sec
    (iii) Typically begin during childhood or adolescence, but may persist into adulthood
    (iv) EEG during absence seizures consists of 3 to 5 Hz generalised spike and slow wave complexes
  (b) Primary generalised tonic–clonic seizures
    (i) 'Grand mal' seizures
    (ii) Generalised tonic extension of the extremities lasting for few seconds, followed by clonic rhythmic movements and prolonged postictal confusion
    (iii) No aura
    (iv) EEG shows generalised (bilateral) spike or polyspike and slow wave complexes
  (c) Tonic seizures
    (i) Sudden-onset tonic extension or flexion of the head, trunk, and/or extremities for several seconds
  (d) Clonic seizures
    (i) Rhythmic, motor, jerking movements with impairment of consciousness
  (e) Myoclonic seizures
    (i) Brief, arrhythmic, jerking motor movements that last less than a second. Often cluster within a few minutes
    (ii) Myoclonus is not always epileptic, and can occur normally in sleep
    (iii) EEG consists of fast polyspike and slow wave complexes
  (f) Atonic seizures
    (i) Brief loss of postural tone

Mechanism of action of antiepileptics

1 Na channels
  (a) Blockage leads to stabilisation of neurones, preventing repetitive firing and seizures
2 Calcium channels
  (a) Thalamic calcium channel inhibition reduces absence seizures
3 GABA
  (a) Inhibitory neurotransmitter
  (b) GABA-A receptors can be activated by benzodiazepines and barbiturates

(c) GABA is produced by glutamic acid decarboxylase – activation of this enzyme will ↑ GABA

(d) GABA metabolised by GABA transaminase – inhibition will ↑ GABA

4 Glutamate
   (a) Excitatory neurotransmitter
   (b) Inhibition will reduce neuroexcitability

[See Table 51, opposite]

DVLA regulations on driving with epilepsy

1 A person who has suffered an epileptic attack while **awake** must refrain from driving for **1** year from the date of the attack

2 A person who has suffered an attack while **asleep** must also refrain from driving for **1** year from the date of the attack, unless they have had an attack while asleep more than 3 years ago and have not had any awake attacks since that asleep attack

HGV

1 Free from **any** epileptic attack for 10 years and not required medication to treat epilepsy

Pregnancy and epilepsy

1 All pregnancies should be planned

2 OCP is less effective in those on enzyme-inducing drugs, eg phenytoin or carbamazepine

3 Epileptic drugs are not contraindicated

4 Risk of fetal malformation also higher in epileptics not on treatment (25%↑)

5 All drugs have teratogenic effects (3 × risk)

6 Risks of uncontrolled epilepsy is greater than adverse effects of drugs

7 Those who have been seizure free for 2 years may have trial off drugs 3–6 months pre-pregnancy

8 Aim to have patients on monotherapy at lowest dose

9 Slow-release valproate should be used (lower peak drug levels) if on valproate

10 Seizure rate predicted by rate prior to pregnancy

Table 51

Drug	Mechanism	Indications	Side effects
Valproate	Uncertain	All forms of epilepsy Drug of choice for tonic–clonic Absence Myoclonic	N+V Tremor Weight gain Sedation ↑ Ammonia Hair loss Hepatotoxicity Pancreatitis
Phenytoin	Blocks Na channels	Tonic–clonic Partial Status epilepticus	Rash Hirsutism Coarsening of facies Gingival hyperplasia Hepatotoxicity Cerebellar symptoms Drowsiness Vitamins D, K and folate deficiency
Carbamazepine	Blocks Na channels	Tonic–clonic Partial Secondary generalised	Rash Dizziness Ataxia Hepatotoxicity Blood dyscrasias
Lamotrigine	Blocks Na channels Glutamate inhibitor	Monotherapy and adjuvant for tonic–clonic Partial Secondary generalised Some myoclonic	Rash Steven–Johnson syndrome Headache Ataxia Dizziness Tremor
Topiramate	Blocks Na channels ↑ GABA Inhibits glutamate	Monotherapy or adjuvant therapy for tonic–clonic and partial and secondary generalised	Ataxia ↓ Concentration Drowsiness
Levetracetam	Unknown	Adjuvant therapy for partial and secondary generalised	Drowsiness Dizziness Ataxia

continued

NEUROLOGY

Table 51 (cont.)

Drug	Mechanism	Indications	Side effects
Vigabatrin	GABA transaminase inhibitor ↑ GABA	Adjuvant treatment for partial or secondary generalised Infantile spasms	Visual field defects Drowsiness
Tiagabine	Inhibits GABA transporter-1 ↑ GABA	Adjuvant for partial or secondary generalised	Diarrhoea Tremor Emotional lability May exacerbate status epilepticus
Phenobarbitone	GABA-A agonist	Status epilepticus All forms except absence	Cognitive slowing Sedation Osteomalacia Dupuytren's contracture Folate deficiency
Primidone	Metabolised to phenobarbitone	All forms of epilepsy except absence	As above
Gabapentin	Enhances GAD ↑ GABA May inhibit glutamate	Adjuvant in partial or secondary generalised Neuropathic pain	Drowsiness Rash
Ethosuxamide	Inhibits thalamic calcium channels	Absence seizures	GI disturbance Blood dyscrasias
Benzodiazepines	GABA-A agonist	Termination of seizures	Respiratory depression Sedation Dizziness Blurred vision

11 Current drug used if starting treatment is lamotrigine
12 Folic acid supplements decrease malformation
13 Those on enzyme-inducing drugs should be given vitamin K to reduce risk of haemorrhagic disease of the newborn (vitamin K deficiency)
14 No contraindication to breastfeeding in those on antiepileptics
15 Child's risk of epilepsy is 3%

ALCOHOL AND THE BRAIN

Wernicke's encephalopathy

1 Acute thiamine deficiency
2 Microvascular lesions in third and fourth ventricles, periaqueductal grey matter, mamillary bodies, brainstem and cerebellum
3 Features
   (a) Ataxia
   (b) Nystagmus
   (c) Ophthalmoplegia
   (d) Global confusional state
   (e) Neuropathy
4 Causes
   (a) Chronic alcohol abuse
   (b) Hyperemesis gravidarum
   (c) Dialysis
   (d) Gastric cancer
5 Treatment with intravenous thiamine
6 80% develop Korsakoff's syndrome

Korsakoff's syndrome

1 Usually as consequence of Wernicke's
2 Features
   (a) Markedly impaired short-term recall
   (b) Anterograde amnesia
   (c) Variable retrograde amnesia
   (d) Registration normal
   (e) Lack of insight
   (f) Confabulation common
3 Other causes
   (a) Carbon monoxide poisoning
   (b) HSV encephalitis

SPINAL CORD AND PERIPHERAL NERVE ANATOMY

Carpal tunnel syndrome

1 Median nerve palsy (nerve compressed at wrist)
2 Features
   (a) Pain and paraesthesias (worse at night)
   (b) Paraesthesia of lateral 3½ fingers
   (c) Weakness of LOAF muscles
       (i) **L**ateral two lumbricals
       (ii) **O**pponens pollicis
       (iii) **A**bductor pollicis
       (iv) **F**lexor pollicis brevis
3 Associations (PHARO)
   (a) **P**regnancy
   (b) **H**ypothyroidism
   (c) **A**cromegaly
   (d) **A**myloidosis
   (e) **R**A
   (f) **O**besity
4 Investigation
   (a) Tinel's sign – tapping on nerve causes tingling
   (b) Phalen's sign – prolonged flexion of wrist leads to tingling
   (c) Nerve conduction studies
5 Treatment
   (a) Splinting of wrist
   (b) Steroid injection to flexor retinaculum
   (c) Surgical decompression

Ulnar nerve palsy

1 Lesion at the elbow
   (a) Wasting of the medial side of the forearm
   (b) Claw hand deformity
   (c) Weakness of
       (i) Hypothenar eminence
       (ii) Abductor digiti minimi
       (iii) Median two lumbricals (weak finger flexion)
       (iv) All interossei (weak adduction and abduction)
   (d) Sensory loss of medial 1½ fingers
   (e) Causes

      (i) Fracture dislocation at elbow
      (ii) Occupational (leaning on elbows etc.)
      (iii) OA
      (iv) Mononeuritis multiplex (See page 342)
2 Wrist lesions
    (a) Weakness of all hand muscles as above
    (b) Sparing of sensory loss on dorsum of the hand

Radial nerve palsy

1 Wrist drop due to weakness of extensor compartment of forearm
2 Sensory loss over first dorsal interosseus
3 No muscles of hand
4 Causes
    (a) Fracture of humerus
    (b) Saturday night palsy
    (c) Mononeuritis multiplex (below)

Causes of small hand muscle wasting

1   Arthritis
2   Old age
3   Cervical cord pathology (C8/T1).
    (a) Spondylosis
    (b) Tumour
4   Cervical rib
5   Pancoast tumour
6   Brachial plexus injury
7   Motor neurone disease (usually fasciculation)
8   Combined ulnar and median nerve palsy
9   Polyneuropathy
10 HSMN (Charcot–Marie–Tooth disease)
11 Old polio
12 Syringomyelia

Common peroneal nerve palsy

1 Features
    (a) Foot drop
    (b) Weakness of inversion of foot (L4)
    (c) Weakness of dorsiflexion, tibialis anterior (L5)

NEUROLOGY

(d) Weakness of eversion, peronei (S1)
(e) Sensory loss dorsum of foot.
2 Causes
(a) Compression at fibular neck
(b) Mononeuritis multiplex (below)

Causes of mononeuritis multiplex

Multiple isolated mononeuropathies

1 DM
2 RA
3 Carcinoma
4 SLE
5 PAN
6 Sjögren's syndrome
7 Churg–Strauss
8 Wegener's granulomatosis
9 Sarcoidosis
10 Amyloidosis
11 Leprosy
12 Lyme disease

Polyneuropathies

Common

1 DM
2 Alcohol (thiamine deficiency and direct neurotoxic effects)
3 Vitamin B deficiency
4 Vitamin B_{12} deficiency
5 Drugs (See page 63)
6 Paraneoplastic
7 Uraemia

Rare

1 Connective tissue disorders
(a) RA
(b) PAN
(c) Wegener's granulomatosis
(d) Sjögren's

2 Guillain–Barré syndrome
3 Porphyria
4 Lead intoxication
5 Arsenic poisoning
6 Vitamin E deficiency
7 Diphtheria
8 Leprosy
9 HIV
10 Lyme disease
11 Amyloidosis
12 Paraproteinaemia
13 Sarcoidosis
14 HSMN (Charcot–Marie–Tooth)
15 Chronic inflammatory demyelinating polyneuropathy (CIDP)

Causes of fasciculation

1 Motor neurone disease
2 Syringomyelia
3 Thyrotoxicosis
4 Cervical spondylosis
5 Acute poliomyelitis
6 HSMN
7 Hyponatraemia
8 Hypomagnesaemia
9 Exercise
10 Drugs
   (a) Lithium
   (b) Salbutamol
   (c) Anticholinesterase

Autonomic neuropathy

1 Features
   (a) Postural hypotension
   (b) Sluggish or absent papillary light response
   (c) Anhidrosis
   (d) Defective piloerection
   (e) Impotence
   (f) Urinary incontinence
   (g) Nocturnal diarrhoea

(h) Constipation
(i) Absent cardiovascular responses
2 Causes
(a) DM
(b) Gullain–Barré syndrome
(c) Amyloidosis
(d) Porphyria
(e) HIV
(f) Craniopharyngioma
(g) Multiple system atrophies (eg Shy–Drager syndrome)

Guillain–Barré syndrome (acute inflammatory demyelinating polyneuropathy: AIDP)

1 Acute infective progressive polyneuropathy
2 Autoimmune injury to the myelin sheath
3 Autoantibodies to central or peripheral nerve proteins, eg GM1, GD1a, GD1b
4 Features
  (a) Ascending symmetrical muscle weakness, paraesthesia and hyporeflexia
  (b) Leads to paralysis
  (c) Cranial nerve involved in 50%
  (d) Autonomic dysfunction
5 60% report recent infection, eg CMV, EBV, *Campylobacter, Mycoplasma*
6 Investigations
  (a) Raised CSF protein with normal white cell count
  (b) Nerve conduction studies show slowing conduction
  (c) Autoantibodies (above)
  (d) FVC 4-hourly as deterioration can occur quickly, requiring ventilation
7 Poor prognosis if
  (a) Older age
  (b) Rapid onset of symptoms
  (c) Axonal neuropathy on nerve conduction studies
  (d) *Campylobacter jejuni* infection
8 Treatment
  (a) Intravenous immunoglobulin
  (b) Plasma exchange

(c) Ventilation
(d) DVT prophylaxis

Miller–Fisher syndrome

1 Variant of GBS (5%)
2 Most patients have GQ1b autoantibody
3 Ophthalmoplegia
4 Ataxia
5 Areflexia

Motor neurone disease (amyotrophic lateral sclerosis)

1 Progressive neurodegenerative disease affecting anterior horn cells
2 10% are AD (SOD I gene on chromosome 21)
3 Features
   (a) Upper and lower motor neurone signs
   (b) Wasting and weakness of limbs particularly hands
   (c) Fasciculation
   (d) Foot drop
   (e) Bulbar symptoms
      (i)   Nasal speech (bulbar palsy)
      (ii) Spastic dysarthria (pseudobulbar palsy)
      (iii) Dysphagia and aspiration
   (f) Respiratory failure
   (g) No sensory signs
4 Diagnosis
   (a) Clinical diagnosis
   (b) Electromyography and nerve conduction studies reveal anterior
      horn cell damage
   (c) MRI to rule out other causes, eg compressive lesion in neck, or
      demyelination
   (d) Investigations to rule out other neurodegenerative conditions,
      eg syphilis, HIV etc.
5 Treatment
   (a) Riluzole (glutamate antagonist) provides modest benefit
   (b) Muscle relaxants
   (c) PEG for feeding
   (d) Tracheostomy
   (e) CPAP

(f) Computer-assisted communication devices
(g) Multidisciplinary team approach
6 Prognosis
   (a) 2 years if bulbar symptoms
   (b) 4 years if peripheral symptoms
7 Variants
   (a) Progressive muscular atrophy
      (i) 10% show only lower motor neurone signs
      (ii) Better prognosis than classic MND
   (b) Progressive bulbar palsy
      (i) Bulbar musculature only
      (ii) Poor prognosis
   (c) Primary lateral sclerosis:
      (i) Upper motor neurone signs only
      (ii) Variant of MND but better prognosis

Hereditary motor and sensory neuropathy (Charcot–Marie–Tooth disease)

1 Several types (various genes identified)
2 Pes cavus and clawing of toes
3 Distal atrophy and muscle weakness – 'inverted champagne bottle legs'
4 Distal sensory loss
5 Hyporeflexia
6 Fasciculation
7 Palpable popliteal nerves (25%)

Spinal cord anatomy

1 Corticospinal (pyramidal) tract
   (a) Descending motor pathway
   (b) Decussates in midbrain
2 Two ascending pathways
   (a) Dorsal columns (posterior columns)
      (i) Joint position sense and vibration
      (ii) Synapse in brainstem, then decussate
   (b) Spinothalamic tracts
      (i) Pain and temperature
      (ii) Decussates immediately or within a few segments
      (iii) Lamination of fibres

Spastic paraparesis

1 Signs
   (a) Increased tone and clonus
   (b) Weakness
   (c) Atrophy and contractures
   (d) Extensor plantars
2 Causes
   (a) Demyelination (MS)*
   (b) Cord compression
      (i)   Spondylosis*
      (ii) Neoplasia*
      (iii) Disc prolapse*
      (iv) RA*
      (v) Pott's disease of the spine*
      (vi) Epidural haemorrhage*
      (vii) Epidural abscess*
   (c) Cerebral palsy
   (d) Motor neurone disease
   (e) Spinal cord infarction*
   (f) Vasculitis*
   (g) Myelitis*
   (h) Subacute combined degeneration of the cord*
   (i) Sarcoidosis*
   (j) Friedreich's ataxia
   (k) Syringomyelia
   (l) Syphilis*
   (m) HIV*
   (n) HTLV-1 infection (tropical spastic paraparesis)
   (o) Radiation myelopathy
   (p) Parasagittal meningioma

* Also cause acute paraparesis (medical emergency)

Anterior cord syndrome (spinal cord infarction)

1 Anterior spinal artery
2 Flaccid/spastic paraparesis (corticospinal tracts)
3 Loss of pain and temperature sensations bilaterally (spinothalamic)
4 Dorsal columns intact

Brown–Séquard syndrome

1 Lateral hemisection of cord
2 Ipsilateral upper motor neurone weakness below lesion
3 Contralateral pain and temperature loss
4 Ipsilateral joint position sense and vibration loss

Tabes dorsalis

1 Syphilis (occurs 15–35 years after infection)
2 Degeneration of dorsal columns
3 Features
    (a) Loss of joint position sense and pain fibres
    (b) Sensory ataxia
    (c) Argyll Robertson pupil
    (d) Bilateral ptosis
    (e) Charcot joints
    (f) Absent reflexes and plantars

Subacute combined degeneration of the cord

1 Secondary to vitamin B_{12} deficiency (See page 187 for causes)
2 Features
    (a) Sensory ataxia (dorsal column loss)
    (b) Peripheral neuropathy (glove and stocking)
    (c) Spastic paraparesis (corticospinal loss)
    (d) Absent reflexes
    (e) Extensor plantars

Absent knee jerks and extensor plantars

1 DM
2 B_{12} deficiency
3 Friedreich's ataxia
4 Motor neurone disease
5 Taboparesis (neurosyphilis)
6 Conus medullaris lesion

Cauda equina lesions

1 Bilateral leg weakness
2 Numbness
3 Loss of sphincter control

4 Weakness most marked at the ankles
5 Sensory loss most marked in the sacral region
6 Causes
  (a) Central lumbar disc protrusion
  (b) Degenerative spondylolisthesis
  (c) Tumour – usually external compression
  (d) Spinal stenosis

Friedreich's ataxia

1 Hereditary spinocerebellar ataxia
2 Autosomal recessive (chromosome 9) frataxin protein
3 Trinvalleoside repeat disorder (See page 182)
4 Average age at onset 12
5 Features
  (a) Kyphoscoliosis
  (b) Pes cavus
  (c) High arched palate
  (d) Ataxia
  (e) Spastic paraparesis
  (f) Peripheral neuropathy
  (g) Cerebellar signs (See page 324)
  (h) Cardiomyopathy
  (i) DM
  (j) Mild dementia
  (k) Optic atrophy

Syringomyelia

1 Fluid-filled cavity in the spinal cord (variable size and position)
2 Mostly cervical
3 Anterior horn cells, sensory fibre decussation and lateral corticospinal tracts affected
4 Associated with type 1 Chiari malformation (cerebellar tissue extends into cervical spinal canal)
5 Features
  (a) Wasting of the hand muscles (asymmetrical)
  (b) Weakness (more extensive than single peripheral nerve)
  (c) May develop spastic paraparesis
  (d) Sensory loss (dissociated)
    (i) Preservation of light touch and proprioception
    (ii) Loss of pain and temperature

(e) Scars from injuries
(f) Scoliosis
(g) Develop Charcot joints
(h) May get Horner's if sympathetic neurones involved
(i) Syringobulbia if medulla involved
(i) Facial sensory loss
(ii) Bulbar palsy

CRANIAL NERVE ANATOMY AND LESIONS

Visual field loss

1 Central scotoma
(a) Ipsilateral optic nerve disease, eg neuritis
2 Ipsilateral complete visual loss
(a) Optic nerve transection
3 Bitemporal hemianopia – chiasmal lesion
(a) Pituitary tumour
(b) Craniopharyngioma
(c) Carotid aneurysm
(d) Parasellar meningioma
(e) Dilated third ventricle
4 Homonymous superior quadrantanopia
(a) Temporal lobe lesion
5 Homonymous Inferior quadrantanopia
(a) Parietal lobe lesion
6 Homonymous hemianopia
(a) Incongruous – optic tract
(b) Congruous – behind the lateral geniculate body
(c) Macular sparing – occipital cortex

Pupil

1 Pupilloconstrictor (parasympathetic) fibres
2 Pupillodilator (sympathetic) fibres

Pupillary light reflex

Afferent loop: retina→optic nerve→lateral geniculate body→
midbrain →Efferent loop: ipsilateral and contralateral

Edinger–Westphal nucleus (midbrain) →third nerve→ciliary ganglion→iris and ciliary muscles

Causes of small pupil (miosis)

1 Senile miosis
2 Horner's syndrome
3 Argyll Robertson pupil – don't react to light but normal accommodation reaction
4 Pontine haemorrhage
5 Myotonic dystrophy
6 Drugs, eg opiates, pilocarpine

Horner's syndrome

1 Features
   (a) Ptosis
   (b) Miosis
   (c) Anhidrosis
   (d) Enophthalmos
2 Causes
   (a) Brainstem or spinal cord
       (i) Vascular
       (ii) Trauma
       (iii) Neoplastic
       (iv) Demyelination
       (v) Syringomyelia
   (b) Preganglionic lesion
       (i) Chest – carcinoma (Pancoast), cervical rib, mediastinal mass
       (ii) Cervical – lymphadenopathy, trauma, thyroid neoplasm
       (iii) Surgical – thyroidectomy, carotid angiography, endarterectomy
   (c) Postganglionic
       (i) Internal carotid artery dissection
       (ii) Cavernous sinus lesion
       (iii) Orbital apex disease

Large pupil (mydriasis)

1 Adie's pupil – idiopathic, poorly reacts to light. Decreased tendon reflexes (Holmes–Adie pupil)

2   Third-nerve palsy
3   Drugs – amphetamines, antidepressants, tropicamide, atropine
4   Trauma or previous surgery

Third-nerve palsy

1   Third nerve supplies all the extraocular muscles except superior
    oblique and lateral rectus
2   Carries parasympathetic pupilloconstrictor fibres
3   Nucleus in pons
4   Features
    (a)   Dilated unreactive pupil
    (b)   Ptosis
    (c)   Inability to move superiorly, inferiorly, medially
    (d)   Eye down and out
5   Causes
    (a)   Medical
        (i)   Atherosclerotic*
        (ii)   DM*
        (iii) Mononeuritis multiplex* (See page 342)
    (b)   Surgical
        (i)   Posterior communicating artery aneurysm
        (ii)   Cavernous sinus syndrome*
        (iii) Orbital tumour or granuloma*
        (iv)   Thyroid eye disease*
        (v)   Trauma*
        (vi)   Uncal herniation (coning)
    (c)   Lesions of nucleus
        (i)   Demyelination*
        (ii)   Infarction*
        (iii) Tumour*

Fourth-nerve palsy

1   Supplies superior oblique (SO4)
2   Nucleus in midbrain
3   Exits dorsal aspect of brainstem (only one to do so)
4   Diplopia on looking down and medially
5   Causes – all those with * above

Sixth-nerve palsy

1 Supplies lateral rectus (LR6)
2 Nucleus in pons
3 Diplopia on lateral gaze
4 Affected eye deviates medially
5 Causes
   (a) All those with * above
   (b) Raised intracranial pressure (false localising sign)

Internuclear ophthalmoplegia

1 Lesion of medial longitudinal fasciculus, which connects third, fourth and sixth nuclei
2 Abnormal conjugate eye movement
3 Features
   (a) Adduction of eye ipsilateral to lesion unpaired
   (b) Horizontal nystagmus in abducting eye contralateral to lesion
   (c) Normal convergence
   (d) May have nystagmus on vertical gaze
4 Causes
   (a) Multiple sclerosis
   (b) Vascular disease
   (c) Pontine glioma
   (d) Miller–Fisher syndrome
   (e) Drug overdose – (barbiturates, phenytoin or amitriptyline)
   (f) Wernicke's encephalopathy

Impaired vertical conjugate gaze

1 Progressive supranuclear palsy
2 Thyroid eye disease
3 Myasthenia gravis
4 Miller–Fisher syndrome
5 Parinaud's syndrome – damage to midbrain and superior colliculus

Structures found in cavernous sinus

1 Cranial nerve III
2 Cranial nerve IV
3 Cranial nerve VI
4 Fifth nerve ophthalmic branch

5 Sympathetic carotid plexus
6 Intracavernous carotid artery

Causes of cavernous sinus syndrome

1 Trauma
2 Vascular
   (a) Posterior communicating artery aneurysm
   (b) Intracavernous carotid artery
   (c) Cavernous sinus thrombosis
   (d) Aortocavernous fistula
3 Neoplasia
   (a) Intracranial tumours
   (b) Nasopharyngeal tumours
   (c) Metastases
4 Infection
   (a) Sinusitis
   (b) TB
5 Granulomatous
   (a) Wegener's granulomatosis

Facial nerve (CN VII)

1 Innervation (**face, ear, taste, tear**)
   (a) Motor nerves to muscles of facial expression (**face**)
   (b) Supplies stapedius in **ear** (palsy leads to hyperacusis)
   (c) Cutaneous sensation to external auditory meatus (**ear**)
   (d) Chorda tympani to anterior 2/3 of tongue (**taste**)
   (e) Parasympathetic fibre to lacrimal gland (**tear**)
2 Causes of facial nerve palsy
   (a) UMN
      (i)   Stroke
      (ii) Multiple sclerosis
      (iii) Tumour
   (b) LMN
      (i)   Bell's palsy
      (ii) Ramsay Hunt syndrome – herpes zoster infection
      (iii) Acoustic neuroma
      (iv) Parotid tumours
      (v)   Mononeuritis multiplex (See page 342)
      (vi) Pontine tumour

(vii)   Cholesteatoma
(viii) Guillain–Barré syndrome
(c) Bilateral facial nerve palsy
   (i)   Myasthenia gravis
   (ii)   Bilateral Bell's palsies
   (iii) Sarcoidosis
   (iv)   Guillain–Barré syndrome
   (v)   Lyme disease
   (vi)   Myotonic dystrophy

Vestibulocochlear nerve (CN VIII)

Rinne's test

1 Normal ear – air conduction greater than bone conduction
2 Nerve deafness – air conduction > bone conduction
3 Middle ear conduction defect – air conduction < bone conduction

Weber's test

1 Tuning fork middle of forehead
2 If sound heard to one side:
   (a) Middle ear deafness on that side
   (b) Opposing ear has nerve deafness

Causes of deafness

1 Conduction
   (a) Ear wax
   (b) Middle ear disease
2 Sensorineural
   (a) Cochlear
      (i)   Otosclerosis
      (ii)   Noise induced
      (iii) Drug induced – aminoglycosides, frusemide, lead
      (iv)   Menière's disease
      (v)   Paget's
   (b) Nerve
      (i)   Acoustic neuroma
      (ii)   Head trauma
      (iii) Meningitis
   (c) Nucleus in pons

(i) Multiple sclerosis
(ii) CVA
(iii) Tumour
(d) Congenital

Causes of vertigo

1 Central (brainstem)
(a) Multiple sclerosis
(b) Space-occupying lesion, eg glioma
(c) Vascular disease
(d) Migraine
(e) Encephalitis
(f) Hypoglycaemia
(g) Alcohol
(h) Drugs
2 Peripheral (labyrinthine)
(a) Trauma
(b) Menière's disease
(c) Viral infection
(d) Benign positional vertigo
(e) Internal auditory artery occlusion
(f) Chronic otitis media

Nystagmus

1 Problem with control of ocular position
2 Three types
(a) Pendular – no fast or slow phase
(b) Jerk
(i) distinct fast/slow phase
(ii) amplitude increases on gaze toward fast phase
(c) Rotatory – combined horizontal and vertical nystagmus
3 Causes
(a) Congenital
(i) X-linked or autosomal dominant
(ii) Second-degree to poor vision, eg cataract, albinism
(b) Acquired
(i) Vestibular: fast phase away from side of lesion
(ii) Cerebellar: fast phase toward side of lesion
(iii) Drug-induced: alcohol, barbiturates, phenytoin

Acoustic neuroma

1 Tumour of eighth cranial nerve (benign schwannoma)
2 Presents with headache, deafness and unsteadiness
3 Causes cerebellopontine angle syndrome
   (a) Fifth-, sixth-, seventh- and eighth-nerve palsies
   (b) Cerebellar signs
4 Associated with neurofibromatosis type 2
5 Treat by surgical removal

Bulbar palsy

1 Bilateral impairment of function of cranial nerves IX, X and XII
2 Lower motor neurone (*cf.* psuedobulbar palsy UMN)
3 Features
   (a) Tongue atrophy with fasciculations
   (b) Weakness of pharynx and larynx
   (c) Dysarthria
   (d) Dysphagia (often with choking episodes and nasal regurgitation of fluids)
   (e) Dysphonia
   (f) Poor cough
   (g) Susceptibility to aspiration pneumonia
4 Causes
   (a) Motor neurone disease
   (b) Guillain–Barré syndrome
   (c) Meningitis
   (d) Polio
   (e) Neurosyphilis
   (f) Syringobulbia

Pseudobulbar palsy

1 UMN impairment of cranial nerves IX, X and XII
2 Features
   (a) Dysarthria ('Donald Duck')
   (b) Small spastic tongue
   (c) Exaggerated jaw jerk
   (d) Emotionally labile
3 Causes
   (a) Commonest bilateral internal capsule CVA

(b) Demyelination (MS)
(c) Motor neurone disease
(d) Brainstem tumours
(e) Trauma

MOVEMENT DISORDERS

Benign essential tremor

1 Affects hands, arms and head
2 No tremor at rest
3 Autosomal dominant
4 Worse with stress
5 Improves with alcohol
6 Treat with propranolol, 30% respond

Causes of myoclonus

1 Generalised
    (a) Physiological (falling asleep)
    (b) Familial myoclonic epilepsy
    (c) Metabolic
        (i)   Hepatic failure
        (ii) Renal failure
        (iii) Hypocalcaemia
        (iv) Drug-induced, eg amitriptyline
        (v) Alcohol and drug withdrawal
        (vi) Cerebral anoxia
    (d) Progressive myoclonic encephalopathies
        (i)   Alzheimer's disease
        (ii) CJD
        (iii) Gaucher's disease
        (iv) Tay-Sachs disease
        (v) Subacute sclerosing leukoencephalopathy
2 Focal
    (a) Cortical/brainstem/spinal
        (i)   Tumour
        (ii) Infarct
        (iii) Demyelination

Causes of chorea

1 Huntington's disease
2 Sydenham's chorea (rheumatic)
3 Polycythaemia rubra vera
4 SLE
5 Thyrotoxicosis
6 Wilson's disease
7 Hypernatraemia
8 Drugs
    (a) OCPs
    (b) Phenytoin
    (c) Neuroleptics (dopamine blocking)
9 During pregnancy (chorea gravidarum)
10 Neuroacanthocytosis
11 Hemiballismus (hemi chorea)
    (a) Tumour
    (b) Infarct
    (c) Demyelination

Huntington's chorea

1 Autosomal dominant – chromosome 4
2 Trinucleoside repeat disorder (See page 182)
3 Symptoms begin 30–50 yrs of age
4 Chorea
5 Cognitive decline and dementia
6 Positive family history
7 Chlorpromazine to relieve chorea

Parkinsonism

1 Dopamine deficiency in striatal pathway of substantia nigra
2 Lewy bodies in brain
3 Main features
    (a) Resting tremor (pill rolling, asymmetric, disappears during sleep, 3–5 Hz)
    (b) Bradykinesia
    (c) Rigidity (cogwheel or lead pipe)
4 Other features
    (a) Expressionless face

    (b) Festinant gait
    (c) Micrographia
    (d) Dysphagia
    (e) Postural hypotension
    (f) Depression (30%)
5 Causes
    (a) Idiopathic Parkinson's disease
    (b) Drug-induced parkinsonism (dopamine antagonists)
    (c) Diffuse Lewy body disease
    (d) Parkinson plus syndromes
        (i) Progressive supranuclear palsy (PSP)
        (ii) Multiple system atrophy, eg Shy–Drager syndrome
    (e) Dementia pugilistica – due to chronic head injury, eg boxing
    (f) Post encephalitis
    (g) Normal-pressure hydrocephalus
    (h) Toxins (narcotics, MPTP, carbon monoxide, manganese)
    (i) Wilson's disease

[See Table 52, opposite]

MUSCULAR DISORDERS

Duchenne muscular dystrophy

1 X-linked, absence of dystrophin protein
2 Features
    (a) Delay in motor milestones
    (b) Girdle muscle weakness – 'waddling' gait
    (c) Axial muscle weakness, particularly proximal limbs
    (d) Pseudohypertrophy of calf muscles
    (e) Contractures
    (f) Raised CK
    (g) Ability to walk lost – 12 years old
    (h) Death by respiratory/cardiac failure 20s or early 30s
3 Genetic counselling
    (a) Female carriers have raised CK
    (b) More advance PCR techniques also available to detect carriers
4 Becker's muscular dystrophy
    (a) X-linked, abnormal dystrophin (*cf.* DMD)

Table 52

Drug	Mechanism	Side effects
Levodopa (given with peripheral dopa-decarboxylase inhibitor, eg carbidopa to reduce peripheral side effects of dopamine)	Precursor of dopamine to replenish striatal dopamine Improves rigidity and bradykinesia	N+V Postural hypotension Somnolence 'On' and 'off' periods Dyskinesia Hallucinations
Dopamine agonists Bromocriptine Pergolide Ropinerole Pramipexole	D$_2$ receptor agonists (also have varying effects on other dopamine receptors) Improve tremor, rigidity and bradykinesia May be used alone or in combination with levodopa	N+V Hypotension Dyskinesia Hallucinations Fibrotic reactions
Selegiline	MAO B inhibitor May slow progression of disease and reduce tremor May be used with levodopa to reduce end of dose deterioration	Hypotension (particularly with levodopa) Hallucinations
Apomorphine	Dopamine agonist Advanced disease with unpredictable off periods	Severe vomiting (need domperidone) As for other dopamine agonists
Entacapone	Catechol-O-methyltransferase inhibitor Inhibits peripheral metabolism of levodopa to increase levels in brain Useful for those with end dose deterioration	Diarrhoea Brown urine
Anticholinergics Benztropine Procyclidine	Antimuscarinic Useful for drug-induced parkinsonism Reduce tremor and rigidity but not bradykinesia	Dry mouth Urinary retention Constipation Tachycardia Psychiatric disturbance
Amantadine	NMDA inhibitor Some benefit in tremor, rigidity and bradykinesia	Confusion Hallucinations

(b) Manifests later
(c) Milder disease

Myotonic dystrophy (dystrophia myotonica)

1 Trinucleotide repeat disorder (See page 182)
2 Features
    (a) Myotonic facies
    (b) Bilateral ptosis
    (c) Frontal balding
    (d) Facial muscle weakness
    (e) Sternomastoid wasting
    (f) Myotonia – unable to relax muscles following contraction
    (g) Progressive muscular weakness and wasting starting distally
    (h) Cataracts
    (i) Insulin resistance
    (j) Cardiac conduction defects
    (k) Bulbar weakness
    (l) Respiratory muscle weakness
    (m) Mental retardation (in severe cases)
    (n) Testicular/ovarian atrophy

Myasthenia gravis

1 Autoimmune disorder leading to fatiguable muscle weakness
2 Autoantibodies to acetylcholine receptors on postsynaptic membrane of neuromuscular junction
3 Penicillamine is a cause
4 Features
    (a) Ptosis
    (b) Ophthalmoplegia
    (c) Dysarthria
    (d) Fatigable weakness of striated muscle
    (e) Respiratory muscle involvement life-threatening
    (f) Bulbar symptoms and nasal regurgitation
    (g) Head drooping (weakness of neck musculature)
5 Investigations
    (a) Acetylcholine receptor antibodies (~90%)
    (b) Antistriated muscle antibody in 80% with thymoma
    (c) Electromyography (EMG) – decreasing muscle action potential with rapid stimulation

(d) Tensilon test – iv edrophonium (short-acting anticholinesterase) leads to rapid improvement in weakness
(e) CT thorax – ?associated thymoma
(f) Thyroid function – 10% coexistent thyrotoxicosis

6 Treatment
(a) Pyridostigmine (cholinesterase inhibitors)
(b) Thymectomy
(c) Steroids
(d) Cyclophosphamide, ciclosporin (immunosuppression)
(e) Plasmapheresis
(f) Intravenous immunoglobulins

Lambert–Eaton myasthenic syndrome

1 Autoimmune destruction of voltage gated calcium channel on motor nerve terminal
2 Paraneoplastic syndrome most common with small cell carcinoma of lung
3 May occur without neoplasia
4 Features
(a) Muscle weakness proximal > distal
(b) Weakness improves with exercise (*cf.* myasthenia) but worsens with sustained exercise
(c) Hyporeflexia
(d) Autonomic symptoms (function difficulty, dry mouth, constipation, impotence)
(e) Ophthalmoplegia and ptosis in < 25%
(f) EMG shows greater response with repetitive stimulation

MULTIPLE SCLEROSIS (MS)

1 Inflammatory demyelinating disease of CNS
2 Cell-mediated autoimmune disease associated with immune activity against myelin
1 CNS lesions disseminated in time and place (anatomically)
2 Diagnosis not possible at time of first neurological event
3 Four subtypes
(a) Relapsing/remitting disease – 80–85% of patients
(b) Secondary progressive disease – 30–50% of patients with relapsing/remitting

(c) Primary progressive disease – 10–15% deterioration from onset
(d) Progressive relapsing disease – superimposed relapses
4 Symptoms
(a) Weakness (40%)
(b) Optic neuritis (22%)
(c) Paraesthesiae (21%)
(d) Diplopia (12%)
(e) Disturbance of micturition (5%)
(f) Vertigo (5%)
5 Diagnosis
(a) MRI scan – high signal white matter lesions on T_2-weighted scanning
(b) Delayed visual evoked response potentials
(c) Oligoclonal bands in CSF (not in serum, non-specific)
6 Management
(a) Multidisciplinary team
(b) Intravenous methylprednisolone for acute attacks
(c) Interferon-β
(i) Reduces frequency and severity of relapses
(ii) Used in relapsing/remitting or secondary progressive
(d) Glatiramer – immunomodulating drug
(e) Linoleic acid may slow progression
(f) Antispasmodics, eg baclofen/tizanidine
(g) Oxybutinin (anticholinergic) for urinary continence

NEUROLOGICAL INVESTIGATIONS

CSF normal values

1 Pressure – 60–200 mmH$_2$O (8–12 cm saline)
2 Protein – 0.2–0.4 g/l
3 Cell count
(a) Zero red cells
(b) < 5/mm^3 white cells
4 Glucose – > 2/3 blood glucose (2.8–4.0 mmol/l)

Lumbar puncture – complications

1 Herniation of brain or spinal cord
2 Headache
3 Meningitis or epidural abscess

4 Intrathecal bleeding
5 Damage or infection of intervertebral disc

Causes of raised pressure

1 Space-occupying lesions or acute brain swelling
2 Benign intracranial hypertension
3 Hydrocephalus
4 TB meningitis
5 High venous pressure, eg dural sinus thrombosis

Increased protein concentration in CSF

Markedly raised: approx 2–6 g/l

1 Guillain–Barré syndrome
2 Spinal block (2° to tumour)
3 TB meningitis
4 Fungal meningitis

Raised

1 Bacterial meningitis
2 Viral encephalitis
3 Cerebral abscess
4 Multiple sclerosis
5 Cerebral tumours (primary and metastases)
6 Cerebral infarction
7 Subdural haematoma
8 Dural sinus thrombosis

Polymorphs in CSF

1 Bacterial meningitis

Lymphocytes in CSF

1 Viral encephalitis/meningitis
2 Partially treated bacterial meningitis
3 CNS vasculitis
4 HIV associated
5 Lymphoma
6 Leukaemia

7 Lyme disease
8 SLE
9 Behçet's
10 Polio
11 Multiple sclerosis
12 Dural sinus thrombosis
13 Stroke

Reduced or absent glucose in CSF

1 Bacterial meningitis
2 TB meningitis
3 Malignant meningitis, ie atypical – fungal, mumps
4 HSV encephalitis
5 Subarachnoid haemorrhage

Oligoclonal bands in CSF

1 Multiple sclerosis
2 Neurosarcoidosis
3 Neurosyphilis
4 Neurological – AIDS
5 CNS lymphoma
6 Subacute sclerosing panencephalitis
7 Guillain–Barré syndrome
8 Subarachnoid haemorrhage
9 Neuro-Lyme disease

[See Table 53, opposite]

Intracranial calcification on head CT/skull X-ray

1 Craniopharyngioma
2 Meningioma
3 Tuberculoma
4 Oligodendroglioma
5 Pineal gland
6 Tuberous sclerosis
7 Sturge–Weber syndrome
8 Toxoplasmosis
9 Hypoparathyroidism
10 Aneurysm

Table 53

	Normal CSF	Acute bacterial meningitis	Acute viral meningitis	Mycobacterium tuberculosis	Multiple sclerosis
Appearance	Crystal clear, colourless	Turbid/ purulent	Clear/turbid	Turbid/viscous	Normal
Glucose	⅔–⅓ of blood glucose	Low	Normal or high	Low	Normal
Protein	0.2–0.4g/l	Very high	High	Very high	High
Cell count – mononuclear	5/mm³	< 50/mm³	10–100/mm³	100–300/mm³	5–60/mm³ typically
Polymorphs	Nil	200–3000/mm³	Nil (early ↑)	0–200/mm³	mononuclear
Microbiology	Nil	Gram stain and blood culture etc.	Throat swab and serology etc.	AAFB on ZN staining	IgG >15% of normal Oligoclonal band positive
Pressure	60–150 mm of H₂O with patient lying	Normal or raised	Normal or raised	Raised	Normal or raised

Electroencephalography (EEG)

Diagnosis of epilepsy

1 Interictal epileptiform discharges (IEDs)
2 Focal or generalised IEDs (start focally) in partial epilepsy
3 Generalised symmetrical IEDs in generalised epilepsy
4 3 Hz spike and wave complexes in absence seizures

Other characteristic EEG patterns
1 CJD: short-interval periodic discharges
2 Subacute sclerosing panencephalitis: long-interval periodic discharges
3 Encephalitis: diffuse slow wave activity

Electromyography (EMG)

Typical findings

1 Myasthenia gravis: decreased response to repetitive stimulation
2 Lambert–Eaton syndrome: increased response to repetitive stimulation
3 Myotonia: 'dive bomber' discharge
4 Polymyositis: fibrillation potentials, low amplitude polyphasic motor unit action potentials
5 Motor neurone disease: fibrillation (degeneration); shape of motor unit action potential (MUAP) changes (reinnervation)

Ophthalmology

EYE SIGNS IN MEDICAL DISORDERS

Table 54

Sign	Disorder
Lisch nodules	Neurofibromatosis
Brushfield's spots	Down's syndrome
Kayser–Fleischer rings	Wilson's disease
Band keratopathy	Hypercalcaemia
	Chronic uveitis
Bitot's spots	Vitamin A deficiency
Corneal arcus	Hypercholesterolaemia (types 2a and 2b)
	Old age
Blue sclera	Osteogenesis imperfecta
	Pseudoxanthoma elasticum
	Ehlers–Danlos syndrome
	Marfan's syndrome
	Hyperthyroidism
Angioid streaks	Pseudoxanthoma elasticum
	Ehlers–Danlos syndrome
	Paget's disease
	Sickle cell disease
Corneal calcification	Sarcoidosis
	Hyperparathyroidism
	Chronic renal failure
	Vitamin D abuse

Diabetic eye disease

Most common cause of blindness in patients aged 30–60

1 Background retinopathy
   (a) Visual acuity unaffected
   (b) Microaneurysms
   (c) Haemorrhages (dot and blot)
   (d) Hard exudates

369

2 Preproliferative retinopathy
   (a) Cottonwool spots
   (b) Dilatation and beading of retinal veins
   (c) Intraretinal microvascular abnormalities
3 Proliferative retinopathy (more common in type 1 diabetics)
   (a) Neovascularisation
   (b) Treated cases will have panretinal laser burns
4 Advanced diabetic eye disease
   (a) Vitreous haemorrhage
   (b) Tractional retinal detachment
   (c) Rubeotic glaucoma
5 Maculopathy (more common in type 2 diabetics)
   (a) Oedema and exudates
   (b) Macular stars (multiple exudates)
   (c) Loss of central vision (peripheral spared)
6 Treatment
   (a) Good diabetic control
   (b) Treat hypertension
   (c) Stop smoking
   (d) Treat hyperlipidaemia
   (e) Regular fundal examination
   (f) Focal retinal photocoagulation
   (g) Panretinal photocoagulation

Criteria for referral to an ophthalmologist

1 Sudden loss of vision
2 Retinal detachment
3 New vessel formation
4 Preretinal or vitreous haemorrhage
5 Rubeosis iritidis
6 Unexplained reduced acuity
7 Hard exudate within 1 disc diameter of the fovea
8 Macular oedema
9 Unexplained retinal findings
10 Preproliferative or more advanced findings

HYPERTENSIVE RETINOPATHY

1 Grade 1
  (a) Silver wiring
2 Grade 2
  (a) A-V nipping
  (b) Focal arteriolar attenuation
3 Grade 3
  (a) Haemorrhages
  (b) Hard exudates
  (c) Cotton wool spots
4 Grade 4
  (a) Papilloedema

CAUSES OF COTTONWOOL SPOTS

1 Diabetes
2 Hypertension
3 Vasculitis
4 HIV retinopathy
5 Septicaemia
6 Haemoglobinopathy
7 Radiation retinopathy
8 Myeloproliferative disorders
9 Fat emboli

ESSENTIAL FEATURES OF THYROID EYE DISEASE

1 Signs
  (a) **NO SPECS**
    (i) **N**o signs or symptoms
    (ii) **O**nly upper lid retraction and stare
    (iii) **S**oft tissue swelling
    (iv) **P**roptosis
    (v) **E**xtraocular muscle involvement (lymphocytic infiltration of inferior and medial recti)
    (vi) **C**orneal involvement (keratoconjunctivitis)
    (vii) **S**ight loss due to optic nerve damage (optic neuropathy)

2 Management
  (a) Severe
    (i)   High-dose steroids
    (ii) Orbital irradiation
    (iii) Plasma exchange
    (iv) Orbital decompression
  (b) Mild and moderate
    (i)   Symptomatic
    (ii) Artificial tears
    (iii) Prisms for diplopia
    (iv) Tarsorrhaphy

CAUSES OF PAPILLOEDEMA

1 Raised intracranial pressure
  (a) Space-occupying lesion
    (i)   Tumour
    (ii) Haematoma
    (iii) Abscess
  (b) Meningitis/encephalitis
  (c) Subarachnoid haemorrhage
  (d) Cerebral oedema
  (e) Aqueduct stenosis
  (f) A-V malformation
2 Hypertensive retinopathy
3 Benign intracranial hypertension
4 Metabolic causes
  (a) CO_2 retention
  (b) Vitamin A intoxication
  (c) Lead poisoning
  (d) Graves' disease
  (e) Hypoparathyroidism
5 Oral contraceptives
6 Tetracyclines
7 Central retinal vein thrombosis
8 Cavernous sinus thrombosis
9 Severe anaemia
10 Polycythaemia rubra vera
11 Paget's disease

CAUSES OF OPTIC ATROPHY

1 Congenital
  (a) Leber's optic atrophy
  (b) DIDMOAD syndrome (diabetes insipidus, diabetes mellitus, optic atrophy and deafness)
  (c) Friedreich's ataxia
2 Multiple sclerosis
3 Compression of the optic nerve
  (a) Tumour (craniopharyngioma, pituitary adenoma)
  (b) Aneurysm
  (c) Orbital cellulitis
4 Glaucoma
5 Chronic papilloedema
6 Ischaemia
  (a) Retinal artery occlusion
  (b) Temporal arteritis
  (c) Tabes dorsalis
7 Diabetes mellitus
8 Nutritional deficiency
  (a) Vitamins B_1, B_2, B_6, B_{12}
  (b) Alcohol–tobacco amblyopia
9 Toxic
  (a) Methanol
  (b) Alcohol
  (c) Arsenic
  (d) Lead
10 Dysthyroid eye disease
11 Toxoplasmosis
12 Syphilis
13 Paget's disease
14 Retinitis pigmentosa
15 Drugs
  (a) Ethambutol
  (b) Isoniazid
  (c) Digitalis
  (d) Chlorpropamide

ESSENTIAL FEATURES OF OPTIC NEURITIS

1 Inflammation of the optic nerve
   (a) Causes
       (i)   Idiopathic
       (ii) MS
       (iii) Infective
             (1) VZV
             (2) EBV
             (3) TB
             (4) Syphilis
       (iv) Sarcoidosis
2 Unilateral reduction of acuity over hours to days
3 Colours (particularly red) appear less intense
4 Painful eye movements
5 Relative afferent pupillary defect present
6 Optic disc swollen
7 Recovery over 2–6 weeks
8 45–80% develop MS over the next 15 yrs
9 Treat with high-dose methylprednisolone for 3 days – reduces risk of developing recurrence and reduces time of visual loss

CAUSES OF CHOROIDORETINITIS

1 CMV
2 Toxoplasmosis
3 Toxocariasis
4 AIDS
5 Sarcoidosis
6 TB
7 Syphilis
8 Behçet's disease
9 Trauma
10 Idiopathic

ESSENTIAL FEATURES OF RETINAL VEIN THROMBOSIS

1 Central retinal vein occlusion or branch retinal vein occlusion
2 Presents with loss of vision or reduced acuity
3 Can be treated with panretinal photocoagulation
4 Fundoscopy may reveal
   (a) Multiple retinal haemorrhages
   (b) Retinal venous dilatation
   (c) Cottonwool spots
   (d) Neovascularisation
5 Causes
   (a) Hypertension
   (b) Diabetes
   (c) Glaucoma
   (d) Hyperviscosity (myeloma and macroglobulinaemia)
   (e) Polycythaemia
   (f) Vasculitides

ESSENTIAL FEATURES OF RETINAL ARTERY OCCLUSION

1 Presents with sudden painless loss of vision
2 Afferent pupillary defect present
3 Leads to pale fundus
4 Cherry red spot may be present for up to 10 days
5 Causes
   (a) Embolus (AF, carotid artery stenosis)
   (b) Thrombosis
   (c) Vasculitides (particularly giant cell arteritis)
   (d) Increased orbital pressure
   (e) Sickle cell disease
   (f) Syphilis
   (g) Spasm (cocaine, retinal migraine)

CAUSES OF CATARACTS

1 Congenital
   (a) Autosomal dominant
   (b) Maternal infection
      (i) Rubella
      (ii) CMV
      (iii) Toxoplasmosis
      (iv) HSV
      (v) Varicella zoster
   (c) Metabolic
      (i) Galactosaemia
      (ii) Galactokinase deficiency
      (iii) Hypocalcaemia
      (iv) Hypoglycaemia
   (d) Chromosomal abnormalities
      (i) Down's syndrome
      (ii) Turner's syndrome
2 Senile
3 UV light
4 Drugs
   (a) Steroids
   (b) Chlorpromazine
   (c) Chloroquine
   (d) Gold
   (e) Amiodarone
5 Ocular disease
   (a) Uveitis
   (b) High myopia
6 Metabolic
   (a) Diabetes
   (b) Cushing's syndrome
   (c) Hypoglycaemia
   (d) Wilson's disease
   (e) Hypoparathyroidism
7 Trauma
8 Radiation
9 Myotonic dystrophy
10 Retinitis pigmentosa

CAUSES OF LENS DISLOCATION

1 Trauma
2 Marfan's syndrome (upwards)
3 Homocystinuria (downwards)
4 Uveal tumours

CAUSES OF UVEITIS

1 Idiopathic
2 Ankylosing spondylitis
3 Reiter's syndrome
4 Psoriatic disease
5 Inflammatory bowel disease
6 Sarcoidosis
7 Behçet's disease
8 Juvenile chronic arthritis
9 Malignancy
   (a) Non-Hodgkin's lymphoma
   (b) Retinoblastoma
   (c) Ocular melanoma
10 Trauma
11 Infections
   (a) TB
   (b) Syphilis
   (c) HSV
   (d) VZV
   (e) Toxoplasmosis
   (f) Toxocariasis
   (g) HIV
   (h) Leprosy
   (i) Brucellosis
   (j) Histoplasmosis
   (k) Onchocerciasis

CAUSES OF SCLERITIS

1 Rheumatoid arthritis
2 Ankylosing spondylitis
3 Sarcoidosis
4 Inflammatory bowel disease
5 PAN
6 SLE
7 Wegener's granulomatosis
8 Relapsing polychondritis
9 Dermatomyositis
10 Behçet's disease
11 Gout
12 Infections
   (a) VZV
   (b) HSV
   (c) TB
   (d) Syphilis
   (e) Toxoplasmosis
   (f) *Pseudomonas*
   (g) *Streptococcus*
   (h) *Staphylococcus*
13 Trauma
14 Chemicals

ESSENTIAL FEATURES OF RETINITIS PIGMENTOSA

1 Degenerative disease of the retina
2 AR, AD, X-linked inheritance
3 Mainly affects rods (cones may be involved late in the disease)
4 Presents with night blindness
5 Peripheral vision lost first (tunnel vision)
6 Most patients are registered blind by the age of 40
7 Characterised by perivascular 'bone spicule pigmentation', arteriolar narrowing and optic atrophy
8 Associated with:
   (a) Laurence–Moon–Bardet syndrome
   (b) Bassen–Kornzweig syndrome (abetalipoproteinaemia)
   (c) Refsum's disease

(d) Kearns–Sayre syndrome
(e) Usher's disease
(f) Friedreich's ataxia

ESSENTIAL FEATURES OF RETINOBLASTOMA

1 Malignant tumour of retina
2 Usually affects children < 3yrs
3 Bilateral in 30%
4 Patients inherit one abnormal RB1 gene (tumour suppressor); when the other normal gene spontaneously mutates, retinoblastoma forms
5 Presents with
 (a) White pupil
 (b) Squint
 (c) Inflammation
 (d) Loss of red reflex
6 Increased incidence of osteosarcoma
7 Treatment with enucleation

ESSENTIAL FEATURES OF GLAUCOMA

1 Acute (closed angle)
 (a) Uniocular
 (b) Caused by blockage of drainage of aqueous from the anterior chamber via the canal of Schlemm
 (c) Most likely to occur when the pupil is semidilated in the dark
 (d) Presents with
  (i) Red eye
  (ii) Pain
  (iii) Vomiting
  (iv) Reduced vision
  (v) Dilated pupil
  (vi) Hazy cornea
 (e) Treatment
  (i) Acetazolamide (reduces formation of aqueous)
  (ii) Topical pilocarpine (constricts pupil to open canal)
  (iii) Topical β-blockers, eg timolol (reduces secretion of aqueous)

    (iv) Topical steroids
    (v) Peripheral iridectomy (laser or surgery)
2 Chronic (open angle)
   (a) Increased intraocular pressure (> 21 mmHg)
   (b) Insidious asymptomatic onset
   (c) Leads to cupping of the optic disc and nerve damage
   (d) Arcuate scotomas near blind spot
   (e) Risk factors
     (i) Family history
     (ii) Afro-Caribbean origin
     (iii) Diabetes
     (iv) Myopia
     (v) Thyroid eye disease
   (f) Treatment (reduces intraocular pressure)
     (i) Topical β-blockers
     (ii) Topical pilocarpine
     (iii) Topical carbonic anhydrase inhibitors, eg dorzolamide
     (iv) Acetazolamide
     (v) Latanoprost (prostaglandin $F_{2\alpha}$ analogue that increases outflow of aqueous)
     (vi) Iridectomy
     (vii) Laser trabeculoplasty
     (viii) Trabeculectomy

CAUSES OF PTOSIS

1 Unilateral
   (a) Congenital
   (b) Idiopathic
   (c) Third-nerve palsy
   (d) Horner's syndrome
   (e) Myasthenia gravis
   (f) Lid tumour
2 Bilateral
   (a) Myasthenia gravis
   (b) Dystrophia myotonica
   (c) Ocular myopathy
   (d) Mitochondrial dystrophy
   (e) Tabes dorsalis
   (f) Bilateral Horner's (syringomyelia)

Psychiatry

SCHIZOPHRENIA

1 Disorder of thought and perceptions
2 Hallmark is auditory hallucinations
3 Cause unknown
4 Incidence equal in social classes, but prevalence higher in lower social classes
5 Prevalence 1%, M = F
6 Onset age 15–45, males younger than females
7 Risk factors
  (a) Genetic predisposition
    (i) Risk of schizophrenia in first-degree relatives of people with schizophrenia is 10%
    (ii) If both parents have schizophrenia the child has 40% chance of having it
8 Symptoms
  (a) Positive – psychotic symptoms, delusions and hallucinations
  (b) Negative – loss of emotion, poverty of speech, loss of interests
  (c) Cognitive – deficits in memory and attention
9 Diagnosis: two or more of the following must have been present over the previous month for > 6 months
  (a) Delusions
    (i) False beliefs (often paranoid, grandiose or persecutory)
    (ii) False interpretation of normal perceptions
    (iii) Passivity (delusion that one's actions are controlled by some outside agency)
  (b) Hallucinations
    (i) Typically auditory (visual or tactile strongly suggest organic aetiology)
    (ii) Voices commenting on the patient's actions or character or giving commands (third-person auditory hallucinations)
    (iii) Thought echo (audible thoughts)

      (iv) Thought withdrawal (feeling that thoughts are being removed from head)

      (v) Thought broadcasting (experience that thoughts are being known to others)

      (vi) Thought insertion (subjective feeling that thoughts are not one's own)

    (c) Disorganised speech

      (i) Tangential, incoherent, rambling speech

      (ii) Neologisms (new word creation)

      (iii) Loosening of associations

    (d) Behaviour – grossly disorganised or catatonic

    (e) Negative symptoms

      (i) Poverty of speech

      (ii) Emotional and/or social withdrawal

      (iii) Blunting of affect

    (f) Loss of a previously held level of occupational, social or self-care functioning must have occurred since the onset of illness

    (g) Presence of an affective disorder (major depression, bipolar disorder or schizoaffective disorder) or an organic aetiology must be excluded

10 Schneider's symptoms are not accurate in the diagnosis of schizophrenia

    (a) 8% with the symptoms don't have schizophrenia

    (b) 20% with schizophrenia don't have Schneider's symptoms

11 10% successfully commit suicide, especially in early stages

12 Good prognostic factors

    (a) Acute onset

    (b) Precipitating stressful event

    (c) No family history of schizophrenia

    (d) Older age

    (e) No previous episodes

    (f) Normal intelligence

    (g) Mainly affective symptoms

    (h) No loss of emotion

    (i) Family history of depression

13 Treatment

    (a) Antipsychotics: useful for positive symptoms i.e delusions, hallucinations and to prevent relapse

      (i) Neuroleptics (daily or depot injections)

      (ii) Atypical antipsychotics

(b) Electroconvulsive therapy (ECT) for stupor
(c) Cognitive behavioural therapy

BIPOLAR AFFECTIVE DISORDER

1 Disorder characterised by prolonged deep depression that alternates with manic episodes
2 Aetiology unknown
3 Lifetime prevalence of 1%, with slight female preponderance
4 Features of mania
   (a) Elevated, elated mood
   (b) Irritability
   (c) Insomnia
   (d) Loss of inhibitions
   (e) Increased appetite
   (f) Weight loss
   (g) Increased libido
   (h) Flight of ideas
   (i) Pressure of speech
   (j) Poor attention span
   (k) Delusions of grandeur
5 Treatment
   (a) Lithium to stabilise mood
   (b) Atypical antipsychotics needed in acute phase
   (c) Carbamazepine or valproate are alternatives for those who do not respond to lithium

DEPRESSION

1 Lifetime incidence up to 20%
2 Twice as common in females
3 Depression more prevalent in physically ill patients
4 Patients with depression may present with physical symptoms (somatisation)
5 Clinical features
   (a) Diurnal variation (worse in morning)
   (b) Low mood

(c) Sad facial appearance
(d) Impaired capacity for enjoyment
(e) Loss of confidence
(f) Pessimism
(g) Guilt
(h) Suicidal ideas
(i) Delusions and hallucinations (psychotic depression)
(j) Biological symptoms
   (i) Sleep disorder (early morning wakening)
   (ii) Loss of appetite
   (iii) Weight loss
   (iv) Decreased libido
   (v) Loss of concentration
6 Prognosis
(a) Most episodes last 3–9 months untreated
(b) 10–15% of severe or recurrent depression eventually die of suicide
7 Treatment
(a) Antidepressants (below)
(b) ECT (below)

EATING DISORDERS

Anorexia nervosa

1 Severe weight loss secondary to reduced intake
2 Usually occurs in adolescence
1 Commoner in higher social classes
3 5% of patients are male
4 Diagnostic features
(a) Self-induced loss of > 15% of body weight
(b) Morbid fear and avoidance of 'fattening' foods
(c) Ideas of and overestimation of body size
(d) Overuse of exercise or purgatives
(e) Amenorrhoea for > 3 months
5 Other features
(a) Emaciation
(b) Lethargy
(c) Constipation

(d) Abdominal bloating
(e) Dry skin
(f) Cold hands and feet
(g) Low sexual appetite
(h) Lanugo hair

Bulimia nervosa

1 Clinical features
   (a) Binge eating and vomiting
   (b) Preoccupation with eating
   (c) Most are within normal weight range
   (d) Usually older than anorexics (20s)
   (e) Binges usually kept secret
   (f) Depression and anxiety prevalent
   (g) Salivary gland enlargement
   (h) Increased amylase (salivary)
   (i) Calluses on dorsum of dominant hand from stimulating gag reflex (Russell's sign)
   (j) Erosion of dental enamel

Medical complications (both)

1 Cardiac
   (a) Bradycardia and hypotension
   (b) Arrhythmias
2 Endocrine
   (a) Low FSH/LH/oestrogens and amenorrhoea
   (b) Osteoporosis and fractures
   (c) Delayed TSH response, leading to reduced T_3 and clinical evidence of hypothyroidism
   (d) ↑ Cortisol
   (e) Hypoglycaemia
   (f) Hypercholesterolaemia
   (g) Metabolic alkalosis, hypochloraemia (vomiting, laxatives, diuretics)
3 Haematological
   (a) Normochromic normocytic anaemia
   (b) Pancytopenia and hypoplastic bone marrow
4 GI
   (a) GI erosions and ulceration
   (b) Delayed gastric emptying

5 Others
  (a) Proximal myopathy, cramps and tetany
  (b) Hypothermia
  (c) Dehydration
  (d) Electrolyte disturbances (especially hypokalaemia)
  (e) Reversible brain atrophy and seizures
  (f) Nephropathy

ANXIETY DISORDERS

Physical symptoms of anxiety

1 Cardiovascular
  (a) Palpitations
  (b) Awareness of ectopic beats
  (c) Discomfort in chest
2 Respiratory
  (a) Hyperventilation
  (b) Sense of dyspnoea
3 GI
  (a) Dry mouth
  (b) Difficulty swallowing
  (c) Epigastric discomfort
  (d) Excessive wind
  (e) Frequent or loose motions
4 GU
  (a) Urinary frequency or urgency
  (b) Impotence
  (c) Amenorrhoea
  (d) Menstrual discomfort
5 Neuromuscular
  (a) Tremor
  (b) Headache
  (c) Dizziness and tinnitus
  (d) Prickling sensations
  (e) Aching muscles

Obsessive–compulsive disorder

1 An anxiety disorder characterised by distressing intrusive thoughts and/or repetitive actions that interfere with the individual's daily functioning
2 Obsessions are recurrent persistent ideas that the patient recognises as abnormal, but resistance to which causes upset
3 Compulsions are thoughts to carry out an action, triggered by obsession
4 Thought to be a an abnormality in 5HT transmission in the CNS
5 Slight female preponderance
6 30% have associated depression
7 Also associated with anorexia nervosa, schizophrenia and organic brain disease
8 Treatment
   (a) Serotonin reuptake inhibitors (TCAs, SSRIs)
   (b) Antipsychotics if antidepressants ineffective
   (c) Cognitive behavioural therapy
   (d) Neurosurgery may be effective

Post-traumatic stress disorder

1 Intense prolonged reaction to a very stressful event, eg accident
2 Symptoms last > 1 month
3 Risk increases if
   (a) Very severe experience
   (b) Past history of stress disorder
   (c) Child or elderly
4 Clinical features
   (a) Anxiety
   (b) Depression
   (c) Poor concentration
   (d) Insomnia and nightmares
   (e) Panic attacks
   (f) 'Flashbacks'
5 Usually lasts a few months, but can last years
6 Treatment
   (a) Antidepressants
   (b) Cognitive behavioural therapy

SUICIDE AND PARASUICIDE

Risk factors for suicide

1 Male
2 Young or late middle age
3 Social class I or V
4 Chronic illness
5 Chronic pain
6 Physical handicap
7 Psychiatric illness
8 Depression
9 Alcoholism
10 Unemployment
11 Farmers and doctors

Risk factors for deliberate self-harm

1 Female
2 Age < 35
3 Social classes IV and V
4 History of depression
5 May have antisocial personality

ALCOHOL

Acute alcohol withdrawal

1 Clinical features
   (a) Symptoms appear within 6 hrs, peak at 48 hrs and subside over
       1 week
   (b) Nausea
   (c) Sweating
   (d) Tremor
   (e) Anxiety and agitation
   (f) Tachycardia
   (g) Visual hallucinations
   (h) Acute confusion
   (i) Insomnia
   (j) Pyrexia (may be associated infection)

(k) Seizures (between 12 and 24 hrs)
(l) Electrolyte deficiencies often seen (potassium, magnesium and phosphate)
2 5% mortality
3 Treatment
  (a) Nurse in a well lit room
  (b) Oral chlordiazepoxide or diazepam
  (c) Intravenous diazepam or lorazepam for seizures
  (d) Haloperidol for severe agitation
  (e) Intravenous Pabrinex to help prevent Wernicke's encephalopathy

Alcohol-dependence syndrome

1 CAGE
  (a) Has tried to **c**ut down alcohol
  (b) **A**nger at criticism of drinking
  (c) **G**uilt at drinking
  (d) **E**arly morning drinking
2 Others
  (a) Drinking usually in fixed pattern
  (b) Repeated absenteeism from work
  (c) Aware of compulsion to drink
  (d) Increased tolerance to alcohol
  (e) Frequent symptoms of withdrawal

THE ACUTE CONFUSIONAL STATE (DELIRIUM)

1 Organic causes for cognitive and behavioural symptoms need to be excluded before a psychiatric diagnosis can be made
2 Usually reversible
3 Causes
  (a) Intracranial
    (i) Head injury
    (ii) CNS infection (encephalitis, meningitis)
    (iii) Epilepsy
    (iv) Space-occupying lesion
    (v) Intracranial bleed (subarachnoid, intracerebral, subdural)
    (vi) Cerebrovascular disease

(b) Extracranial
  (i) Infection (UTI, chest etc)
  (ii) Toxic (alcohol, drugs – prescribed or illicit)
  (iii) Endocrine (thyroid, diabetes, adrenal especially Cushing's)
  (iv) Electrolyte disorder (sodium, calcium)
  (v) Metabolic (hypoglycaemia, uraemia, hepatic encephalopathy)
  (vi) Systemic (SLE)

DRUGS AND PSYCHIATRY

Antidepressants

Tricyclic antidepressants (TCA)

1 **Drugs:** Amitriptyline, dothiepin, imipramine, lofepramine, trazodone
2 **Pharmacology:** Inhibit neuronal uptake of 5HT and noradrenaline (NA; norepinephrine)
3 **Uses:** Depression, panic disorder, neuropathic pain, IBS
4 **Side effects:** Anticholinergic (dry mouth, constipation, urinary retention, blurred vision), lower seizure threshold, drowsiness, arrhythmias, sexual dysfunction, hypotension, hyponatraemia, hepatotoxicity and blood dyscrasias

Selective serotonin reuptake inhibitors (SSRI)

1 **Drugs:** Citalopram, fluoxetine, paroxetine, sertraline
2 **Pharmacology:** Inhibition of neuronal 5HT uptake
3 **Uses:** Depression, panic disorder, bulimia nervosa, obsessive–compulsive disorder, post-traumatic stress disorder
4 **Side effects:** Nausea, vomiting, anxiety, sweating and rash. Less toxic than TCAs, therefore preferred for those at risk of suicide. Good for patients who have side effects of TCAs

Serotonin and noradrenaline reuptake inhibitor (SNRI)

1 **Drug:** Venlafaxine
2 **Pharmacology:** Inhibits both 5HT and NA reuptake
3 **Uses:** Depression, generalised anxiety disorder

4 **Side effects:** Nausea, headache, insomnia, sexual dysfunction, seizures and hypertension

Monoamine oxidase inhibitors

1 **Drug:** Phenelzine
2 **Pharmacology:** Blocks monoamine oxidase leading to ↑ 5HT, NA and dopamine
3 **Uses:** Depression in those who have failed other therapies
4 **Side effects**
   (a) Tyramine reaction – caused by certain foods high in tyramine, leads to hypertensive episode. Treat with α_1 blockade, eg phentolamine
   (b) Others – dizziness, confusion, insomnia, postural hypotension, hypertension, anticholinergic side effects, hepatotoxicity and leukopenia
5 **Interactions:** Amphetamine, ephedrine and opiates all potentiate MOAI, leading to rise in BP. Insulin and hypoglycaemics (hypoglycaemic effect enhanced)

Mood-stabilising drugs

1 **Drug:** Lithium
2 **Pharmacology:** Affects receptor transduction systems that may prevent excessive intracellular signalling. Also produces increase in brain 5HT function
3 **Uses:** Prophylaxis of bipolar affective disorder and mania, treatment of acute mania (less effective than antipsychotics). May also be used with antidepressant in recurrent depression
4 **Side effects**
   (a) Endocrine – hypothyroidism, hyperglycaemia, hyperparathyroidism
   (b) CNS – tremor, headache lethargy, memory impairment, convulsions
   (c) GI – nausea, vomiting, diarrhoea
   (d) GU – polydipsia, polyuria, nephrogenic diabetes insipidus, renal failure
   (e) Other – rash, leukocytosis, weight gain
5 **Interactions:** Thiazides, NSAIDs, metronidazole, erythromycin and ACEIs may increase levels, leading to toxicity

Antipsychotic drugs

1 **Drugs:** Chlorpromazine, haloperidol, fluphenthixol, trifluoperazine
2 **Pharmacology:** Block dopaminergic transmission at D_2 receptors
Can be given as a depot to improve compliance
3 **Uses:** Schizophrenia, mania, psychotic depression, acute confusional states, hiccup, nausea and vomiting
4 **Side effects**
(a) Movement disorders – parkinsonism, acute dystonic reactions, akathisia, tardive dyskinesia (treat with anticholinergic such as benztropine)
(b) Neuroleptic malignant syndrome – fever, rigidity, coma, tachycardia and labile blood pressure and death. Treat with bromocriptine or dantrolene
(c) Others – anticholinergic side effects, raised prolactin levels, rashes, weight gain, cardiac arrhythmias, seizures, hepatotoxicity

Atypical antipsychotics

1 **Drugs:** Olanzapine, risperidone, quetiapine
2 **Pharmacology:** Weak D_2 antagonist, binds strongly to $5HT_2$ receptor
3 **Uses:** Schizophrenia, psychosis, mania
4 **Side effects**
(a) Less increase in prolactin than conventional antipsychotics
(b) Fewer extrapyramidal side effects than conventional antipsychotics
(c) Increased risk of stroke in elderly or patients with dementia
(d) Possible prolongation of QT interval
(e) Others – weight gain, dizziness, postural hypotension, hyperglycaemia

Clozapine

1 **Pharmacology:** Weak D_2 antagonist, binds strongly to $5HT_2$ receptor
2 **Uses**
(a) Schizophrenia unresponsive to or intolerant of conventional antipsychotic drugs
(b) 50% of those unresponsive to conventional antipsychotics will respond to clozapine
(c) May improve negative symptoms also

3 **Side effects**
   (a) Leukopenia and agranulocytosis (monitoring required)
   (b) Rebound psychosis on withdrawal
   (c) Less increase in prolactin than with conventional antipsychotics
   (d) Fewer extrapyramidal side effects
   (e) Others – hypersalivation, drowsiness, weight gain, postural hypotension, seizures, myocarditis and cardiomyopathy

ELECTROCONVULSIVE THERAPY

1 Electric current passed briefly through the brain to induce a generalised seizure
2 Unknown mechanism of action
3 Indicated for treatment of
   (a) Marked depressive illness with biological symptoms
   (b) Catatonia
   (c) Prolonged severe manic episode
4 Side effects: headache, impaired short-term memory, confusion, fractures, dislocations
5 Contraindications: raised intracranial pressure (absolute), recent MI/CVA, cardiac arrhythmia, brain tumour (relative)

Respiratory Medicine

PHYSIOLOGY

Pulmonary blood flow — approximately 5000 ml/min
Alveolar ventilation — approximately 5250 ml/min

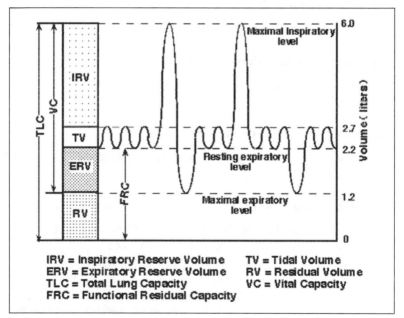

Figure 5 Physiology

Tests of pulmonary function

Total lung capacity (TLC)

1 Volume of gas in the lungs after a maximal inspiration
2 TLC = RV + VC
3 Measured by body plethysmography or helium dilution technique
4 Approximately 6–7 litres in the normal adult

Vital capacity (VC)

1 Change in volume of gas in the lungs from complete inspiration to complete expiration
2 75% of TLC
3 Decreases with age
4 Dependent on age, sex and ethnic origin

Residual volume (RV)

1 Volume of gas in the lungs at the end of maximal expiration

Expiratory reserve volume (ERV)

1 Volume of gas expired from resting expiratory level to maximal expiration

Functional residual capacity (FRC)

1 Volume of gas in the lungs at the resting expiratory level
2 FRC = RV + ERV

Peak expiratory flow (PEF)

1 The greatest flow that can be sustained for 10 ms on forced expiration, starting from full inflation of the lungs
2 It is expressed in litres/minute with a peak flow meter
3 Valuable for individual self-monitoring of changes in airflow in asthma
4 Not effective as a diagnostic test – can be reduced for reasons other than asthma, and sometimes PEF can be preserved even when there is severe lung damage (e.g. emphysema)

Compliance

A measure of the distensibility of lung tissue and airways
1 ↑ in emphysema
2 ↓ in fibrosis or pulmonary oedema

Spirometry

1 Forced expiratory volume in one second (FEV_1) is the volume of air expelled in the first second of forced expiration, starting from full inspiration
2 Forced vital capacity (FVC) is the total volume of air expelled in a forced expiration, starting from full inspiration
3 FEV_1/FVC ratio is helpful in determining the pattern of spirometric abnormality
   (a) In an *obstructive disorder* the FEV_1 and FVC are both reduced, the FEV_1 to a greater extent, leading to FEV_1/FVC < 0.75
   (b) In a *restrictive disorder* the FVC is reduced, with the FEV_1 reduced in proportion and the FEV_1/FVC ratio > 0.75

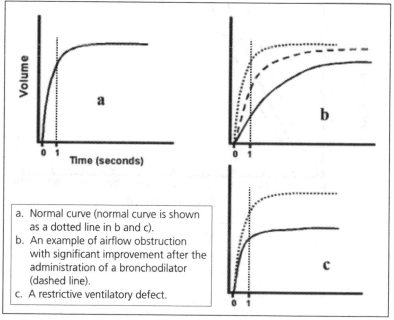

a. Normal curve (normal curve is shown as a dotted line in b and c).
b. An example of airflow obstruction with significant improvement after the administration of a bronchodilator (dashed line).
c. A restrictive ventilatory defect.

Figure 6 Spirograms

Gas exchange

Oxygenation of haemoglobin

1 Hb is changed from ferric to ferrous form
2 Fetal haemoglobin (HbF) has greater affinity for O_2
3 Partial pressure of O_2 and saturation (SaO_2) follows oxygen dissociation curve
4 Increased affinity for O_2 represents shift of curve to the RIGHT

NB: These are all things that occur in working muscle

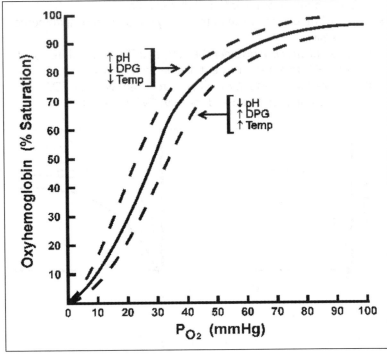

Figure 7 Oxygenation of haemoglobin

Causes of increased O_2 affinity

1 ↑ Temperature
2 ↑ H^+ (i.e. pH)
3 ↑ $Pa\text{CO}_2$
4 ↑ 2,3 DPG (adaptation to altitude, chronic anaemia)

NB: These are all things that occur in working muscle

Gas transfer factor

Causes of decreased transfer factor

1 Pulmonary
  (a) Emphysema
  (b) Interstitial lung disease
  (c) Pneumonia
  (d) Pulmonary embolus
  (e) Loss of lung tissue (eg pneumonectomy)
2 Cardiovascular
  (a) Low cardiac output
  (b) Pulmonary oedema
3 Haematological
  (a) Anaemia

Causes of increased transfer factor

1 Pulmonary
  (a) Pulmonary haemorrhage (eg Goodpasture's syndrome)
2 Cardiovascular
  (a) Exercise
  (b) Hyperkinetic circulation (eg thyrotoxicosis)
  (c) Left-to-right shunt
3 Haematological
  (a) Polycythaemia

RESPIRATORY MEDICINE

RESPIRATORY FAILURE

Type I

1 Hypoxemic respiratory failure – secondary to a ventilation–perfusion mismatch
2 Po_2 < 8 kPa (60 mmHg) with normal Pco_2
3 Causes
   (a) Early stages of severe asthma
   (b) Emphysema
   (c) Pneumonia
   (d) Pulmonary embolus
   (e) Pulmonary oedema
   (f) Interstitial lung disease
   (g) ARDS

Type II

1 Ventilatory failure leading to a raised Pco_2 (> 6.7 kPa) as well as hypoxaemia
2 Causes
   (a) Respiratory
      (i) COPD
      (ii) Severe asthma
      (iii) Bronchiectasis
   (b) Thoracic cage
      (i) Kyphoscoliosis
      (ii) Ankylosing spondylitis
      (iii) Chest trauma/surgery
   (c) Muscular dystrophies
   (d) Peripheral nerve and motor endplate
      (i) Guillain–Barré
      (ii) Myasthenia gravis
   (e) Spinal cord and CNS
      (i) Cord transection
      (ii) Polio
      (iii) CVA
   (f) Drugs
      (i) Opiates
      (ii) Benzodiazepines

ASTHMA

Chronic asthma

1 Incidence 20% in children, 15% in adults
2 Chronic inflammatory disorder with variable airflow obstruction
3 Combination of genetic predisposition and environmental atopy
4 Mediated by IgE, prostaglandin-derived growth factor (PDGF) and interleukins
5 Cells involved
   (a) Mast cells
   (b) Macrophages
   (c) Epithelial cells
   (d) Eosinophils
6 Pulmonary function tests
   (a) > 25% variation in PEFR
   (b) ↓ FEV_1
   (c) ↓ FEV_1/FVC ratio
   (d) PEFR and FEV_1 ↑ post bronchodilator
   (e) ↑ lung volume
7 Acute attack provoked by
   (a) Exposure to allergen (pollen, housedust mite, cat and dog dander)
   (b) Exercise
   (c) Drugs (NSAIDs and aspirin, beta blockers)
   (d) Infection
   (e) Oesophageal reflux
   (f) Smoke
   (g) Non-compliance with medication

Acute asthma

1 1500 deaths per year in UK
2 Markers of severe acute asthma
   (a) Difficulty speaking
   (b) Tachycardia > 110
   (c) Pulsus paradoxus
   (d) Respiratory rate > 30
   (e) PEFR < 33% of best/predicted
   (f) Silent chest
   (g) Hypoxia
   (h) Normal or raised $P\text{CO}_2$

3 Management
   (a) High-flow O_2
   (b) Nebulised bronchodilators
   (c) Steroids
   (d) Antibiotics
   (e) Intravenous aminophylline or salbutamol
   (f) Intravenous magnesium
   (g) Ventilation

Exercise-induced asthma

1 Characteristically occurs 5–10 minutes after exercise
2 Lasts < 1 hour
3 Worse in cold air
4 Prevented by beta-agonist pre exercise

Causes of occupational asthma

1 Isocyanates (paint, plastics, insulation)
2 Flour
3 Grain dusts
4 Soldering flux (colophony)
5 Epoxy resins
6 Proteolytic enzymes (detergents)
7 Platinum salts
8 Laboratory animals

DISEASES CAUSED BY *ASPERGILLUS FUMIGATUS*

(See also page 263)

Allergic bronchopulmonary aspergillosis (ABPA)

Key diagnostic criteria

1 Asthma
2 Blood eosinophilia (>1000/mm^3)
3 History of pulmonary infiltrates
4 Proximal bronchiectasis
5 Precipitins against *A. fumigatus* positive
6 Aspergillus IgE antibody >2x asthma control

7 Aspergillus IgG antibody >2x asthma control
8 Total serum IgE concentration >1000 iu/ml

If three of the tests are positive then ABPA is very likely; if four are positive the diagnosis is established

Features of ABPA

1 Seen in 1–2% of asthmatics
2 Flitting infiltrates on CXR. Also perihilar infiltrate lobar collapse, upper lobe fibrosis and proximal bronchiectasis
3 May see fungal hyphae in sputum/lavage fluid
4 Associated with eosinophilia and positive precipitins
5 Types I and III hypersensitivity reactions

Chronic cavitatory pulmonary aspergillosis (aspergilloma)

1 Fungal ball
2 Patients have underlying lung disease (commonly TB or opportunistic mycobacterium)
3 Smoking history very common
4 Many features similar to neoplastic illness
5 Aspergillus precipitins positive and elevated inflammatory markers
6 May require surgical resection
7 Medical treatment difficult
8 Cavity seen on CXR/CT
9 Can be complicated by haemorrhage

CHRONIC OBSTRUCTIVE PULMONARY DISEASE (COPD)

1 Chronic progressive airflow obstruction, mainly non-reversible
2 Biggest aetiological factor is smoking (approx 1 in 20 are non-smokers)
3 Age > 35 years
4 Exacerbations are one of the commonest reasons for admission to hospital in the UK
5 Marked morbidity/mortality
6 FEV_1/FVC ratio < 0.75; FEV_1 < 80% predicted

Long-term O$_2$ therapy (LTOT)

1 Proven to increase 3-year survival by 50% in eligible patients
2 Need to raise Po_2 to > 60 mmHg for > 15 hours per day
3 Strict criteria for prescription (all of below)
   (a) ABGs must be measured on two occasions, three weeks apart, when patient is free from exacerbation
   (b) Po_2 < 7.3 kPa (55 mmHg), or 7.3–8.0 kPa (55–60 mmHg) with evidence of cor pulmonale
   (c) Pco_2 normal or raised
   (d) FEV$_1$ < 1.5 litres
   (e) Non-smoker
   (f) Po_2 on oxygen should rise to > 8 kPa (60 mmHg) without a significant rise in Pco_2

Alpha-$_1$-antitrypsin deficiency

1 Autosomal codominant (chromosome 14)
2 Alpha-$_1$-antitrypsin is a protective enzyme (inhibits proteolytic enzymes such as elastase)
3 If levels are less than 40% tissue destruction may occur, leading to emphysema
4 MM genotype normal level of alpha-$_1$-antitrypsin
5 MS genotype 80% of normal
6 MZ genotype 60% of normal
7 SZ genotype 40% of normal
8 ZZ genotype 15% of normal
9 Most severe with ZZ deficiency
10 Presents in third to fourth decades
11 Marked panlobular emphysema in basal lung areas
12 Worse in smokers
13 Associated with liver cirrhosis

BRONCHIECTASIS

1 Irreversible dilatation of small airways. Obstructive spirometry due to plugging by secretions. Appearances may be saccular, atelectatic or follicular

2 Causes
   (a) Congenital
        (i)   Selective IgA deficiency
        (ii) Kartagener's syndrome (ciliary dyskinesis associated with infertility, dextrocardia and situs invertus)
        (iii) Primary immotile cilia syndrome
        (iv) X-linked hypogammaglobulinaemia
   (b) Acquired
        (i)   Childhood pneumonia, pertussis, measles
        (ii) Post TB
        (iii) ABPA
        (iv) Distal to obstructed bronchus (foreign body, tumour)
        (v)   Associated with pulmonary fibrosis and sarcoid
        (vi) Idiopathic
3 Features
   (a) Chronic production of purulent sputum
   (b) Exertional breathlessness
   (c) Clubbing
   (d) Early/mid-inspiratory crepitations
4 Diagnosis
   (a) CXR shows thickened bronchial walls and ring shadows
   (b) Obstructive or restrictive spirometry
   (c) High-resolution CT usually diagnostic

CYSTIC FIBROSIS

1 Autosomal recessive
2 1 in 25 adults carriers
3 Incidence 1:2000 live births
4 Gene on long arm of chromosome 7 codes for cystic fibrosis transmembrane regulator protein (CFTR)
5 300+ mutations; commonest is deletion of three bases called Δ508 (68% of cases)
6 Defect of chloride and water transport across epithelial cell membrane
7 Diagnosis by sweat test; sodium and chloride concentrations > 60 mmol/l
8 Life expectancy improving (> 40 years)
9 Prognosis best predicted by spirometry, weight and microbiology

10 Managed in the UK in specialist centres by multidisciplinary teams
11 Respiratory features
  (a) Obstruction of small airways with thick mucus due to ↓ chloride secretion and ↑ sodium resorption
  (b) Colonisation with *S. aureus, H. influenzae* and *Pseudomonas aeruginosa*
  (c) *Burkholderia cepacia* increasingly important: highly transmissible
  (d) Chronic infection and inflammation with bronchiectasis
  (e) Respiratory failure in late stages
  (f) Treat with antibiotics, acutely and prophylactically, oral ± nebulised
  (g) Transplantation
12 Gastrointestinal features
  (a) Pancreatic insufficiency in 80% (steatorrhoea, vitamin deficiency); oral pancreatic supplements given
  (b) Meconium ileus in infancy, small bowel obstruction in adults
  (c) Chronic liver disease seen due to biliary tree obstruction (< 5%)
  (d) Gallstones
  (e) Pancreatitis
13 Other features
  (a) Diabetes (> 30% of patients in late teens)
  (b) Nasal polyps (30%)
  (c) Pneumothorax (5%)
  (d) Infertility (almost all men)
  (e) Osteoporosis

INTERSTITIAL LUNG DISEASE (PULMONARY FIBROSIS)

Clinical classification of interstitial lung disease

Connective tissue diseases

1 Scleroderma
2 Polymyositis–dermatomyositis
3 Systemic lupus erythematosus
4 Rheumatoid arthritis

5 Mixed connective tissue disease
6 Ankylosing spondylitis

Treatment or drug induced

1 Antibiotics (nitrofurantoin, sulfasalazine)
2 Antiarrhythmics (amiodarone, propranolol)
3 Anti-inflammatory agents (gold, penicillamine)
4 Anticonvulsants (phenytoin)
5 Chemotherapy agents (mitomycin C, bleomycin, busulfan, cyclophosphamide, azathioprine, BCNU, methotrexate)
6 Therapeutic radiation
7 Oxygen
8 Cocaine

Primary diseases

1 Sarcoidosis
2 Eosinophilic granuloma
3 Amyloidosis
4 Lymphangitic carcinoma
5 Bronchoalveolar carcinoma
6 Pulmonary lymphoma
7 Adult respiratory distress syndrome
8 Acquired immunodeficiency syndrome (AIDS)
9 Bone marrow transplantation
10 Post-infectious
11 Respiratory bronchiolitis
12 Eosinophilic pneumonia
13 Diffuse alveolar haemorrhage syndrome

Occupational and environmental

1 Inorganic dusts
2 Asbestosis
3 Silicosis
4 Coal worker's pneumoconiosis
5 Talc pneumoconiosis
6 Organic dusts
  (a) Bird fancier's lung
  (b) Farmer's lung

Idiopathic interstitial pneumonia

This term refers to a group of disorders rather than to a single specific diagnosis. It includes, in decreasing order of incidence
1 Usual interstitial pneumonitis (UIP) – cryptogenic fibrosing alveolitis
2 Non-specific interstitial pneumonitis (NSIP)
3 Bronchiolitis obliterans–organizing pneumonia (BOOP)
4 Respiratory bronchiolitis-associated interstitial lung disease (RB-ILD)
5 Desquamative interstitial pneumonitis (DIP)
6 Lymphocytic interstitial pneumonitis (LIP)
7 Acute interstitial pneumonitis (AIP)

Known causes of pulmonary fibrosis and location on CXR

1 Upper lobe fibrosis
  (a) Sarcoidosis
  (b) TB
  (c) Pneumoconiosis
  (d) Silicosis
  (e) Histiocytosis X
  (f) Ankylosing spondylitis
  (g) ABPA
2 Lower lobe fibrosis
  (a) Bronchiectasis
  (b) Asbestosis
  (c) Usual interstitial pneumonia (cryptogenic fibrosing alveolitis).
  (d) RA
  (e) Systemic sclerosis
  (f) Radiation
3 Drug-induced fibrosis
  (a) Amiodarone
  (b) Methotrexate
  (c) Azathioprine
  (d) Nitrofurantoin
  (e) Bleomycin
  (f) Busulphan
  (g) Chlorambucil

USUAL INTERSTITIAL PNEUMONITIS (CRYPTOGENIC FIBROSING ALVEOLITIS)

Classification and features

1 Temporal heterogeneity is the hallmark, with variations in the degree of involvement and appearance of the interstitial infiltrate
2 Alternating zones of inflammation, fibrosis, honeycomb change and normal lung
3 Inflammatory cells usually lymphocytes, plasma cells and mast cells – in general the inflammation is scant and the diagnosis should be questioned if prominent
4 Intimal proliferation and medial thickening of the muscular pulmonary arteries
5 More common in men
6 Clinical features
   (a) Dry cough
   (b) Breathlessness
   (c) Clubbing
   (d) Cyanosis
   (e) Fine late-inspiratory crepitations

Extrinsic allergic alveolitis (EAA)

1 Allergic alveolitis and pneumonitis due to inhaled organic dust particles of fungal, thermophilic actinomycete or other origin
2 IgG-mediated type III and IV hypersensitivity reaction to inhaled particles. Causes pneumonitis
3 Farmer's lung
   (a) Caused by *Micropolyspora faeni* and *Thermoactinomyces vulgaris* in mouldy hay
4 Bagassosis
   (a) Due to *Thermoactinomyces sacchari* in sugar cane
5 Bird-fancier's lung
   (a) Budgerigar fancier's disease
   (b) Pigeon fancier's disease
   (c) Due to keratin in faeces and feather bloom
6 Suberosis
   (a) Corkhandler's disease

7 Malt worker's lung
(a) Alveolitis due to *Aspergillus clavatus*
8 Mushroom worker's lung
9 Maple bark-stripper's lung
10 Clinical features
(a) Fever, cough and breathlessness 4–9 hours after exposure. No wheeze. Settles in 48 hours
(b) CXR may be normal; may have nodular shadows and hazy infiltrate
(c) Chronic disease causes irreversible fibrosis and restrictive spirometry
(d) Serum precipitins helpful in diagnosis
(e) No eosinophilia
(f) Bronchoalveolar lavage shows lymphocytosis and normal/low CD4:CD8 count
(g) Transbronchial biopsy may show mononuclear infiltrate and granulomata
(h) Treatment is avoidance of precipitant and steroids in acute illness (no improvement in outcome in chronic disease)

OCCUPATIONAL LUNG DISEASE

Coal worker's pneumoconiosis (CWP)

1 > 10–20 years after exposure
2 Small particles retained in alveoli and small bronchioles
3 Show as small rounded opacities in lung fields
4 Background CWP may go on to progressive massive fibrosis (PMF)
5 Large opacities > 10 mm. Usually upper lobe. May cavitate
6 Mixed obstructive/restrictive pattern
7 Compensatable (only if CXR changes)
8 Caplan's syndrome – multiple lung nodules in patient with rheumatoid arthritis and CWP

Silicosis

1 Inhaled silicon dioxide in rock-face miners, quarry workers, engineers and sand blasters
2 Subacute phase within a few months of exposure. SOB and dry cough

3 Progresses to upper lobe nodule formation
4 Late stages sees restrictive lung disease
5 Previously marked increase in TB
6 Only treatment is transplant
7 Compensatable

Berylliosis

1 Acute beryllium fume inhalation causes alveolitis. Jobs in which exposure occurs include
   (a) Electronics
   (b) Fibreoptics
   (c) Manufacturing ceramics, bicycle frames, golf clubs, mirrors and microwave ovens
   (d) Mining
   (e) Nuclear weapons and reactors
   (f) Reclaiming scrap metal
   (g) Space and atomic engineering
   (h) Dental and laboratory technology
2 Chronic exposure causes sarcoid-like illness
3 Non-caseating granulomata and fibrous lymph nodes
4 CXR – bilateral hilar lymphadenopathy and diffuse fine nodules
5 Interstitial fibrosis develops

Byssinosis

1 Inhalation of cotton dust, hemp and flax
2 Symptoms worse on Monday morning, improves over week
3 1–6 hours after exposure
4 Cough, SOB and wheeze
5 Commoner in smokers
6 CXR normal
7 Compensatable

Diseases caused by exposure to asbestos

Pleural plaques and thickening

1 20+ years after exposure
2 Plaques on parietal pleura
3 Usually asymptomatic

4 May progress to diffuse confluent thickening, causing exertional SOB
5 Restrictive spirometry, Kco normal

Asbestosis

1 20+ years after exposure
2 Lower lobe fibrosis
3 Dry cough, exertional SOB, lower zone crepitations and clubbing
4 CXR shows irregular shadowing, with ring and honeycomb patterns in later disease
5 Restrictive spirometry and low Kco
6 Associated with increased incidence of lung cancer
7 Compensatable

Mesothelioma

1 85% due to asbestos
2 See page 418

GRANULOMATOUS LUNG DISEASE

Sarcoidosis

1 Multisystem disease
2 Cause unknown
3 Mainly affects young adults
4 Prevalence 25/100 000
5 Three times more common in blacks
6 Characteristic lesion is a non-caseating granuloma
7 Associated with HLA A1, B8 and DR3
8 Symptoms
   (a) No respiratory symptoms
   (b) Dry cough, fever, SOB, weight loss
   (c) Examination often NAD, occasional clubbing
9 Bilateral hilar lymphadenopathy and erythema nodosum almost diagnostic
10 Chest X-ray classification
   (a) Stage 0   normal CXR
   (b) Stage 1   bilateral hilar lymphadenopathy (BHL)

(c) Stage 2   BHL and pulmonary infiltrates
(d) Stage 3   Diffuse infiltration
11 May progress to irreversible fibrosis; upper and mid-zones usually affected
12 May rarely see upper airway involvement, with obstruction and discharge
13 Diagnosis
   (a) Transbronchial biopsy diagnostic in 85% stage 1
   (b) ↑ Ca^{2+} and ACE
   (c) Kveim test positive in 75% (spleen extract from patient with active sarcoid injected under skin and biopsied at 6 weeks – see granulomatous response)
14 Extrapulmonary manifestations
   (a) Liver (40–70%) – subclinical granuloma infiltration
   (b) Cardiac (30–70%) – myocardial infiltration, arrhythmias
   (c) Skin (25%) – erythema nodosum, nodules, plaques, lupus pernio
   (d) Eyes (25%) – anterior uveitis
   (e) Splenomegaly (25%)
   (f) Neurological (5%) – meningitis, hydrocephalus, space-occupying lesions, cranial nerve palsy, spinal cord involvement. May affect posterior pituitary
   (g) Bone – cysts (small bones of hands and feet), arthritis
   (h) Löfgren's syndrome – triad of BHL, polyarthritis and erythema nodosum
15 Treatment
   (a) Symptomatic
   (b) Steroids
   (c) Azathioprine, methotrexate
   (d) Hydroxychloroquine
   (e) Thalidomide
16 Prognosis
   (a) Stage 1 – 80 % spontaneous remission
   (b) Stage 2 – 50% spontaneous remission
   (c) Stage 3 – 30% spontaneous remission
   (d) Bad prognosis if
      (i) Stage 3
      (ii) Age > 40
      (iii) Symptoms > 6 months
      (iv) No erythema nodosum

(v) Three systems involved
(vi) Splenomegaly

Pulmonary histiocytosis X – PHX (Langerhans' cell histiocytosis)

1 Pathophysiology: characterised by abnormal infiltration of the lungs by Langerhans' cells. Langerhans' cells are differentiated cells of the monocyte–macrophage line that are found in the skin, reticuloendothelial system, pleura and lungs
2 An uncommon interstitial lung disease related to tobacco smoking
3 Primarily affects young adults
4 Disorder is similar to paediatric histiocytic disorders (Letterer–Siwe disease and Hand–Schüller–Christian disease). PHX generally involves the lungs and sometimes the bones. Other systems are only rarely affected
5 PHX is more common in whites than in Asians and blacks
6 Spontaneous pneumothorax, which may be recurrent, is a classic presentation found in 25% of patients
7 In order of frequency, the common presenting symptoms are as follows
   (a) Non-productive cough (56–70%)
   (b) Dyspnoea (40%)
   (c) Chest pain (21%)
   (d) Fatigue (30%)
   (e) Weight loss (20–30%)
   (f) Fever (15%)
   (g) Cystic bone lesions (4–20%) – these may be painful and may predispose the patient to pathologic fracture
   (h) Central nervous system involvement: may manifest as central diabetes insipidus (associated with a less favourable prognosis)

CONNECTIVE TISSUE DISEASE AND THE LUNG

Lung involvement seen in
1 Rheumatoid arthritis
   (a) Nodules
   (b) Fibrosis
   (c) Bronchiectasis

(d) Caplan's syndrome
(e) Effusion
2 Systemic lupus erythematosus
  (a) Fibrosis
  (b) Shrinking lung syndrome
3 Systemic sclerosis
  (a) Fibrosis
  (b) Bronchiectasis

Causes of pulmonary vasculitis (See also page 452)

Classification

1 Idiopathic vasculitis *commonly* affecting the lung
  (a) Pulmonary Wegener's granulomatosis
  (b) Churg–Strauss syndrome (Churg–Strauss angiitis and granulomatosis)
  (c) Microscopic polyangiitis
2 Idiopathic vasculitis *uncommonly* affecting the lung
  (a) Necrotising sarcoid granulomatosis
  (b) Polyarteritis nodosa
  (c) Small cell vasculitis
  (d) Giant cell arteritis
  (e) Takayasu's arteritis
  (f) Behçet's syndrome
  (g) Henoch–Schönlein purpura
  (h) Cryoglobulinaemic vasculitis
  (i) Hypocomplementaemic vasculitis
  (j) Giant cell arteritis
  (k) Disseminated visceral giant cell angiitis
3 Miscellaneous systemic disorders
  (a) Sarcoidosis
  (b) Dysimmune vascular diseases
  (c) Inflammatory bowel disease
  (d) Malignancy
4 Secondary or localised vasculitis
  (a) Pulmonary infections
  (b) Bronchocentric granulomatosis
  (c) Pulmonary hypertension
  (d) Interstitial lung diseases
      (i) Chronic eosinophilic pneumonia
      (ii) Langerhans' histiocytosis

(e) Pulmonary inflammatory pseudotumors
(f) Pulmonary pseudolymphomas
(g) Pulmonary sequestration
(h) Embolic material (intravenous drug abuse)
(i) Drug or toxic substances
(j) Pulmonary transplantation
(k) Radiotherapy
5 Vascular involvement in lymphoproliferative disorders
(a) Angiocentric immunoproliferative lesions
(b) Lymphomatoid granulomatosis
(c) Non-Hodgkin's lymphoma

Churg–Strauss syndrome

1 Churg and Strauss, in 1951, described syndrome in patients who had
(a) Asthma
(b) Eosinophilia
(c) Granulomatous inflammation
(d) Necrotising systemic vasculitis
(e) Necrotising glomerulonephritis
2 Granulomata and eosinophilic infiltrates
3 pANCA positive in 50%
4 Clinical features
(a) Asthma (97%)
(i) May precede vasculitis by up to 10 years and is usually persistent
(ii) Patients are usually treated with steroids, which might mask other features of the syndrome
(b) Constitutional symptoms
(i) Malaise
(ii) Flu-like symptoms
(iii) Weight loss (70%)
(iv) Fever (57%)
(v) Myalgias (52%)
(c) Paranasal sinusitis (61%) and allergic rhinitis
(d) Pulmonary symptoms (37%), including cough and haemoptysis
(e) Arthralgias (40%)
(f) Skin manifestations (49%)
(i) Purpura
(ii) Skin nodules

    (iii) Urticarial rash
    (iv) Necrotic bullae
    (v) Digital ischaemia
 (g) Cardiac manifestations
    (i) Heart failure
    (ii) Myocarditis
    (iii) Myocardial infarction
 (h) Gastrointestinal symptoms (31%)
    (i) GI vasculitis
    (ii) GI bleeding
 (i) Peripheral neuropathy – mononeuritis multiplex

LUNG CANCER

1 Causes
 (a) Smoking (95%)
 (b) Industrial (asbestos, arsenic, benzoyl chloride, aluminium salts)
 (c) Atmospheric (pollution, passive smoking)
 (d) Also associated with UIP and systemic sclerosis
2 Cell types
 (a) Non small cell lung carcinoma (NSCLC)
    (i) Squamous (52%) – arise in central airways
    (ii) Adenocarcinoma (11%) – may be peripheral
    (iii) Large cell (10%)
    (iv) Bronchiolar–alveolar cell (6%)
 (b) Small cell (21%) – central airway, rapidly growing and metastasise early
3 Complications
 (a) Metastatic/physical
 (b) Pleural effusion
 (c) Dysphagia
 (d) SVC obstruction
 (e) Recurrent laryngeal nerve palsy → hoarseness
 (f) Phrenic nerve palsy → raised hemidiaphragm
 (g) Pericarditis and effusion
 (h) Spontaneous pneumothorax
4 Non-metastatic
 (a) SIADH (small cell)
 (b) Ectopic ACTH (small cell)

(c) Hypercalcaemia (metastases, squamous cell PTHrP)
(d) Gynaecomastia (large cell)
(e) Clubbing (commonest in non-small cell)
(f) Eaton–Lambert syndrome (small cell): proximal myopathy and reduced tendon reflexes
(g) Hypertrophic pulmonary osteoarthropathy (squamous cell): arthritis, clubbing and periostitis. Commonly affects long bones

5 Treatment
(a) Surgery for non-small cell. Only 20% operable. 5-year survival post surgery only 25%
(b) Palliative/radical radiotherapy
(c) Chemotherapy (small cell): no significant improvement in survival

6 Contraindications to surgery
(a) Small cell histology
(b) Tumour/node/metastasis (TNM) Stage > 3A
(c) Local invasion (laryngeal nerve, oesophagus etc)
(d) Distant metastasis, including mediastinal nodes
(e) Bloody pleural effusion
(f) Poor performance status/poor exercise tolerance
(g) FEV_1 < 1.5 litres
(h) Tumour < 1.5 cm from carina

7 Prognosis
(a) Median survival in small cell is 14 months in limited disease, 10 months in extensive
(b) 5-year survival in non-small cell is 10%

Mesothelioma

1 1000 cases per year in UK
2 Commonest in men
3 85% due to asbestos exposure
4 Blue (crocidolite) > brown (amosite) > white (crysotile)
5 Presents 20–50 years after exposure
6 No cure
7 Median survival 16 months

Bronchial carcinoid

1 1% of lung tumours
2 Cherry red ball in bronchial tree

3 1–2% associated with carcinoid syndrome
4 Histology similar to small cell carcinoma
5 5-year survival 90%

PNEUMONIA

1 Community acquired
  (a) Incidence 3 per 1000 per year
  (b) Causal organisms
    (i) *Streptococcus pneumoniae* (60–75%)
    (ii) Atypicals (5–18%)
      (1) *Mycoplasma pneumoniae*
      (2) *Legionella*
      (3) *Chlamydia psittaci* and *C. pneumoniae*
    (iii) *Haemophilus influenzae* (5%)
    (iv) *Staphylococcus aureus*
    (v) *Moraxella catarrhalis*
    (vi) Viruses (influenza, parainfluenza, varicella, RSV)
2 *Mycoplasma* pneumonia
  (a) Affects young adults
  (b) Epidemics every 3 4 years
  (c) Long prodrome
  (d) May be associated with cold agglutinins
3 *Legionella* pneumonia
  (a) Contaminated air-conditioning, showers, water cooling systems
  (b) Often underlying lung disease
  (c) Jaundice may occur
  (d) WCC may be normal, with lymphopenia
  (e) SIADH and low sodium
  (f) Abnormal LFTs in 50%
  (g) Neurological signs and symptoms common
4 *Staphylococcus* pneumonia
  (a) May complicate influenza
  (b) Common in IVDAs
  (c) Associated with lung abscess and empyema
5 Markers of severity in pneumonia (BTS Guidelines)
  (a) Two or more = severe
  (b) **C**onfusion
  (c) **U**rea > 7 mmol/l

(d) **R**espiratory rate > 30/min
(e) **B**P – diastolic BP < 60 and systolic BP < 90
(f) Age more than **65 years**
6 Hospital-acquired pneumonia
   (a) Organisms
      (i) *Staphylococcus aureus*
      (ii) Gram-negatives (*Klebsiella, Proteus, E. coli, Pseudomonas*)
      (iii) Anaerobes
   (b) Treatment with third-generation cephalosporin
7 *Pneumocystis carinii* pneumonia (PCP)
   (a) Commonest in immunocompromised
   (b) Symptoms of dry cough, fever and breathlessness
   (c) CXR may be normal; diffuse perihilar shadowing
   (d) Diagnosis by bronchoscopy, washings and silver stain or PCR
   (e) Treatment with Septrin ± pentamidine, and steroids if $Po_2 < 9.3$ kPa
   (f) 5% mortality
8 Causes of eosinophilic pneumonia
   (a) Allergic aspergillosis
   (b) Drugs (sulphasalazine, nitofurantoin, imipramine)
   (c) Other infections
   (d) Parasites
   (e) Smoke inhalation

TUBERCULOSIS

1 At-risk groups
   (a) Immigrants from endemic areas
   (b) Alcoholics
   (c) HIV-positive
   (d) Homeless
   (e) Low income
2 Primary TB
   (a) May be entirely asymptomatic
   (b) Infection in person with no immunity
   (c) Ghon focus develops in lung
   (d) Bacilli transported through lymphatics
   (e) Infection arrested
   (f) Tuberculin tests become positive after this
   (g) May cause mild cough, wheeze and erythema nodosum

3 Post-primary TB
   (a) Reactivation of disseminated dormant organisms
4 Miliary TB
   (a) Widespread haematological spread of bacilli
5 Symptoms
   (a) Night sweats
   (b) Weight loss
   (c) Cough
   (d) Haemoptysis
   (e) Pleural effusion
   (f) Meningitis
6 Diagnosis
   (a) CXR (upper lobe shadowing, loss of volume, cavitation)
   (b) Sputum examination for acid–alcohol-fast bacilli (AAFBs)
   (c) Early morning urine for AAFBs
   (d) Lymph node biopsy
   (e) Bone marrow aspirate
   (f) Bronchoscopy and lavage
   (g) Culture takes at least 6 weeks
   (h) PCR available
7 Treatment
   (a) In HIV-negative Caucasian with no previous treatment or
       contact, triple therapy with rifampicin, isoniazid and
       pyrazinamide
   (b) For others add ethambutol
   (c) Triple/quadruple therapy for 2 months, rifampicin/isoniazid
       further 4 months
   (d) Rifampicin, isoniazid, pyrazinamide all bactericidal, ethambutol
       bacteriostatic
   (e) Compliance very important
   (f) Side effects common
       (i) Rifampicin
           (1) Hepatitis
           (2) Nausea
           (3) Pink/orange urine
           (4) Enzyme inducer
           (5) May precipitate addisonian crisis
       (ii) Isoniazid
           (1) Hepatitis
           (2) Peripheral neuropathy (cover with pyridoxine)

(iii) Pyrazinamide
    (1) Hepatitis
    (2) Rash
    (3) Gout
(iv) Ethambutol
    (1) Optic neuritis
    (2) Renal dysfunction
8 Multidrug-resistant TB ≈ 2% of all cases
9 Atypical TB organisms (clinically and radiologically indistinguishable from *Mycobacterium tuberculosis* infection) – 10%
  (a) *Mycobacterium malmoensae*
  (b) *Mycobacterium kansasii*
  (c) *Mycobacterium xenopi*
  (d) *Mycobacterium avium intracellulare*

OBSTRUCTIVE SLEEP APNOEA

1 Incidence 1–2%, middle-aged men
2 10+ episodes of apnoea of at least 10 seconds' duration per hour
3 Occurs in REM sleep
4 Airway obstruction at base of tongue/soft palate owing to loss of muscle tone
5 Symptoms include
  (a) Heavy snoring
  (b) Hypersomnolence
  (c) Restless sleep
  (d) Morning headache
  (e) Poor concentration
  (f) Impotence
6 Symptoms of hypersomnolence in daytime, snoring and headaches
7 Causes are obesity (80%), acromegaly, hypothyroidism, alcohol and Marfan's syndrome
8 Diagnosis with Epworth sleep score and overnight pulse oximetry
9 Treatment is weight loss and nasal CPAP

PLEURAL EFFUSION

Light's criteria

1 Pleural fluid is classified as an exudate if it meets any one of the following criteria
  (a) Pleural fluid protein/serum protein ratio > 0.5
  (b) Pleural fluid lactate dehydrogenase (LDH)/serum LDH ratio > 0.6
  (c) Pleural fluid LDH more than two-thirds the upper limit of normal for serum LDH
2 Causes of a transudative effusion
  (a) Cardiac failure
  (b) Cirrhosis
  (c) Hypoalbuminaemia
  (d) Nephrotic syndrome
  (e) Hypothyroidism
  (f) Dialysis
3 Causes of an exudative effusion
  (a) Malignancy
  (b) Parapneumonia
  (c) TB
  (d) Subphrenic abscess
  (e) PE
  (f) Pancreatitis
  (g) Asbestos
  (h) Rheumatoid disease
  (i) SLE
4 Causes of low glucose in pleural fluid
  (a) RA
  (b) TB
  (c) Malignancy
  (d) Empyema

CAUSES OF HAEMOPTYSIS

1 Lung cancer
2 TB
3 PE
4 Bronchiectasis

5 Aspergilloma
6 Pulmonary abscess
7 Farmer's lung
8 Wegener's syndrome
9 Goodpasture's syndrome
10 PAN
11 Haemosiderosis
12 Endometriosis

CAUSES OF CAVITATION ON CXR

1 Bullae
2 Pneumonias (*Klebsiella*, *Staphylococcus*, anaerobic)
3 TB
4 Abscess
5 Tumour (squamous cell, secondaries)
6 PE
7 Pneumoconiotic nodule
8 Rheumatoid nodule
9 Wegener's syndrome
10 Churg–Strauss syndrome
11 Honeycomb lung (systemic sclerosis)
12 Progressive massive fibrosis

CAUSES OF CALCIFICATION ON CXR

1 Lung
   (a) TB
   (b) Carcinoma
   (c) Chicken pox
   (d) Sarcoidosis
   (e) Asbestos exposure
   (f) Silicosis
   (g) Pneumoconiosis
   (h) Hydatid disease
   (i) Schistosomiasis

2 Pleura
   (a) Asbestos
   (b) Empyema
   (c) Haemothorax
   (d) TB
   (e) Recurrent pneumothorax
3 Lymph nodes
   (a) TB
   (b) Carcinoid
   (c) Silicosis
4 Others
   (a) Pericardium
   (b) Heart valves
   (c) Calcified aorta

Rheumatology

CHARACTERISTICS OF SYNOVIAL FLUID IN HEALTH AND DISEASE

Table 55

Source	Colour culture	Clarity	Viscosity	WCC $\times$ 10^6/l
Normal	Yellow Negative	Clear	High	<200
OA	Yellow Negative	Clear	High	<200
RA	Yellow/green Negative	Clear/turbid	Low	3000–50 000
Bacterial arthritis	Purulent Positive	Turbid	Low	50 000–100 000
Gout	Yellow/white Negative	Clear	Low	100–150 000
Pseudogout	Yellow/white Negative	Clear/ blood-stained	Low	50–75 000

ACUTE ARTHRITIS

Common causes of an acute monoarthritis

1 Acute septic arthritis
2 Gout
3 Pseudogout
4 Trauma
5 Seronegative spondyloarthritides
6 RA
7 Haemarthrosis

Causes of an acute polyarthritis

1 RA
2 OA (generalised)
3 Viral infections
  (a) Rubella
  (b) Mumps
  (c) Parvovirus
  (d) Coxsackie
  (e) Arbovirus (including Dengue fever)
  (f) Hepatitis B and C
4 Reiter's syndrome
5 Seronegative arthritides
6 Gonococcal arthritis
7 Adult – and childhood-onset Still's disease
8 Rheumatic fever
9 SLE
10 Gout (10% are polyarthropathy)
11 Pseudogout
12 Acute sarcoidosis

BACTERIA ASSOCIATED WITH SPECIFIC ARTHRITIDES

Septic arthritis

1 *Staphylococcus aureus*
2 *Streptococcus pyogenes*
3 *Streptococcus pneumoniae*
4 *Mycobacterium tuberculosis*
5 *Neisseria gonorrhoeae*
6 *Salmonella* spp

Osteomyelitis

1 *Staphylococcus aureus*
2 *Bacteroides fragilis*
3 Enterobacteriaceae
4 *Mycobacterium tuberculosis*
5 Non-group A streptococcus

CRYSTAL-RELATED ARTHROPATHIES

Gout

1 Inflammatory arthropathy secondary to urate crystal deposition in joints
2 Negatively birefringent needle-shaped crystals of monosodium urate
3 Causes of hyperuricaemia – which may lead to gout
  (a) Increased production of urate
    (i) Increased purine synthesis
    (ii) Idiopathic
    (iii) Lesch–Nyhan syndrome – X-linked
  (b) Increased turnover of preformed purines
    (i) Lymphoproliferative and myeloproliferative disorders
    (ii) Cytotoxic drugs
    (iii) Carcinomatosis
    (iv) Polycythaemia
    (v) Chronic haemolytic anaemias
  (c) Decreased excretion
    (i) Reduction in fractional urate clearance
    (ii) Idiopathic
    (iii) Chronic renal failure
    (iv) Increased level of organic acids (alcohol, starvation, exercise, ketoacidosis)
    (v) Familial juvenile gouty nephropathy (AD)
  (d) Drug administration
    (i) Diuretics – thiazides and frusemide
    (ii) Salicylates (low dose)
    (iii) Ciclosporin
4 Events provoking gouty arthritis
  (a) Trauma
  (b) Unusual physical exercise
  (c) Surgery
  (d) Severe systemic illness
  (e) Severe dieting
  (f) Dietary excess
  (g) Alcohol
  (h) Drugs (above + allopurinol and probenecid)
5 Treatment
  (a) Acute flare

(b) NSAIDs
(c) Colchicine
(d) Steroids (intra-articular or systemic)
(e) Prophylaxis
   (i) Allopurinol
      (1) Xanthine oxidase inhibitor
      (2) Reduces production of urate
   (ii) Probenecid

Pyrophosphate arthropathy (pseudogout)

1 Arthropathy caused by deposition of calcium pyrophosphate in the joints
2 Leads to acute and chronic arthropathy (chondrocalcinosis)
3 Positively birefringent rhomboid crystals
4 Causes
   (a) Age
   (b) OA
   (c) Familial
   (d) DM
   (e) Acromegaly
   (f) Haemochromatosis
   (g) Hypothyroidism
   (h) Hyperparathyroidism
   (i) Hypophosphataemia
5 Treatment
   (a) NSAIDs
   (b) Steroids (intra-articular or systemic)

RHEUMATOID ARTHRITIS

Revised American College of Rheumatology criteria for the classification of rheumatoid arthritis (1987)

1 Morning stiffness (> 1 hr) for > 6 wks
2 Arthritis of > = three joint areas for > 6 wks
3 Arthritis of the hand joints for > 6 wks
4 Symmetrical arthritis
5 Rheumatoid nodules

6 Serum rheumatoid factor
7 Radiographic changes

RA if at least four of the seven criteria

Joint involvement in RA

Symmetrical polyarthropathy affecting

1	MCP	90%
2	PIP	90%
3	MTP	90%
4	Wrists	80%
5	Knees	80%
6	Ankle/subtalar	80%
7	Shoulder	60%
8	Hip	50%
9	Elbow	50%
10	Acromioclavicular	50%
11	Cervical spine	40%

Extra-articular features of RA

1 Non-organ specific
   (a) Weight loss
   (b) Malaise
   (c) Fever
   (d) Lymphadenopathy
   (e) Rheumatoid nodules
   (f) Felty's syndrome (triad of RA, splenomegaly and
       granulocytopenia)
   (g) Amyloidosis
   (h) Increased susceptibility to infections
   (i) Osteoporosis
2 Organ specific
   (a) Vasculitis
       (i)   Splinter haemorrhages and nailfold infarcts
       (ii) Distal gangrene
       (iii) Peripheral neuropathy
       (iv) Organ vasculitis (eg mesenteric)

(b) Cardiac
  (i) Pericarditis and effusion
  (ii) Constrictive pericarditis
  (iii) Valvular heart disease
(c) Pulmonary
  (i) Pleurisy
  (ii) Pleural effusion
  (iii) Interstitial fibrosis
  (iv) Nodular lung disease
  (v) Bronchiectasis
  (vi) Caplan's syndrome (nodules and progressive massive fibrosis in coal workers)
(d) Renal
  (i) Drug induced
    (1) Second-line agents (gold and penicillamine) – membranous glomerulonephritis
    (2) NSAIDs – interstitial nephritis and minimal change glomerulonephritis
    (3) Renal papillary necrosis secondary to analgesic abuse
  (ii) Amyloidosis
  (iii) Renal tubular acidosis type 1
(e) Neurological
  (i) Compressive neuropathies, eg carpal tunnel syndrome
  (ii) Mononeuritis multiplex (vasculitis)
  (iii) Cervical myelopathies
(f) Ocular
  (i) Episcleritis
  (ii) Scleritis
  (iii) Scleromalacia perforans
  (iv) Sjögren's syndrome
  (v) Extraocular paralysis from mononeuritis multiplex
  (vi) Cataracts from steroid therapy
(g) Other
  (i) Palmar erythema
  (ii) Pyoderma gangrenosum

Factors associated with poorer prognosis in RA

1 Insidious polyarticular onset
2 Female patients

3 Extra-articular manifestations
4 Functional disability at 1 year after start of the disease
5 Substantially raised concentration of rheumatoid factors
6 Presence of HLA DR4
7 Family history of RA
8 Radiographic evidence of erosions within 1 year of disease onset

Laboratory findings in RA

1 Anaemia – normochromic or hypochromic, normocytic
2 Thrombocytosis
3 Raised ESR
4 Raised CRP
5 Raised ferritin
6 Low iron concentration
7 Low TIBC
8 Raised globulins
9 Raised ALP
10 Rheumatoid factor

Features of rheumatoid factor (RF)

1 IgM, IgG or IgA antibodies against the Fc component of IgG antibodies
2 Agglutination tests (latex) detect IgM RF (seropositive disease)
3 ELISA tests detect IgM and IgG RF
4 Found in 80% of patients with RA
5 Found in 5% of the general population (up to 25% in > 75-yr-olds)
6 Role is unclear in the pathogenesis of RA
7 Extra-articular features are commoner in patients with high concentrates of RF
8 Positive RF is poor guide to severity of joint disease
9 Other causes for a positive RF
   (a) Connective tissue diseases (often high titre > 1/160)
(i)	RA	80% (extra-articular 100%)
(ii)	Sjögren's syndrome	75–100%
(iii)	RA + sicca	98%
(iv)	SLE	20–40%
(v)	Systemic sclerosis	5–10%
(vi)	PAN	0–5%
(vii)	Dermatomyositis	0–5%

(b) Chronic infections (usually low titre)
  (i)   Syphilis   10%
  (ii) Leprosy   50%
  (iii) Endocarditis   25%
  (iv) TB   5–20%
(c) Autoimmune liver diseases
(d) Sarcoidosis
(e) Mixed essential cryoglobulinaemia
(f) Paraproteinaemias
(g) Transplant recipients

Causes of anaemia in RA

1 Anaemia of chronic disease
2 Iron deficiency – NSAIDs
3 Bone marrow suppression – gold, penicillamine, sulphasalazine and cytotoxics
4 Folate deficiency – sulphasalazine, methotrexate
5 Vitamin B_{12} deficiency – associated pernicious anaemia
6 Haemolysis – dapsone, sulphasalazine
7 Felty's syndrome

Radiological features in RA

1 Soft tissue swelling
2 Loss of joint space due to erosion of articular cartilage
3 Juxta-articular osteoporosis
4 Marginal bone erosions
5 Joint deformities

Drug treatments for RA

Symptom-modifying drugs

1 Analgesics
2 NSAIDs
3 Corticosteroids

Disease-modifying drugs

Pharmacology of these drugs (See page 463)

  1 Antimalarials (chloroquine, hydroxychloroquine)

2 Sulphasalazine
3 Methotrexate
4 Leflunomide
5 Gold
6 Penicillamine
7 Azathioprine
8 Ciclosporin
9 Cyclophosphamide
10 Infliximab/etanercept (anti-TNF-α)
11 Anakinra (IL-1 receptor antagonist)

SERONEGATIVE SPONDYLOARTHRITIDES

The seronegative spondyloarthritides

Associated with HLA B27, except Behçet's

1 Ankylosing spondylitis
2 Psoriatic arthritis
3 Enteropathic arthritis – Crohn's, UC, Whipple's
4 Reiter's syndrome/reactive arthritis
5 Behçet's syndrome (can also be classified as a vasculitis)

Comparison of seronegative spondyloarthritides and seropositive RA

[See Table 56, overleaf]

Common features of seronegative spondyloarthritides

1 Negative RF
2 Asymmetrical inflammatory peripheral arthritis (oligoarthritis)
3 Radiological sacroiliitis
4 Spondylitis
5 Enthesitis
6 HLA B27 association (96% in AS)
7 Anterior uveitis
8 Evidence of clinical overlap between diseases

Table 56

Feature	Seronegative	Seropositive
Peripheral arthritis	Asymmetrical	Symmetrical
Spinal involvement	Ankylosis	Cervical subluxation
Cartilaginous joints	Commonly affected (SI joints)	Rarely affected
Tissue typing	HLA-B27	(HLA-DR4)
Eye	Anterior uveitis	Scleritis
	Conjunctivitis	Sicca syndrome
Skin	Psoriasis	Cutaneous nodules
	Keratoderma blenorrhagica	Vasculitis
	Mucosal ulceration	
	Erythema nodosum	
Heart	AR	Pericarditis
	Conduction defects	Nodules
Pulmonary	Chest wall ankylosis	Effusions
	Apical fibrosis	Fibrosis
GI	Ulceration of small or large intestine	Drug-induced symptoms
GU	Urethritis	
	Genital ulceration	

Ankylosing spondylitis

European Spondyloarthropathy Study Group diagnostic criteria for ankylosing spondylitis

Inflammatory spinal pain or synovitis and any one of the following:
1 Positive family history
2 Psoriasis
3 Inflammatory bowel disease
4 Alternate buttock pain
5 Enthesopathy
6 Sacroiliitis

Clinical features of AS (the A disease)

1 **A**rthritis
2 **A**tlantoaxial subluxation

3 **A**nterior uveitis
4 **A**pical pulmonary fibrosis
5 **A**myloidosis
6 **A**ortic regurgitation
7 **A**ortitis
8 **A**-V conduction defects
9 Cauda equin**A** syndrome
10 Ig**A** nephropathy
11 **A**chilles tendonitis
12 Plantar f**A**sciitis

Radiological features of AS

1 SI joints
  (a) Irregular joint margins
  (b) Subchondral erosion
  (c) Sclerosis
  (d) Fusion
2 Spine
  (a) Loss of lumbar lordosis
  (b) Vertebral squaring
  (c) Syndesmophyte formation (calcification of the annulus fibrosis)
  (d) Bamboo spine (calcification in anterior and posterior spinal ligaments)
3 Peripheral joints
  (a) Erosive arthropathy
  (b) Enthesopathies

Reiter's syndrome

HLA B-27 in 80%
1 Clinical features
  (a) Classic triad
    (i) Arthropathy
    (ii) Conjunctivitis
    (iii) Urethritis
  (b) Other features
    (i) Sacroiliitis
    (ii) Plantar fasciitis
    (iii) Anterior uveitis
    (iv) Circinate balanitis

     (v)   Keratoderma blenorrhagicum
     (vi)   Oral ulceration
     (vii) Dystrophic nails
     (viii) Pericarditis
     (ix)   Aortitis
     (x)   Cardiac conduction defects
     (xi)   Pleurisy
     (xii) Meningoencephalitis
     (xiii) Peripheral neuropathy

2 Triggers for Reiter's/reactive arthritis
   (a) *Chlamydia trachomatis*
   (b) *Campylobacter jejuni*
   (c) *Salmonella* spp
   (d) *Shigella flexneri*
   (e) *Neisseria gonorrhoeae*
   (f) *Borrelia burgdorferi*
   (g) *Streptococcus pyogenes*
   (h) *Yersinia enterocolitica*
   (i) *Yersinia pseudotuberculosis*

Psoriatic arthropathy

Patterns of disease in psoriatic arthropathy

1 Peripheral oligoarthritis or polyarthritis (60%)
2 Spondylitis (15%)
3 Distal interphalangeal disease (10%)
4 Rheumatoid type (10%)
5 Arthritis mutilans (5%)

Radiological features of psoriatic arthritis in peripheral joints

1 Relative lack of juxta-articular osteoporosis compared with RA
2 Periostitis and bony remodelling within the joints, leading to 'pencil in cup' erosions
3 Osteolysis leading to complete destruction of phalanges in some cases
4 Ankylosis

Treatment for spondyloarthropathies

1 Physiotherapy
2 Local steroid injection

3 NSAIDs
4 Systemic steroids
5 Sulphasalazine
6 Methotrexate
7 Anti-TNF-α drugs
8 Antibiotics – acute infections

Behçet's syndrome

1 Presumed autoimmune multisystem disease
2 Primary lesion is vasculitis
3 HLA B5 and B51 increase risk of Behçet's
4 Clinical features
   (a) Oral ulceration
   (b) Genital ulceration
   (c) Uveitis
   (d) Phlebitis leading to thrombosis
   (e) Synovitis
   (f) Arthralgia/arthritis
   (g) Cutaneous vasculitis
   (h) Erythema nodosum
   (i) Meningoencephalitis
   (j) Large artery aneurysms
   (k) Discrete intestinal ulcers (bloody diarrhoea)
   (l) Pathergy (excessive erythema following skin prick)
   (m) Epididymitis

CONNECTIVE TISSUE DISEASES

SLE

American College of Rheumatology revised criteria for the diagnosis of SLE (1982)

SLE diagnosed with four or more of the following
1 Malar rash
2 Discoid rash
3 Photosensitivity
4 Oral ulcers
5 Arthritis

6 Serositis (pleurisy, pericarditis)
7 Renal disease (persistent proteinuria > 0.5 g/day, cellular casts)
8 Neurological disorder (seizures, psychosis)
9 Haematological disorder (haemolytic anaemia, leukopenia, lymphopenia, thrombocytopenia)
10 Immunological disorder (LE cells, anti-dsDNA antibody, anti-Sm or false positive VDRL)
11 Antinuclear antibody

Clinical features of SLE

1 Constitutional symptoms
  (a) Fever
  (b) Fatigue
  (c) Anorexia
  (d) Nausea
2 Mucocutaneous (81%)
  (a) Rash (malar, discoid, photosensitive)
  (b) Alopecia
  (c) Oral, nasal, or vaginal ulcers
  (d) Raynaud's phenomenon (50%)
  (e) Livedo reticularis
  (f) Cutaneous vasculitis
  (g) Sjögren's syndrome
  (h) Purpura
3 Musculoskeletal (95%)
  (a) Migratory asymmetrical non-erosive (Jaccoud's) arthritis
  (b) Myalgia
  (c) Myositis
  (d) Avascular necrosis of femoral head
4 Renal (53%)
  (a) Glomerulonephritis
  (b) Proteinuria
  (c) Nephrotic syndrome
  (d) Hypertension
  (e) End-stage renal failure (< 5%)
  (f) Tubulointerstitial disease
  (g) Renal vasculitis
5 Respiratory (48%)
  (a) Pleurisy

   (b) Recurrent pneumonitis
   (c) Shrinking lung syndrome
   (d) Cor pulmonale from pulmonary hypertension
6 Cardiovascular (38%)
   (a) Pericarditis
   (b) Cardiomyopathy
   (c) Myocarditis
   (d) Coronary vasculitis-myocardial ischaemia
   (e) Libman–Sacks endocarditis
7 CNS disease (59%)
   (a) Headaches
   (b) Migraine
   (c) Seizures
   (d) Chorea
   (e) Psychosis
   (f) Poor memory
   (g) CVA – vasculitis
   (h) Mononeuritis multiplex
   (i) Aseptic meningitis
8 Haematology
   (a) Neutropenia
   (b) Lymphopenia
   (c) Thrombocytopenia
   (d) Lymphadenopathy
   (e) Splenomegaly
   (f) Hyposplenism
   (g) Antiphospholipid syndrome
9 GI disease
   (a) Abdominal pain
   (b) Mesenteric vasculitis
   (c) Peptic ulcer disease (drugs)
   (d) Autoimmune hepatitis

Typical results in a patient with SLE

1 Normochromic normocytic anaemia with active disease
2 Leukopenia/lymphopenia
3 Raised ESR
4 Normal CRP (unless accompanied by serositis, synovitis or infection)
5 ANA positive in 95%

6 Raised immunoglobulins
7 Low C3 and C4
8 Antiphospholipid antibodies in 30–40%
9 Coombs-positive haemolytic anaemia

Patterns of staining of ANA

Table 57

Staining	Disease
Homogeneous	SLE
Speckled	MCTD, Sjögren's
Nucleolar	Scleroderma
Centromere	Limited systemic sclerosis (CREST)

Causes of a positive ANA

1 SLE 95%
2 Sjögren's 80%
3 Polymyositis/dermatomyositis 80%
4 RA 30%
5 Systemic sclerosis
6 Autoimmune hepatitis
7 Chronic infections
8 Malignancy
9 Old age

Autoantibody associations with clinical syndromes in SLE

Table 58

Clinical syndrome	Autoantibody
Nephritis, photosensitivity, serositis	Anti-dsDNA
Photosensitivity	Anti-Ro/La
Neonatal lupus syndromes	Anti-Ro/La
Coagulopathy, thrombocytopenia, miscarriages, CNS syndromes	Lupus anticoagulant, antiphospholipid
Overlap features such as Raynaud's, myositis, and cardiopulmonary lesions	Anti-RNP
Drug-induced lupus	Antihistone

Causes of drug-induced lupus

1 Hydralazine
2 Procainamide
3 Phenytoin
4 Isoniazid
5 Penicillamine
6 Methyldopa
7 Propylthiouracil
8 Bleomycin
9 Sulphonamides
10 Minocycline
11 OCPs may exacerbate pre-existing SLE

Pregnancy with SLE

1 No evidence of reduced fertility
2 Pre-existing renal disease may worsen during pregnancy
3 Hypertension more difficult to control
4 Pre-eclampsia difficult to distinguish from renal flare
5 Increased fetal loss in patients with antiphospholipid antibodies
6 Overall no increased risk of fetal abnormalities
7 Antimetabolites contraindicated because of teratogenesis
8 Low-dose prednisolone and azathioprine probably safe
9 Neonatal SLE is a rare complication

Treatment of SLE

1 Sunscreens – photosensitivity
2 NSAIDs – symptomatic
3 Chloroquine/hydroxychloroquine – rashes, arthritis, malaise
4 Corticosteroids – severe flare, low dose for maintenance
5 Immunosuppressants (azathioprine, methotrexate, cyclophosphamide) – for severe flare
6 Thalidomide – rash
7 Dapsone – rash
8 Plasma exchange – severe cases
9 Anticoagulation – recurrent thromboses
10 Vasodilators (calcium blockers, prostacyclin) – Raynaud's
11 Antihypertensives
12 Anticonvulsants – cerebral lupus

Essential features of antiphospholipid antibody syndrome

1 IgG or IgM antibodies against phospholipids
2 Antibodies may cause a false positive VDRL
3 In vitro anticoagulant effect – prolonged APTT which fails to correct after addition of normal plasma
4 In vivo predisposes to recurrent thromboses
5 Associations
  (a) SLE
  (b) RA
  (c) Sjögren's
  (d) ITP
  (e) Other CTDs
  (f) Syphilis
  (g) Hepatitis C
  (h) HIV
  (i) Drugs
    (i) Hydralazine
    (ii) Phenytoin
    (iii) Interferon-α
6 Clinical features
  (a) Venous thrombosis
    (i) DVT
    (ii) Major vein thrombosis
    (iii) Ocular thrombosis
    (iv) Renal vein thrombosis
    (v) Budd–Chiari syndrome
    (vi) Pulmonary hypertension
  (b) Arterial thrombosis
    (i) Limb ischaemia
    (ii) Stroke/TIA
    (iii) MI
    (iv) Adrenal infarction
  (c) Other
    (i) Recurrent miscarriage
    (ii) Thrombocytopenia
    (iii) Haemolytic anaemia
    (iv) Livedo reticularis
    (v) Migraine
    (vi) Epilepsy

(vii)   Chorea
(viii) Myelopathy
(ix)   Heart valve disease
(x)   Pulmonary hypertension

Systemic sclerosis (scleroderma)

Systemic disorder that results from excessive production and deposition of type 1 and type 3 collagen in tissues

Classification of systemic sclerosis spectrum of disorders

1 Pre-scleroderma
   (a) Raynaud's phenomenon
   (b) Nailfold capillary changes
   (c) Circulating antinuclear antibodies (Scl-70 (topoisomerase 1), anticentromere)
2 Diffuse systemic sclerosis
   (a) Onset of skin changes within 1 year of onset of Raynaud's phenomenon
   (b) Truncal and forearm skin involvement
   (c) Presence of tendon friction rubs
   (d) Early and significant incidence of
       (i)   Interstitial lung disease
       (ii) Oliguric renal failure
       (iii) Diffuse GI disease
       (iv) Myocardial involvement
   (e) Nailfold capillary dilatation and capillary dropout
   (f) Scl-70 Antibodies in 30%
3 Limited systemic sclerosis
   (a) Raynaud's phenomenon for years
   (b) Skin involvement to hands, face, feet and forearms or absent
   (c) Includes CREST syndrome (calcinosis, Raynaud's, oesophageal involvement, sclerodactyly and telangiectasia)
   (d) A significant (10–15 yrs) late incidence of pulmonary hypertension, with or without interstitial lung disease, skin calcinosis, telangiectasia and GI involvement
   (e) High incidence of anticentromere antibody (70–80%)
   (f) Dilated nailfold capillary loops, usually **without** capillary dropout
4 Scleroderma sine scleroderma

RHEUMATOLOGY

(a) Raynaud's +/–
(b) No skin involvement
(c) Presentation with
  (i) Pulmonary fibrosis
  (ii) Scleroderma renal crisis
  (iii) Cardiac disease
  (iv) GI disease
  (v) Antinuclear antibodies may be present (Scl-70, centromere, nucleolar)
5 Overlap syndromes
  (a) Features of scleroderma coexist with those of other autoimmune disorders
    (i) SLE
    (ii) RA
    (iii) Dermatomyositis
    (iv) Vasculitis
    (v) Sjögren's syndrome
6 Localised forms
  (a) Localised morphoea
  (b) Generalised morphoea
  (c) Linear scleroderma
  (d) *En coup de sabre*

Clinical features of systemic sclerosis

1 Musculoskeletal
  (a) Polyarthralgia
  (b) Polymyositis
2 Skin
  (a) Raynaud's phenomenon
  (b) Abnormal nailfold capillaries
  (c) Sclerodactyly
  (d) Telangiectasia
  (e) Tight smooth waxy pigmented skin
  (f) Skin ulcers
  (g) Vitiligo
  (h) Increased pigmentation
  (i) Subcutaneous calcification
3 Heart
  (a) Cardiomyopathy

(b) Pericarditis
(c) Pericardial effusion
(d) Hypertension
4 Lungs
  (a) Pulmonary fibrosis
  (b) Pulmonary hypertension
  (c) Aspiration pneumonia
  (d) Bronchiectasis
5 GI
  (a) Microstomia and sicca syndrome
  (b) Dysphagia – poor motility, peptic strictures
  (c) GORD – low sphincter pressure, hiatus hernia
  (d) Diverticulae – small bowel, colonic
  (e) Hypomotility + stasis – can lead to pseudo-obstruction
  (f) Bacterial overgrowth
  (g) Malabsorption
  (h) Pneumatosis intestinalis
  (i) PBC and autoimmune hepatitis
6 Renal
  (a) Progressive renal failure
  (b) Hypertensive renal crisis
7 Neurological
  (a) Trigeminal neuralgia
  (b) Autonomic neuropathy

Essential features of Raynaud's phenomenon

1 Episodic event characterised by the digits turning white and numb, then cyanosed and finally red and painful (rebound hyperaemia)
2 3–10% of adults affected
3 1% of Raynaud's sufferers have a connective tissue disorder
4 Causes
  (a) Idiopathic
  (b) Connective tissue disorders
  (c) Hypothyroidism
  (d) Increased plasma viscosity
    (i) Leukaemia
    (ii) Lymphoma
    (iii) Myeloma
    (iv) Polycythaemia
    (v) Cryoglobulinaemia

    (e) Drugs – β-blockers, ergot
    (f) Vibrating instruments
5 Treatments
    (a) Warmth
    (b) No smoking or β-blockers
    (c) Calcium channel blockers
    (d) GTN
    (e) ACE inhibitors
    (f) Prostacyclin infusion
    (g) Amputation

Sjögren's syndrome

1 Disorder characterised by lymphocytic infiltration of exocrine organs mainly affecting the salivary and lacrimal glands
2 Clinical features
    (a) Dryness from atrophy of exocrine glands (eyes, mouth, respiratory tract, vagina) (100%)
    (b) Arthralgia/arthritis (60%)
    (c) Raynaud's phenomenon (37%)
    (d) Lymphadenopathy (14%)
    (e) Vasculitis (11%)
    (f) RTA type 1 (9%)
    (g) Liver involvement (7%)
    (h) Splenomegaly (3%)
    (i) Peripheral neuropathy (2%)
    (j) Myositis (1%)
3 Autoimmune diseases in which Sjögren's syndrome may occur
    (a) RA
    (b) SLE
    (c) Systemic sclerosis
    (d) PBC
    (e) MCTD
    (f) Mixed cryoglobulinaemia
    (g) Hashimoto's thyroiditis
    (h) MS

Essential features of dermatomyositis and polymyositis

1 Idiopathic inflammation of skeletal muscle + cutaneous lesions
2 Polymyositis – similar features without skin lesions

3 Cutaneous lesions
   (a) Heliotrope rash
   (b) Nailfold changes with periungual erythema, cuticular hypertrophy and infarcts
   (c) Gottron's papules (scaly rash on back of hands)
   (d) Sclerodermatous skin changes with cutaneous and muscular calcification
   (e) Raynaud's disease
4 Proximal muscle weakness
5 Elevated serum levels of muscle enzymes
6 Typical muscle biopsy changes
7 EMG changes
   (a) Polyphasic, short, small motor unit potentials
   (b) High-frequency repetitive discharges
   (c) Spontaneous fibrillation
8 Calcification and vasculitis common in childhood form (more severe)
9 Pulmonary fibrosis, cardiomyopathy and arthropathy may be present
   (a) Associated with other connective tissue disorders
   (b) Associated with malignancy in 20% of patients over 50 yrs of age
   (c) ANA and anti-Jo-1 antibodies may be present
   (d) Treatment with steroids and immunosuppressants

MCTD

1 Overlap syndrome with features of
   (a) Polymyositis
   (b) Systemic sclerosis
   (c) SLE
2 High titre of antibodies to RNP
3 Clinical features
   (a) Arthritis > 90%
   (b) Sclerodactyly 90%
   (c) Raynaud's 80%
   (d) Abnormal oesophageal motility 70%
   (e) Myositis 70%
   (f) Lymphadenopathy
   (g) Hepatosplenomegaly
   (h) Serositis
   (i) Hypergammaglobulinaemia

Common autoantibodies seen in connective tissue diseases
Table 59

Antibody	Disease	Specificity	Prevalence (%)
Anti-dsDNA	SLE	H	60
Anti-Sm	SLE	H	4% Caucasian 30–50% Afro-Caribbean
Anti-Ro	Sjögren's SLE Congenital neonatal heart block	L	80 50
Anti-La	Sjögren's SLE	H	50 15
Anti-RNP	MCTD SLE	L	90 5
Anti-Jo-1	Polymyositis lung fibrosis	H	25
Anti-Scl-70 (topoisomerase 1)	Diffuse cutaneous systemic sclerosis	H	25
Anticentromere	Limited cutaneous systemic sclerosis	M	70
Anticardiolipin	Antiphospholipid antibody syndrome, SLE	L	
Antihistones	Drug-induced lupus	L	60

JUVENILE CHRONIC ARTHRITIS

1 Arthritis in at least one joint for > 3 months
2 Onset before 16 years
3 Exclusion of other diseases that may cause arthritis
4 Three types
  (a) Pauciarticular (70%)
    (i) Four or fewer joints affected in first 6 months
    (ii) Commonly associated with ANA
    (iii) Strong association with anterior uveitis
    (iv) Good articular prognosis

  (b) Polyarticular (20%)
      (i)   Five or more joints affected in the first 6 months
      (ii) 10% are RF positive (often progress to severe RA)
  (c) Systemic – Still's disease (10%)
      (i)   Fever
      (ii) Evanescent, macular, erythematous rash (salmon pink)
      (iii) Arthritis (usually systemic features precede arthritis)
      (iv) Organomegaly
      (v)   Lymphadenopathy
      (vi) Can lead to amyloidosis

Diagnostic criteria for adult Still's disease

1 Each of
  (a) Quotidian fever >39
  (b) Arthralgia/arthritis
  (c) Negative RF
  (d) Negative ANA
2 Plus two of
  (a) Leukocytosis > 15
  (b) Evanescent macular/maculopapular rash (salmon pink)
  (c) Serositis (pleuritic/pericardiac)
  (d) Hepatomegaly
  (e) Splenomegaly
  (f) Generalised lymphadenopathy

Rheumatic fever

1 Revised Jones criteria for a diagnosis of acute rheumatic fever
  (a) Major
      (i)   Carditis
      (ii) Polyarthritis
      (iii) Chorea
      (iv) Erythema marginatum
      (v)   Subcutaneous nodules
  (b) Minor
      (i)   Fever
      (ii) Arthralgia
      (iii) Previous history of rheumatic fever or rheumatic heart
            disease
2 Diagnosis requires two major or one major and two minor, plus

evidence of recent streptococcal infection (raised ASO titre or culture of group A *Streptococcus*)
3 Treatment
   (a) Penicillin
   (b) NSAIDs
   (c) Steroids (severe carditis)
   (d) Haloperidol (chorea)
   (e) Long-term prophylaxis with penicillin

ESSENTIAL FEATURES OF VASCULITIS

Large vessel vasculitis

1 Takayasu's arteritis
   (a) Chronic progressive inflammatory occlusive disease of the aorta and its branches
   (b) Most commonly presents in females < 40 yrs
   (c) Ischaemia or aneurysm formation in the aorta or its branches
   (d) Often presents with arm claudication and pulseless vessels
   (e) Diagnosis by angiography
   (f) Treat with steroids, immunosuppressants and surgery
2 Giant cell arteritis
   (a) Vasculitis that typically involves extracranial arteries, leading to ischaemia
   (b) Diagnosis by temporal artery biopsy (negative biopsy does not exclude diagnosis)
   (c) Clinical features
       (i) Unilateral throbbing headache
       (ii) Jaw claudication
       (iii) Amaurosis fugax
       (iv) Diplopia
       (v) Polymyalgia rheumatica symptoms in 50%
   (d) Treat with steroids

Medium vessel vasculitis

Polyarteritis nodosa

1 Systemic vasculitis leading to necrotising inflammatory lesions of medium vessels

2 Associated with hepatitis B infection
3 American College of Rheumatology criteria for PAN
   (a) Weight loss of > 4 kg
   (b) Livedo reticularis
   (c) Testicular pain
   (d) Myalgia/leg tenderness
   (e) Mono-/polyneuropathy
   (f) Hepatitis Bs Ag positive
   (g) Arteriographic abnormality
   (h) Positive biopsy
2 Treatment with steroids and cyclophosphamide

Features of Kawasaki disease

1 Occurs primarily in children under 5 yrs
1 Clinical features
   (a) Fever for 5 days or more
   (b) Bilateral congestion of conjunctiva without conjunctivitis
   (c) Dryness, redness and fissuring of the lips and inflammation of the oral cavity
   (d) Acute non-purulent swelling of the cervical lymph nodes
   (e) Skin rash comprising morbilliform, scarlatiniform, urticarious or erythema multiforme-like lesions
   (f) Reddening of the palms and soles with oedema, fading to produce desquamation
   (g) Coronary artery lesions (aneurysms) in 40% can lead to sudden death, MI or papillary muscle dysfunction
2 Treatment is with aspirin and high-dose immunoglobulin (reduces mortality from 30% to < 1%)

Small vessel vasculitis

Churg–Strauss syndrome

1 Allergic granulomatous vasculitis of small vessels
2 Asthma (usually precedes vasculitis symptoms)
3 Eosinophilia
4 25% cANCA positive, 50% pANCA positive
5 Systemic vasculitis which may lead to
   (a) Myocarditis
   (b) Coronary arteritis

   (c) Pulmonary infiltrate or haemorrhage
   (d) Stroke
   (e) Mononeuritis multiplex
   (f) GI involvement
   (g) Renal disease – focal segmental necrotising glomerulonephritis
        may develop
6 Diagnosis with biopsy
7 Treatment with steroids

Wegener's granulomatosis

1 Necrotising granulomatous systemic vasculitis
2 cANCA positive (proteinase 3) in > 95%
3 Characterised by upper respiratory tract lesions, pulmonary disease
   and glomerulonephritis
4 Clinical features
   (a) Upper respiratory tract (90%)
        (i)   Epistaxis
        (ii)   Purulent nasal discharge
        (iii) Sinusitis
        (iv)   Destruction of nasal septum
   (b) Lower respiratory tract (90%)
        (i)   Pulmonary infiltrates
        (ii)   Pulmonary haemorrhage
   (c) Kidney
        (i)   Proteinuria
        (ii)   Haematuria
        (iii) Focal necrotising GN
        (iv)   Renal failure
   (d) Others
        (i)   Polyarthralgia
        (ii)   Myalgia
        (iii) Vasculitic rash
        (iv)   Nailfold infarcts
        (v)   Pericarditis
        (vi)   Arrhythmias
        (vii) Scleritis
        (viii) Uveitis
        (ix)   Proptosis – retro-orbital granuloma formation
        (x)   Mononeuritis multiplex

Microscopic polyangiitis

1 Vasculitis affects single organ or multisystems
2 ANCA positive in 80% (60% pANCA/MPO, 40% c ANCA/PR3)
3 Clinical features
   (a) Kidney (almost 100%)
      (i) Glomerulonephritis
      (ii) Microscopic haematuria
   (b) Lung
      (i) Pulmonary haemorrhage
      (ii) Pleurisy
      (iii) Pleural effusions
   (c) Others
      (i) Purpuric rash
      (ii) Arthralgia
      (iii) Mononeuritis multiplex
      (iv) GI symptoms
      (v) Pericarditis
      (vi) Arrhythmias
4 Diagnosis with biopsy
5 Treatment with steroids and immunosuppressants

Henoch–Schönlein purpura

1 IgA leukocytoclastic vasculitis
2 Most common systemic vasculitis in children
3 IgA deposited in skin and kidney
4 Preceded by upper respiratory tract infection in 90%
5 Clinical features
   (a) Purpuric rash (100%) – lower limbs and buttocks
   (b) Arthralgia
   (c) Glomerulonephritis
   (d) GI bleeding
   (e) Intussusception

Essential features of polymyalgia rheumatica

1 Most common in patients aged 60–70
2 One-third of patients are under 60
3 25% have giant cell arteritis
4 Raised ESR and ALP (30%)

5 Symptoms and ESR respond rapidly to steroids
6 Clinical features (often sudden onset)
   (a) Proximal muscle weakness worse in the morning
   (b) Malaise
   (c) Weight loss
   (d) Joint pain
   (e) Depression
   (f) Symptoms of giant cell arteritis (above)

ANCA (antineutrophil cytoplasmic antibody)

Table 60

Autoantibody	Staining	Antigen	Diseases
cANCA	Cytoplasm	Proteinase 3 (PR3)	Wegener's Granulomatosis
pANCA	Perinuclear	Myeloperoxidase (MPO)	Microscopic polyangiitis Idiopathic GN
pANCA	Perinuclear	Non-specific subset bind Elastase Lactoferrin Lysozyme	SLE MCTD UC RTA CFA

Essential features of familial Mediterranean fever

1 Polyserositis
2 Affects Arabs, Jews, Armenians and Turks
3 Clinical features
   (a) Abdominal pain from peritonitis
   (b) Vomiting
   (c) Constipation
   (d) Pyrexia
   (e) Pleurisy
   (f) Large joint arthritis
   (g) Rash
   (h) Cutaneous vasculitis
   (i) Myalgia
   (j) Episcleritis

(k) Headaches
(l) Pericarditis
(m) Splenomegaly
4 Often develop amyloidosis
5 Treated with colchicine (long term)

Essential features of cryoglobulinaemia

1 Immunoglobulins that reversibly precipitate in the cold < 4° C
2 Types:

Table 61

	Type 1	Type 2	Type 3
Composition	Monoclonal immunoglobulin Usually IgM or IgG	Monoclonal IgM RF + polyclonal IgG	Polyclonal IgM RF + polyclonal IgG
Disease associations	Myeloma, Waldenstrom's Lymphoproliferative disease	Bacterial endocarditis Hep C Hep B EBV CMV	Lyme disease Syphilis Malaria SLE RA Sjögren's Systemic sclerosis Mixed essential cryoglobulinaemia

3 Clinical features
  (a) Purpura
  (b) Arthralgia
  (c) Leg ulcers
  (d) Raynaud's
  (e) Abdominal pain
  (f) Sjögren's syndrome
  (g) Sensorimotor peripheral neuropathy
  (h) Liver disease
  (i) Renal disease – mesangiocapillary nephritis
4 Treat with interferon-α if hepatitis C positive

MISCELLANEOUS CONDITIONS

Risk factors for OA

1 Age
2 Female gender
3 Genetic predisposition
4 Obesity
5 Hypermobility
6 Joint trauma – particularly fractures through the joint
7 Chondrocalcinosis
8 Infection
9 Hereditary type 2 collagen defects
10 Developmental conditions
   (a) Congenital dislocation of the hip
   (b) Perthes' disease
   (c) Joint dysplasias
11 Bone disease
   (a) Paget's disease
   (b) Avascular necrosis of bone
   (c) Osteopetrosis
12 Endocrine conditions
   (a) Acromegaly
   (b) Ochronosis
   (c) Haemochromatosis
   (d) Wilson's disease
13 Charcot's joints

OSTEOPOROSIS

1 Reduced bone mass and density
2 Abnormal bone architecture
3 Increase risk of fracture (particularly hip, vertebrae and wrist)
4 Causes
   (a) Postmenopausal
   (b) Elderly
   (c) Immobility
   (d) Long-term steroids
   (e) Familial or racial

   (f) Smoking
   (g) Alcohol
   (h) Endocrine
       (i)   Lack of oestrogen
            (1) Oophorectomy
            (2) Hysterectomy
            (3) Obsessive athletes
            (4) Early menopause
       (ii) Lack of testosterone in men
       (iii) Cushing's syndrome
       (iv) Thyrotoxicosis
       (v) Hypopituitarism
   (i) Gastrointestinal
       (i)   Anorexia nervosa
       (ii) Starvation
       (iii) Coeliac disease
       (iv) IBD
       (v) Partial gastrectomy
       (vi) Liver disease
   (j) Bone disease
       (i)   Osteogenesis imperfecta
       (ii) RA
   (k) Multiple myeloma
   (l) Metastatic carcinoma
  (m) Drugs
       (i)   Heparin
       (ii) Cytotoxics
       (iii) Anticonvulsants
5 Treatment
   (a) Exercise
   (b) Stop smoking and reduce alcohol
   (c) Calcium and vitamin D
   (d) Bisphosphonates
   (e) Calcitonin
   (f) Strontium ranelate
   (g) Recombinant PTH

Essential features of fibromyalgia

1 Symptoms
  (a) Pain
      (i) Predominantly neck and back (may be all over)
      (ii) Aggravated by stress, cold, activity
  (b) Generalised morning stiffness
  (c) Paraesthesiae of hands and feet
  (d) Fatiguability
  (e) Non-restorative sleep
  (f) Headache
  (g) Diffuse abdominal pain and variable bowel habit
  (h) Urinary frequency
  (i) Dysmenorrhoea
2 Signs
  (a) Discordance between symptoms, disability and objective findings
  (b) No objective weakness, synovitis or neurological abnormality
  (c) Multiple hyperalgesic sites
  (d) Pronounced tenderness to rolling the mid-trapezius skin fold
  (e) Cutaneous hyperaemia after palpation of tender sites
  (f) Negative control sites

Malignant tumours of bone

[See Table 62, opposite]

Causes of avascular necrosis of bone

1 Corticosteroids/Cushing's
2 Fractured neck of femur
3 Severe OA/RA
4 Sickle cell disease
5 Heparin therapy
6 SLE
7 Pregnancy
8 Chronic exposure to raised barometric pressure (divers)
9 Alcohol
10 Diabetes
11 Obesity
12 Polycythaemia rubra vera

Table 62

Tumour	Age	Common sites	Behaviour	Treatment and prognosis
Osteosarcoma	Young adults	Long bones, especially distal femur and proximal tibia	Rapid growth, pain and swelling, lung mets	Surgery and chemotherapy 40% cure rate
Chondrosarcoma	35–60	Pelvis, ribs, spine, long bones	Slow enlargement, eventual vascular invasion	Surgery 75% cure rate
Fibrosarcoma and malignant fibrous histiocytoma	Any age, peak 30–40	Femur, tibia, humerus, pelvis	Local growth, vascular invasion	Surgery 40% cure rate
Ewing's sarcoma	Children and teenagers	Long bones, pelvis and ribs	Widespread mets	Chemotherapy 10% cure rate

13 Neuropathic joint
14 Bacterial endocarditis
15 Perthes' disease
16 Theimann's disease (AD, small joints of hands and feet)

Causes of Charcot's joints

1 Neurosyphilis
2 Syringomyelia
3 Myelomeningocoele
4 Leprosy
5 Diabetes
6 Charcot–Marie–Tooth disease

Rheumatological diseases associated with malignancy

1 Dermatomyositis – carcinoma
2 Scleroderma – adenocarcinoma
3 Primary Sjögren's syndrome – lymphoma
4 RA – lymphoma, myeloma

Causes of a very high ESR (> 100)

1 Multiple myeloma
2 Giant cell arteritis/PMR
3 Sepsis
4 Occult malignancy
5 SLE

DRUGS AND RHEUMATOLOGY

NSAIDs

1 Analgesic, antipyretic and anti-inflammatory action
2 Block cyclo-oxygenase (COX), which blocks the production of prostaglandins and thromboxanes
3 Varying degrees of COX 1 and COX 2 inhibition between drugs
4 COX 1 present in most tissues (largely responsible for side effects)
5 COX 2 present on inflammatory cells
6 Full analgesic effect after 1 week
7 Full anti-inflammatory effect after 3 weeks

8 Side effects
  (a) GI
    (i) Dyspepsia/gastritis/peptic ulceration
    (ii) Diarrhoea (including microscopic colitis)
    (iii) Hepatitis
  (b) CNS
    (i) Headache and dizziness
    (ii) Tinnitus
    (iii) Aseptic meningitis
  (c) CVS
    (i) Oedema
    (ii) Hypertension
    (iii) Heart failure
  (d) Respiratory
    (i) Asthma
    (ii) Pneumonitis
  (e) Blood
    (i) Neutropenia
    (ii) Thrombocytopenia
    (iii) Aplastic anaemia
    (iv) Haemolytic anaemia
  (f) Kidney
    (i) ARF
    (ii) Haematuria
    (iii) Nephrotic syndrome
    (iv) Papillary necrosis
    (v) Interstitial nephritis
  (g) Skin
    (i) Erythema multiforme
    (ii) Fixed drug eruption

COX 2 inhibitors (See page 71)

DMARDs

1 Hydroxychloroquine
  (a) Inhibits chemotaxis of eosinophils
  (b) Inhibits locomotion of neutrophils
  (c) Impairs complement-dependent antigen–antibody reactions
  (d) Side effects
    (i) Pruritic skin rash

    (ii) Pigmentation
    (iii) Maculopathy
    (iv) Leukopenia

2 Gold
  (a) Gold is taken up by macrophages
  (b) Inhibits phagocytosis of macrophage
  (c) Stabilises lysosomal membrane
  (d) Decreasing prostaglandin synthesis and lysosomal enzyme activity
  (e) Side effects
    (i)   Dermatitis (30%)
    (ii)   Stomatitis
    (iii) Proteinuria
    (iv) Thrombocytopenia
    (v)   Leukopenia
    (vi) Aplastic anaemia
    (vii) Diarrhoea

3 Penicillamine
  (a) Depresses circulating IgM rheumatoid factor and T-cell activity
  (b) Side effects
    (i)   Maculopapular rash
    (ii)   Nausea
    (iii) Loss of taste
    (iv) Mouth ulcers
    (v)   Proteinuria
    (vi) Nephrotic syndrome
    (vii) Drug-induced lupus
    (viii) Myasthenia gravis
    (ix) Pemphigus
    (x)   Goodpasture's syndrome
    (xi) Thrombocytopenia
    (xii) Pancytopenia

4 Sulphasalazine
  (a) Sulphasalazine is cleaved in the colon by bacterial enzymes to release acetylsalicylic acid and sulphapyridine
  (b) Sulphapyridine decreases inflammatory reactions and systemically inhibits prostaglandin synthesis
  (c) Side effects
    (i)   Nausea
    (ii) Skin rashes

   (iii) Allergic reactions
   (iv) Hepatitis
   (v) Pulmonary eosinophilia
   (vi) Macrocytosis
   (vii) Haemolytic anaemia
   (viii) Pancytopenia
   (ix) Reduced sperm (reversible)

5 Methotrexate
  (a) Folic acid antagonist cytotoxic drug
  (b) Binds to dihydrofolate reductase and interferes with DNA synthesis and cell replication
  (c) Side effects
    (i) Nausea
    (ii) Mouth ulcers
    (iii) Hepatic fibrosis
    (iv) Bone marrow suppression

6 Leflunomide
  (a) Inhibits replication of activated lymphocytes by blocking the synthesis of pyrimidines and DNA
  (b) Also has a weak anti-inflammatory action.
  (c) Side effects
    (i) Nausea
    (ii) Diarrhoea
    (iii) Skin rash
    (iv) Reversible alopecia
    (v) Hepatitis
    (vi) Bone marrow suppression

7 Anti-TNF-α drugs (See page 68)

Immunosuppressants

1 Cyclophosphamide
  (a) Alkylating agent
  (b) Powerful immunosuppressant that reduces both antibody-mediated and cell-mediated response
  (c) Side effects
    (i) Nausea and vomiting
    (ii) Haemorrhagic cystitis
    (iii) Bone marrow suppression

2 Ciclosporin (See page 66)

3 Azathioprine
   (a) Converted to 6-mercaptopurine (active)
   (b) Enzyme TPMT metabolises azathioprine, those with low TMPT levels at high risk of myelosuppression
   (c) Inhibits nucleic acid synthesis, suppressing cell-mediated hypersensitivity and altering antibody production
   (d) Side effects
      (i) Hypersensitivity reactions
      (ii) Nausea and vomiting
      (iii) Bone marrow suppression
      (iv) Pancreatitis
      (v) Alopecia
      (vi) Hepatotoxicity
      (vii) Increased susceptibility to infection

Self Assessment: Best of Five Questions and Answers

QUESTIONS

1 A 64-year-old patient presents with heartburn and has severe oesophagitis diagnosed by endoscopy. Which of the following is most likely to be the cause?
   □ (A) Nifedipine
   □ (B) Isosorbide mononitrate
   □ (C) Ramipril
   □ (D) Aspirin 75 mg
   □ (E) Alendronate

2 A 40-year-old patient has dysphagia for solids and liquids. Oesophageal manometry shows lack of relaxation of the lower oesophageal sphincter. What is the most appropriate treatment?
   □ (A) Omeprazole
   □ (B) Nifedipine
   □ (C) Isosorbide mononitrate
   □ (D) Endoscopic dilatation
   □ (E) Laparoscopic fundoplication

3 A 62-year-old patient presents with lethargy, diarrhoea and weight loss over the past month. He has had pains on and off in several of his large joints. Which of the following is most likely?

- ❑ (A) Whipple's disease
- ❑ (B) Chronic pancreatitis
- ❑ (C) Bacterial overgrowth
- ❑ (D) Lymphoma
- ❑ (E) Coeliac disease

4 A 60-year-old patient presents with gradually increasing abdominal girth. On examination he has ascites. An ascitic tap is taken and results are as follows: ascitic fluid protein 14 g/l, ascitic fluid albumin 4 g/l, serum albumin 26 g/l. Which of the following diagnoses can be ruled out?

- ❑ (A) Congestive cardiac failure
- ❑ (B) Liver cirrhosis
- ❑ (C) Constrictive pericarditis
- ❑ (D) Budd–Chiari syndrome
- ❑ (E) Malnutrition

5 A 12-week pregnant patient presents with severe vomiting and dehydration for the last 2 weeks. Blood results are as follows: bilirubin 16 µmol/l, ALT 90 u/l, albumin 36 g/l, ALP 216 u/l, prothrombin time 14 seconds, platelets 223 × 10^9, haemoglobin 11.3 g/dl. Which of the following is the most likely diagnosis?

- ❑ (A) Acute fatty liver of pregnancy
- ❑ (B) Pre-eclampsia
- ❑ (C) HELLP syndrome
- ❑ (D) Intrahepatic cholestasis of pregnancy
- ❑ (E) Hyperemesis gravidarum

6 A 43-year-old man recently had a flare-up of ulcerative colitis treated with steroids. He was commenced on azathioprine 3 weeks ago. He presents with a 2-day history of vomiting and severe abdominal pain. Which of these is the most likely diagnosis?

- ❑ (A) Small bowel obstruction
- ❑ (B) Pancreatitis
- ❑ (C) Toxic megacolon
- ❑ (D) Constipation
- ❑ (E) Gastroenteritis

7 A 31-year-old woman presents with anaemia. The following results are available: Hb 9.6 g/dl, ferritin 7 mg/l, B_{12} 390 pmol/l, folate 1.0 mg/l. Antiendomysial antibody negative. Which of the following investigations should be done first?
- ❏ (A) Barium follow-through
- ❏ (B) Colonoscopy and ileoscopy
- ❏ (C) Gastroscopy and duodenal biopsy
- ❏ (D) PABA test
- ❏ (E) Glycocholate breath test

8 A 39-year-old patient with long-standing ulcerative colitis presents with 2-week history of jaundice. The following results are available: bilirubin 96 μmol/l, ALP 1026 u/l, ALT 263 u/l, prothrombin time 13 seconds, albumin 35 g/l. Ultrasound shows a normal-sized liver. The common bile duct is normal and there are no gallstones. No abdominal masses are noted. Which would be the most appropriate next investigation?
- ❏ (A) ERCP
- ❏ (B) MRCP
- ❏ (C) Liver biopsy
- ❏ (D) CT abdomen
- ❏ (E) pANCA

9 A 16-year-old female is referred by her GP with jaundice that was noted by her family. She is otherwise asymptomatic. Blood results are as follows: total bilirubin 39 μmol/l, conjugated bilirubin 11 μmol/l, ALT 14 u/l, ALP 63 u/l, albumin 43 g/l. Hb 15.3 g/dl, reticulocytes 1.6%. What is the most likely diagnosis?
- ❏ (A) Gilbert's syndrome
- ❏ (B) Rotor syndrome
- ❏ (C) Dubin–Johnson syndrome
- ❏ (D) Gallstones
- ❏ (E) Autoimmune haemolytic anaemia

10 A patient presents with jaundice. The following results are available: HBs Ag +ve, HBeAg +ve, HBeAb –ve, HBc IgM –ve. Which of the following interpretations is correct?
- ❏ (A) Acute hepatitis B
- ❏ (B) Chronic hepatitis B with low infectivity
- ❏ (C) Chronic hepatitis B with high infectivity
- ❏ (D) Previous vaccination against hepatitis B
- ❏ (E) Natural immunity against hepatitis B

11 **A 43-year-old woman presents with a collapse and loss of consciousness while running for a bus. In addition, she complains of shortness of breath on exertion. She has no history of lung disease. On examination her BP is 110/90. What are the most likely findings on auscultation?**
   - ❑ (A) Pansystolic murmur loudest at the apex
   - ❑ (B) Pansystolic murmur at the left sternal edge
   - ❑ (C) Normal heart sounds
   - ❑ (D) Ejection systolic murmur that radiates to the neck
   - ❑ (E) Mid-diastolic murmur at the apex

12 **A 34-year-old man is admitted for a second time with atrial fibrillation. Last time he reverted to sinus rhythm spontaneously. He drinks a bottle of whisky every day. Which of the following treatments is most appropriate?**
   - ❑ (A) Amiodarone
   - ❑ (B) Digoxin and warfarin
   - ❑ (C) Digoxin
   - ❑ (D) Sotalol
   - ❑ (E) Sotalol and warfarin

13 **A 46-year-old woman is admitted following a collapse. She has recently noticed a reduced exercise capacity. Heart sounds are normal. ECG shows right axis deviation and tall R waves with T wave inversion in V1–V3. Chest X-ray is normal. What is the next most appropriate investigation?**
   - ❑ (A) V/Q scan
   - ❑ (B) Echocardiogram
   - ❑ (C) Exercise test
   - ❑ (D) Pulmonary function tests
   - ❑ (E) 24-hour tape

14 **A 35-year-old IV drug user is admitted with fever, cough and SOB. On examination he has a soft pansystolic murmur at the left sternal edge and a raised JVP with large V waves. Which of the following organisms is most likely to be grown in blood culture?**
   - ❑ (A) *Mycoplasma pneumoniae*
   - ❑ (B) *Pneumocystis carinii*
   - ❑ (C) *Staphylococcus aureus*
   - ❑ (D) *Pseudomonas aeruginosa*
   - ❑ (E) *Legionella pneumophila*

15 A 46-year-old man with known acute intermittent porphyria is found to be hypertensive. Which of the following antihypertensives is indicated?
- [ ] (A) Atenolol
- [ ] (B) Verapamil
- [ ] (C) Nifedipine
- [ ] (D) Ramipril
- [ ] (E) Frusemide

16 A 43-year-old patient who is known to have Wolff–Parkinson–White syndrome is admitted with palpitations. The pulse is 180/min, BP 101/62. ECG shows a narrow complex tachycardia. There was no response to carotid sinus massage. What is the most appropriate next step?
- [ ] (A) DC cardioversion
- [ ] (B) Adenosine
- [ ] (C) Verapamil
- [ ] (D) Amiodarone
- [ ] (E) Digoxin

17 A 41-year-old woman presented to her GP with shortness of breath. On auscultation she has fixed splitting of the second heart sound. ECG shows partial RBBB and right axis deviation. Chest X ray shows prominent pulmonary vasculature. What is the most likely diagnosis?
- [ ] (A) Fallot's tetralogy
- [ ] (B) VSD
- [ ] (C) PDA
- [ ] (D) Ostium secundum ASD
- [ ] (E) Ostium primum ASD

18 A 28-year-old patient is found to have a BP of 206/122 during a work medical. Urine dipstick is negative. ECG shows left ventricular hypertrophy. Blood results are as follows: Na 143 mmol/l, K 2.5 mmol/l, HCO_3 40 mmol/l, urea 4.1 mmol/l, creatinine 87 µmol/l. Which of the following tests should be done to determine the underlying diagnosis?
- [ ] (A) Echocardiogram
- [ ] (B) Serum renin and aldosterone
- [ ] (C) Urinary catecholamines
- [ ] (D) Renal biopsy
- [ ] (E) Glucose tolerance test

19 An 86-year-old woman is admitted with epistaxis. She had been on warfarin for 10 years for atrial fibrillation. INR is >10. She had been seen by her GP 5 days earlier for a cough and was started on an antibiotic, but she can't remember which one. Which of the following is most likely?

- ☐ (A) Erythromycin
- ☐ (B) Rifampicin
- ☐ (C) Penicillin V
- ☐ (D) Doxycycline
- ☐ (E) Amoxicillin

20 Regarding the treatment of breast cancer, which of the following statements is correct?

- ☐ (A) All patients with breast cancer should be offered treatment with tamoxifen
- ☐ (B) Anastrazole is more effective at preventing recurrence but has more menopausal side effects than tamoxifen
- ☐ (C) Hypocalcaemia is a recognised side effect of tamoxifen
- ☐ (D) Tamoxifen should be continued indefinitely for oestrogen receptor-positive tumours
- ☐ (E) Patients on tamoxifen are at increased risk of thromboembolism

21 A 48-year-old woman is a diet-controlled diabetic. Sugars have been running at 13 mmol/l. HbA_{1c} is 7.9%, BMI 32. Which of the following is most appropriate?

- ☐ (A) Metformin
- ☐ (B) Gliclazide
- ☐ (C) Further dietary advice
- ☐ (D) Insulin
- ☐ (E) Rosiglitazone

22 A 23-year-old man is admitted 6 hours after taking an overdose of an unknown quantity of tablets. He is sweating and hyperventilating. ECG shows sinus tachycardia with U waves. Blood gases are as follows: pH 7.21, Po_2 14.0 kPa, Pco_2 2.1 kPa, HCO_3 10 mmol/l. Blood glucose is 2.3 mmol/l. What is the most likely substance that has been ingested?

- ☐ (A) Paracetamol
- ☐ (B) Aspirin
- ☐ (C) Aminophylline
- ☐ (D) Iron
- ☐ (E) Amitriptyline

23 **A 42-year-old Afro-Caribbean man presents with fever, dry cough and joint pains. On examination his chest is clear. He has multiple tender warm erythematous nodules on both shins. Which of the following tests is most likely to provide a diagnosis?**
- ❑ (A) Blood culture
- ❑ (B) Chest X-ray
- ❑ (C) Sputum culture and TB smear
- ❑ (D) Heaf test
- ❑ (E) Skin biopsy

24 **A 62-year-old man presents with a lump in the anterior neck. He has no symptoms of thyrotoxicosis. He also has a hoarse voice. Fine-needle aspiration suggests papillary carcinoma. Which of the following is correct?**
- ❑ (A) Hoarse voice suggests invasion of the larynx
- ❑ (B) Calcitonin is typically raised
- ❑ (C) Most patients have distant metastases at presentation
- ❑ (D) Histology may show psammoma bodies
- ❑ (E) Most cases are familial

25 **A patient presents with weight gain, diabetes and hypertension. Bloods show: Na 146 mmol/l, K 2.4 mmol/l, urea 6.2 mmol/l, creatinine 112 μmol/l. Urinary free cortisol is elevated. Which of the following is correct?**
- ❑ (A) Low ACTH suggests pituitary adenoma
- ❑ (B) No suppression following high-dose dexamethasone suppression test suggests ectopic ACTH production
- ❑ (C) ACTH level is useful at differentiating pituitary adenoma from ectopic ACTH
- ❑ (D) All pituitary adenomas will be seen with MRI scanning
- ❑ (E) Patients with low ACTH should have an MRI pituitary

26 **A patient is 24 weeks pregnant and presents with weight loss. Examination reveals a goitre. Bloods show TSH 0.01 mu/l, FT$_4$ 29 pmol/l. Which of the following statements is correct?**
- ❑ (A) Radioiodine treatment should be given as soon as possible
- ❑ (B) Carbimazole may cause fetal hypothyroidism
- ❑ (C) Propranolol should be given for symptomatic relief
- ❑ (D) Carbimazole treatment will lead to rapid improvement in symptoms
- ❑ (E) Thyroxine is the treatment of choice

27 **Regarding pemphigus, which of the following statements is correct?**
☐ (A) Blistering is usually widespread
☐ (B) Mucous membranes are rarely involved
☐ (C) Treatment with low-dose steroids is effective
☐ (D) IgM autoantibodies against the epidermis are present in 90%
☐ (E) Blisters are typically tense

28 **A 6-year-old girl is referred for genetic counselling. Her mother had a thyroid cancer removed. Histology showed medullary carcinoma. Which of the following statements are correct?**
☐ (A) Medullary carcinoma of the thyroid is associated with Bcl-1 oncogene
☐ (B) Most patients with MEN2 develop medullary carcinoma of the thyroid
☐ (C) Phaeochromocytoma is not associated with medullary carcinoma of thyroid
☐ (D) Patients with medullary carcinoma of thyroid may have hyperprolactinaemia
☐ (E) MEN1 patients should have prophylactic thyroidectomy

29 **A 27-week pregnant patient is admitted with diarrhoea and vomiting. She was noted to have pigmentation around the mouth. BP is 90/60, blood glucose 3.5 mmol/l, Na 126 mmol/l, K 4.9, urea 8.2 mmol/l, creatinine 117 μmol/l. Which of the following tests is most likely to provide a diagnosis?**
☐ (A) Stool culture
☐ (B) Short synacthen test
☐ (C) 24-hour urinary cortisol
☐ (D) Urinary porphyrins
☐ (E) Endomysial antibody

30 **A patient is admitted with a collapse. On arrival the blood glucose is 2.1 mmol/l. The patient is taking no medications. Which of the following is correct?**
☐ (A) High serum insulin with high C peptide suggests insulin overdose
☐ (B) High serum insulin and high C peptide suggests insulinoma
☐ (C) Urinary catecholamines may be raised
☐ (D) 24-hour urinary cortisol may be raised
☐ (E) Insulin antibodies may be present in the blood

31 A patient is found unconscious following an overdose of an unknown drug. On arrival at A & E the patient has a seizure, which self-terminates after 30 seconds. GCS is 3/15, respiratory rate 5/min, oxygen saturation 78%. The patient is intubated. Initial ECG showed wide QRS complex of 140 ms and a prolonged QTc interval with tachycardia of 110/min. Blood gases before intubation are pH 7.12, P_{O_2} 7.6 kPa, P_{CO_2} 7.7 kPa, HCO_3 12 mmol/l. The patient develops a broad complex tachycardia 180/min after intubation and BP drops to 90/45. What is the most appropriate management?
- [ ] (A) IV amiodarone
- [ ] (B) IV lignocaine
- [ ] (C) IV bicarbonate
- [ ] (D) IV magnesium
- [ ] (E) IV potassium

32 A patients presents with deafness in the right ear. On examination there are three *café-au-lait* spots. He has a spastic paraparesis following spinal surgery for a 'tumour'. Which of the following other features could he have?
- [ ] (A) Peripheral schwannomas
- [ ] (B) Lisch nodules
- [ ] (C) Ash leaf macules
- [ ] (D) Subungal fibromas
- [ ] (E) Adenoma sebum

33 A 18-year-old patient has short stature and is being investigated for amenorrhoea. Buccal smear shows absent Barr body. Which of these features is most likely to be present?
- [ ] (A) Webbed neck
- [ ] (B) Rocker-bottom feet
- [ ] (C) Clinodactyly
- [ ] (D) Fallot's tetralogy
- [ ] (E) Ptosis

34 Regarding the HIV virus, which of the following statements is true?
- [ ] (A) HIV is a reovirus
- [ ] (B) HIV has an affinity for T-helper cells
- [ ] (C) HIV is a DNA virus with the enzyme reverse transcriptase
- [ ] (D) Leads to depletion of CD8 cells
- [ ] (E) HIV2 is the most common in the UK

35 **A 20-year-old patient complains of ankle swelling and breathlessness. Blood tests show urea 7 mmol/l, creatinine 80 µmol/l, Na 138 mmol/l, K 4.2 mmol/l, ALT 20 u/l, bilirubin 16 µmol/l, albumin 20 g/l, total cholesterol 9.2 mmol/l. What is the next best investigation?**
   - ❑ (A) Urine dipstick
   - ❑ (B) ANA
   - ❑ (C) 24-hour urinary protein
   - ❑ (D) Urine microscopy
   - ❑ (E) 24-hour creatinine clearance

36 **A patient is admitted with confusion. Results are as follows: Na 123 mmol/l, K 3.5 mmol/l, urea 1.2 mmol/l, creatinine 46 µmol/l, serum osmolality 243 mmol/kg, urine osmolality 726 mmol/kg, urine Na 46. Which of the following is the most appropriate initial treatment?**
   - ❑ (A) Hypertonic saline
   - ❑ (B) DDAVP
   - ❑ (C) Fluid restriction
   - ❑ (D) Rehydrate with normal saline
   - ❑ (E) Chlorpropamide

37 **A 16-year-old boy presents with central abdominal pain and haematuria for the last week. He has also had pain in both knees. Examination reveals a non-blanching rash on his legs. Urine dipstix blood ++, protein +. Bloods show urea 26.3 mmol/l, creatinine 289 µmol/l. What is the renal biopsy most likely to show?**
   - ❑ (A) Podocyte formation
   - ❑ (B) Mesangial IgA deposition
   - ❑ (C) Thickening of the basement membrane
   - ❑ (D) Focal segmental glomerulosclerosis
   - ❑ (E) Crescent formation

38 **A patient presents after a collapse 24 hours earlier. Bloods show Na 143 mmol/l, K 7.2 mmol/l, urea 11.1 mmol/l, creatinine 980 µmol/l, PO_4 2.1 mmol/l. Which is the test most likely confirm the diagnosis?**
   - ❑ (A) Ultrasound abdomen
   - ❑ (B) ANCA
   - ❑ (C) CK
   - ❑ (D) Urinary myoglobin
   - ❑ (E) Urine dipstick for blood

39 **A patient is admitted with oliguria. Bloods show Na 128 mmol/l, K 7.2 mmol/l, urea 42.6 mmol/l, creatinine 828 μmol/l. ECG shows tenting of the T waves. Which of the following treatment should be given first?**
- ❑ (A) Calcium gluconate
- ❑ (B) Calcium resonium
- ❑ (C) Insulin and dextrose
- ❑ (D) Salbutamol nebulisers
- ❑ (E) Intravenous saline

40 **A patient presents with oliguria. Bloods show urea 42 mmol/l and 734 μmol/l. Bloods were normal 2 weeks previously. Urine microscopy shows numerous eosinophils. Which of the following is most likely?**
- ❑ (A) Wegener's granulomatosis
- ❑ (B) Interstitial nephritis secondary to drug reaction
- ❑ (C) Goodpasture's syndrome
- ❑ (D) Mesangiocapillary glomerulonephritis
- ❑ (E) Post-streptococcal glomerulonephritis

41 **A 42-year-old woman is admitted with SOB and hypoxia. Chest X-ray shows bilateral pneumonia. BP was 82/54 on admission and remained at this level despite aggressive fluid resuscitation. Blood cultures grew *Streptococcus pneumoniae*. 24 hours after admission bloods show Na 142 mmol/l, K 3.9 mmol/l, urea 20.4 mmol/l, creatinine 280 μmol/l. Which of the following is the most likely cause?**
- ❑ (A) Acute tubular necrosis
- ❑ (B) Mesangioproliferative glomerulonephritis
- ❑ (C) Diffuse proliferative glomerulonephritis
- ❑ (D) Rapidly progressive glomerulonephritis
- ❑ (E) Membranous glomerulonephritis

42 **A patient is under investigation for polyuria. Plasma osmolality is 301 mmol/kg. Following water deprivation urine osmolality is 264 mmol/kg, post DDAVP urine osmolality is 696 mmol/kg. What is the diagnosis?**
- ❑ (A) Normal
- ❑ (B) Nephrogenic diabetes insipidus
- ❑ (C) Cranial diabetes insipidus
- ❑ (D) Primary polyuria
- ❑ (E) SIADH

43 A patient is admitted with wheeze and an urticarial rash 20 minutes after the ingestion of ciprofloxacin for a urinary tract infection. Which of the following is correct?

☐ (A) This is a type 2 hypersensitivity reaction

☐ (B) Serum IgE will be low

☐ (C) Antihistamines are of no benefit

☐ (D) Intravenous adrenaline is the treatment of choice

☐ (E) Binding of IgE to mast cells leads to a release of histamine

44 A 22-year-old man presents with swelling of the right leg. DVT is confirmed. He had a previous DVT 2 years ago with no obvious precipitant. He also complains of dark urine. Blood shows a total bilirubin of 36 μmol/l, with other liver function tests normal. Reticulocyte count is 4% (0.5–2%). Which of the following is most likely?

☐ (A) Paroxysmal nocturnal haemoglobinuria

☐ (B) Homocystinuria

☐ (C) Protein C deficiency

☐ (D) Protein S deficiency

☐ (E) Factor V Leiden deficiency

45 A 24-year-old IV drug user presents with gradually increasing shortness of breath and a dry cough over the last 2 weeks. He has had fevers at night. He has had no chest pain. Temperature is 38.1°C. Saturations on air are 82%, Respiratory rate is 28/min. Chest is clear on examination. Chest X-ray shows bilateral perihilar shadowing. Which of the following tests should be performed next?

☐ (A) Sputum for TB

☐ (B) Bronchoscopy and BAL

☐ (C) CTPA

☐ (D) Blood culture

☐ (E) Induced sputum for *Pneumocystis*

46 A 28-year-old woman has recently been diagnosed with migraine. She has two episodes per week, with limited relief from sumatriptan. Which of the following should be prescribed next?

☐ (A) Carbamazepine

☐ (B) Valproate

☐ (C) Paracetamol

☐ (D) Propranolol

☐ (E) Tramadol

47 An 82-year-old man is admitted 'off legs'. He has a history of type 2 diabetes, but no other past history. Examination reveals ⅕ power in both legs. Pain and temperature sensation is lost, but vibration and joint position sense is preserved. What is the diagnosis?
   - (A) Brown–Séquard syndrome
   - (B) Subacute combined degeneration of the cord
   - (C) Syringomyelia
   - (D) Anterior spinal artery occlusion
   - (E) Spinal cord compression

48 A 42-year-old patient presents with double vision on looking to the right. On examination, there is nystagmus at rest. On looking to the right the right eye abducts normally but the left eye fails to adduct. Otherwise eye movements are normal. What is the diagnosis?
   - (A) Lesion of the left medial longitudinal fasciculus
   - (B) Sixth-nerve palsy
   - (C) Third-nerve palsy
   - (D) Lesion of the right medial longitudinal fasciculus
   - (E) Cerebellopontine angle tumour

49 Regarding COX 2 inhibitors, which of the following statements is correct?
   - (A) COX 2 inhibitors should be used instead of non-selective NSAIDs in those with heart failure
   - (B) COX 2 inhibitors are safe to use in those with active peptic ulceration
   - (C) Stevens–Johnson syndrome is a recognised side effect
   - (D) COX 2 inhibitors should be used instead of non-selective NSAIDs in renal failure
   - (E) COX 2 inhibitors should be used in those patients who are on aspirin, as GI side effects are reduced compared to those taking non-selective NSAIDs

50 A patient presents with bilateral leg weakness and urinary incontinence. Ankle jerks are lost. There is loss of sensation around the perineum. Which is the most likely diagnosis?
   - (A) Normal pressure hydrocephalus
   - (B) Cauda equina compression
   - (C) Syringomyelia
   - (D) Subacute combined degeneration of the cord
   - (E) CJD

51 A 62-year-old patient presents with weakness of the hands. On examination there is wasting of the small muscles of the hand with fasciculation. There is no sensory loss. Which of the following is most likely?

- ❑ (A) Motor neurone disease
- ❑ (B) Hereditary motor and sensory neuropathy
- ❑ (C) Cervical spondylosis
- ❑ (D) Bilateral combined ulnar and median nerve palsies
- ❑ (E) Syringomyelia

52 A patient is admitted with a seizure and reduced conscious level. Lumbar puncture reveals protein 0.8 g/l, glucose 3.5 mmol/l (blood 5). White cell count 80/mm³, 90% lymphocytes. Which of the following tests will provide a diagnosis?

- ❑ (A) HSV PCR
- ❑ (B) CSF Gram stain and culture
- ❑ (C) CSF for TB
- ❑ (D) Blood culture
- ❑ (E) CT brain

53 A 46-year-old man presents with severe headache and pyrexia. He has no rash. Lumbar puncture shows protein 1.0 g/l, glucose 2.1 mmol/l (blood 6) White cell count 160/mm³, 90% polymorphs. Gram stain shows Gram-negative diplococci. What is the cause?

- ❑ (A) *Pneumococcus*
- ❑ (B) *Meningococcus*
- ❑ (C) *Listeria*
- ❑ (D) *Mycobacterium tuberculosis*
- ❑ (E) *Haemophilus influenzae*

54 An 82-year-old diabetic patient presents with dysphagia and dysphonia. On examination there is a right-sided Horner's syndrome and nystagmus. There is loss of pain and temperature on the right side of the face and left-sided loss of pain and temperature on the body. Which of the following arteries is occluded?

- ❑ (A) Left posterior inferior cerebellar
- ❑ (B) Right posterior inferior cerebellar
- ❑ (C) Left posterior superior cerebellar
- ❑ (D) Right posterior superior cerebellar
- ❑ (E) Middle cerebral

55 A patient is noted to have ptosis of the right eye with a small pupil. Which of the following is the most likely?
- ❑ (A) Myotonic dystrophy
- ❑ (B) Pilocarpine eye drops
- ❑ (C) Myasthenia gravis
- ❑ (D) Third-nerve palsy
- ❑ (E) Tropicamide eye drops

56 A patient presents with sudden loss of vision in the right eye. On examination there is a pale fundus and an afferent pupillary defect. What is the most likely cause?
- ❑ (A) Retinal artery occlusion
- ❑ (B) Retinal vein thrombosis
- ❑ (C) Optic neuritis
- ❑ (D) Anterior uveitis
- ❑ (E) Acute glaucoma

57 A 40-year-old man is admitted with severe right-sided headache and vomiting. He complains of blurring of vision and pain is behind the right eye. On examination there are prominent vessels around the cornea. What is the most appropriate next step?
- ❑ (A) CT head
- ❑ (B) Reassure and treat with sumatriptan
- ❑ (C) Measure ocular pressure
- ❑ (D) Lumbar puncture
- ❑ (E) Reassure and treat with diclofenac

58 Which of the following statements is correct regarding acute alcohol withdrawal?
- ❑ (A) Pyrexia usually suggests underlying infection
- ❑ (B) Seizures are rare
- ❑ (C) Visual hallucinations suggest coexistent psychiatric disorder
- ❑ (D) Hypophosphataemia is commonly seen
- ❑ (E) All patients who have a seizure should be commenced on an antiepileptic

59 Regarding sulfasalazine, which of the following statements is correct?
- ❑ (A) 5-ASA is the active component which is absorbed to have systemic anti-inflammatory activity
- ❑ (B) Irreversible azoospermia is a side effect
- ❑ (C) Can safely be given to those with aspirin allergy
- ❑ (D) Acetylator status is important in its metabolism
- ❑ (E) Black females are at risk of haemolysis

60 A 20-year-old intravenous drug user presents with a painful swollen right knee. On examination he is pyrexial and the knee is hot and has a large effusion. Frank pus is aspirated and the Gram stain is positive. Which is the most likely organism?

- ❑ (A) *Staphylococcus aureus*
- ❑ (B) *Pseudomonas*
- ❑ (C) *Escherichia coli*
- ❑ (D) *Haemophilus influenzae*
- ❑ (E) *Neisseria gonorrhoeae*

61 A 30-year-old man presents with pain affecting the right knee and left ankle. On further questioning he complained of dysuria and had woken with both eyes 'stuck together' for the last 3 days. He had diarrhoea the week before. Which of the following is most likely to be the cause?

- ❑ (A) *E. coli*
- ❑ (B) *Staphylococcus aureus*
- ❑ (C) *Clostridium perfringens*
- ❑ (D) *Pseudomonas*
- ❑ (E) *Salmonella*

62 A patient presents with tetany. ECG shows a prolonged QT interval. The patient had been taking ciclosporin for 2 months for severe ulcerative colitis. Which of the following is the most likely cause?

- ❑ (A) Hypokalaemia
- ❑ (B) Hypocalcaemia
- ❑ (C) Hypomagnesaemia
- ❑ (D) Hypophosphataemia
- ❑ (E) Zinc deficiency

63 A 40-year-old woman is referred for investigation of hypertension. On examination she has a beaked nose and telangiectasia of the face. There is evidence of tight waxy skin of the fingers, with calcification on one finger. She has had Raynaud's for many years. Which of the following autoantibodies is most likely to be positive?

- ❑ (A) Anticentromere antibody
- ❑ (B) Anti-Scl-70
- ❑ (C) Anti-RNP antibody
- ❑ (D) Anti-Ro antibody
- ❑ (E) Anti-Jo-1 antibody

64 A 4-year-old child presents with a fever. On examination there is conjunctival injection and cervical lymphadenopathy. Over the body there is a generalised macular rash and desquamation of the hands. Which is the most likely diagnosis?

- ❑ (A) Scalded skin syndrome
- ❑ (B) Kawasaki's disease
- ❑ (C) Parvovirus B_{19} infection
- ❑ (D) Scarlet fever
- ❑ (E) Henoch–Schönlein purpura

65 A patient with known hepatitis C presents with arthralgia for 4 weeks. On examination there is a purpuric rash on the legs. He has a history of Raynaud's disease and dry eyes. Which of the following is the most likely diagnosis?

- ❑ (A) Meningococcal septicaemia
- ❑ (B) Cryoglobulinaemia
- ❑ (C) Scurvy
- ❑ (D) Henoch–Schönlein purpura
- ❑ (E) Lymphoma

66 A 32-year-old woman presents with progressive weakness of the arms and legs over 1 week. Three weeks earlier she had diarrhoea. Examination confirms distal weakness and 'glove and stocking' sensory loss. Which of the following statements is correct?

- ❑ (A) CSF will show very raised protein and white cell count
- ❑ (B) GD1a antibodies may be present
- ❑ (C) Nerve conduction studies usually show axonal loss
- ❑ (D) Regular peak flows should be performed 4 hourly
- ❑ (E) MRI of the spine is the investigation of choice

67 A patient complains that over the last year he has had a constant 'runny nose' and recurrent nosebleeds. For the last week he has been coughing up blood. Blood results show: CRP 160 mg/l, ESR 79 mm/h, Hb 10.6 g/dl, urea 32 mmol/l, creatinine 364 µmol/l. What is the next most appropriate investigation?

- ❑ (A) Bronchoscopy
- ❑ (B) CT chest
- ❑ (C) ANCA
- ❑ (D) Sputum for cytology and TB
- ❑ (E) Pulmonary function tests

68 A 24-year-old man presents with jaundice. On examination he has signs of chronic liver disease and has a tremor and dysarthria. Bloods show bilirubin 364, AST 114 u/l, ALT 68 u/l, ALP 42 u/l, albumin 24 g/l, PT 41 seconds. Which of the following results would you expect?

- ❑ (A) Ferritin 1268 mg/l
- ❑ (B) ANA 1:320
- ❑ (C) α_1-Antitrypsin 0.2
- ❑ (D) PANCA +ve
- ❑ (E) Caeruloplasmin <0.1

69 A 24-year-old woman presents with severe abdominal pain and vomiting. She was started on the oral contraceptive pill 3 days earlier. She is confused, hypertensive and tachycardic. Blood tests show Na 118 mmol/l. Which of the following can be given to control the pain?

- ❑ (A) Diclofenac
- ❑ (B) Morphine
- ❑ (C) Mebeverine
- ❑ (D) Buscopan
- ❑ (E) Ketorolac

70 As part of a routine medical, bloods are taken from a 40-year-old man. He has xanthelasma around his eyes. Results show total cholesterol 11.2 mmol/l, triglycerides 1.8 mmol/l. Which of the following is the most likely cause?

- ❑ (A) Familial hypercholesterolaemia
- ❑ (B) Alcohol excess
- ❑ (C) Familial hypertriglyceridaemia
- ❑ (D) Lipoprotein lipase deficiency
- ❑ (E) Familial combined hyperlipidaemia

71 An 82-year-old woman is admitted with dysuria and confusion. She is treated with ciprofloxacin for 3 days and develops diarrhoea. Pulse is 82/min. BP 140/78, temperature 37.4°C. Abdomen is mildly tender throughout, but no guarding. Bloods show WCC 28.7 × 10⁹ (was 11.6). Which of the following is most likely?

- ❑ (A) Antibiotic-associated diarrhoea
- ❑ (B) MRSA enteritis
- ❑ (C) *Clostridium difficile*
- ❑ (D) Quinolone-resistant UTI
- ❑ (E) Overflow diarrhoea

72 A 2-year-old patient presents with a large bruise on the thigh following a fall. Investigations show Hb 11.2 g/dl, platelets 186 × 10^9/l, PT 13.6 seconds, APTT 70 seconds, Factor VIII:C levels are low, bleeding time normal. Which of the following is most likely?

- (A) Haemophilia A
- (B) Von Willebrand's disease
- (C) Vitamin K deficiency
- (D) Childhood cirrhosis
- (E) Haemophilia B

73 A 50-year-old patient is found collapsed and confused. No history is available. Blood results are as follows: Na 130 mmol/l, K 4.0 mmol/l, urea 6.0 mmol/l, creatinine 78 μmol/l, glucose 6.0 mmol/l, Cl 97 mmol/l, HCO$_3$ 13 mmol/l, serum osmolality 300 mmol/kg. Which of the following is the most likely cause?

- (A) Salicylate overdose
- (B) Paraquat poisoning
- (C) Amitriptyline
- (D) Digoxin overdose
- (E) Ethylene glycol

74 A 16-year-old diabetic is investigated for poor mobility and reduced coordination. Examination reveals dysarthria, pes cavus and kyphoscoliosis. She has a wide-based gait and past pointing. Which of the following statements is correct?

- (A) Autosomal dominant inheritance is typical
- (B) Inheritance of the fibrillin gene is responsible
- (C) Children of this patient who inherit the disease will have more severe disease
- (D) Inheritance is by mitochondrial genes
- (E) Non-disjunction is responsible for this condition

75 An 18-year-old woman presents with acute shortness of breath with stridor, facial oedema and severe abdominal pain. She was recently started on the oral contraceptive pill. What is the likely diagnosis?

- (A) Anaphylaxis
- (B) Cl esterase deficiency
- (C) Drug reaction
- (D) Polycystic ovarian disease
- (E) Epiglottitis

76 Regarding antibiotics, which of the following antibiotics is correctly paired with its mechanism of action?
   □ (A) Erythromycin, inhibits DNA gyrase
   □ (B) Ciprofloxacin inhibits transpeptidase
   □ (C) Trimethoprim inhibits dihydrofolate reductase
   □ (D) Isoniazid inhibits RNA polymerase
   □ (E) Penicillin inhibits bacterial protein synthesis

77 An 82-year-old woman is admitted with confusion and dysuria. Urine dipstick for leukocytes is positive. Which of the following is the most likely organism?
   □ (A) *Proteus*
   □ (B) *Klebsiella*
   □ (C) MRSA
   □ (D) *Enterococcus*
   □ (E) *E. coli*

78 A patient presents with excessive thirst and abdominal pain. Bloods show Ca 3.02 mmol/l, PO$_4$ 0.42 mmol/l ALP 324 u/l. Which of the following is the most likely cause?
   □ (A) Excess vitamin D
   □ (B) Renal failure
   □ (C) Primary hyperparathyroidism
   □ (D) Bone metastases
   □ (E) Pseudohyperparathyroidism

79 A patient presents with fever, rigors and confusion 14 days after returning from Nigeria. Examination reveals mild jaundice and splenomegaly. Some of the bloods show: WCC 9.8 × 10^9, Hb 9.8 g/l, platelets 54 × 10^9, bilirubin 54 µmol/l, glucose 3.6 mmol/l. Which of the following is most likely?
   □ (A) Dengue fever
   □ (B) Yellow fever
   □ (C) Typhoid
   □ (D) HIV
   □ (E) Malaria

80 Regarding amoebic liver abscess, which of the following is correct?
   □ (A) Daughter cysts are characteristic
   □ (B) Metronidazole alone is the treatment of choice
   □ (C) Amoebic abscesses are more common in the right lobe
   □ (D) Most patients are asymptomatic
   □ (E) Stool culture is the investigation of choice

81 **Which of the following is correct regarding syphilis?**
- [ ] (A) Chancre is characteristic of tertiary syphilis
- [ ] (B) In primary syphilis VDRL, TPHA and FTA are positive
- [ ] (C) Generalised lymphadenopathy is a feature of secondary syphilis
- [ ] (D) The incubation period for syphilis is around 8 weeks
- [ ] (E) Gummas are characteristic of primary syphilis

82 **A patient presents with shortness of breath. Chest X-ray shows pleural effusion. The aspirate has a protein content of 38 g/l. Which of the following is least likely?**
- [ ] (A) Pancreatitis
- [ ] (B) Hypothyroidism
- [ ] (C) Rheumatoid arthritis
- [ ] (D) Pulmonary embolism
- [ ] (E) Tuberculosis

83 **Regarding drug-induced pulmonary disease, which of the following statements is true?**
- [ ] (A) Methotrexate may cause pulmonary eosinophilia
- [ ] (B) Amiodarone causes asthma
- [ ] (C) Carbamazepine may cause bronchospasm
- [ ] (D) Paraquat ingestion causes pulmonary fibrosis
- [ ] (E) Azathioprine causes pulmonary eosinophilia

84 **Regarding Goodpasture's syndrome, which of the following is true?**
- [ ] (A) There is a strong association with HLA DR2
- [ ] (B) The antigen for anti-GBM antibody is type 3 collagen
- [ ] (C) Membranous glomerulonephritis is typical
- [ ] (D) Eosinophilic pulmonary infiltrate is typical
- [ ] (E) Pulmonary haemorrhage is more common in non-smokers

85 **A patient presents with a dry cough and shortness of breath for 3 days. He complains of a severe headache, joint pain and muscle aches. There are multiple 'target lesions' on the skin. Chest X-ray shows bilateral patchy consolidation. Which of the following is most likely to be present?**
- [ ] (A) Low CD4 count
- [ ] (B) Cryoglobulins
- [ ] (C) Cold agglutinins
- [ ] (D) Malarial parasites
- [ ] (E) Raised serum ACE

86 Regarding blood films, which of the following statements is true?
- ☐ (A) Helmet cells are typical of myelofibrosis
- ☐ (B) Target cells can be seen in thalassaemia
- ☐ (C) Sickle cells are seen following splenectomy
- ☐ (D) Pencil cells are seen in B_{12} deficiency
- ☐ (E) Burr cells are seen in haemolysis

87 Regarding lung cancer, which of the following statements is true?
- ☐ (A) Hypercalcaemia mediated by PTHrP occurs in small cell lung cancer
- ☐ (B) Voltage gated calcium channel antibodies are a feature of squamous cell cancer
- ☐ (C) Small cell cancer leads to hypertrophic pulmonary osteoarthropathy
- ☐ (D) SIADH is common in squamous cell cancer
- ☐ (E) Cavitating tumours are mostly squamous cell carcinoma

88 A 60-year-old man presents with haemoptysis for the last 2 days. He has had a productive cough for 7 years, which has gradually worsened. He is particularly bad in the winter and has had several courses of antibiotics from his GP. He had TB aged 20. On examination, he is clubbed and has florid crepitations in both lower zones. Which of the following test is most likely to provide the diagnosis?
- ☐ (A) Spirometry
- ☐ (B) CXR
- ☐ (C) Bronchoscopy and biopsy
- ☐ (D) High-resolution CT chest
- ☐ (E) Staging CT chest

89 The following spirometry results are:

	Measured	Expected
FEV_1	2.59 litres	3.46 litres
FVC	3.16 litres	4.21 litres
Ratio	82%	81%

Which of the following is the most likely cause?
- ☐ (A) Asthma
- ☐ (B) Emphysema
- ☐ (C) Bronchiectasis
- ☐ (D) ABPA
- ☐ (E) Asbestosis

90 **Regarding thrombophilia, which of the following statements is correct?**
   - ❑ (A) Skin necrosis may occur in patients with protein C deficiency on warfarin
   - ❑ (B) Protein C production is independent of vitamin K
   - ❑ (C) Most patients with anticardiolipin antibody have SLE
   - ❑ (D) Thrombosis, thrombocytosis and recurrent miscarriage suggests antiphospholipid antibody syndrome
   - ❑ (E) Antithrombin III deficiency is the most common inherited cause of thrombosis

91 **A 64-year-old smoker presents with a 6 kg weight loss in the last 2 months. He has a chronic cough. Chest X-ray shows a right pleural effusion. Pleural aspirate shows protein 42 g/dl and LDH 642 Iu/l. What is the best next investigation?**
   - ❑ (A) CT chest
   - ❑ (B) Bronchoscopy
   - ❑ (C) Sputum for cytology
   - ❑ (D) Thoracoscopy and biopsy
   - ❑ (E) Spirometry

92 **Which of the following statements is correct regarding haemolysis?**
   - ❑ (A) Hereditary spherocytosis is autosomal recessive
   - ❑ (B) Erythromycin may cause haemolysis in those with G6PD deficiency
   - ❑ (C) Methyldopa causes haemolysis in those with G6PD deficiency
   - ❑ (D) Malaria typically causes an immune-mediated haemolytic anaemia
   - ❑ (E) Haemolysis occurs in pyruvate kinase deficiency

93 **A 60-year-old man complains of several lumps in the neck and groin that have appeared over the last month. On further questioning he complains of night sweats and some weight loss. He complains of neck and groin pain after drinking alcohol. Which of the following is the most likely diagnosis?**
   - ❑ (Λ) Toxoplasmosis
   - ❑ (B) HIV
   - ❑ (C) Low-grade lymphoma
   - ❑ (D) Hodgkin's disease
   - ❑ (E) Syphilis

94 A 64-year-old patient complains presents with multiple
bruises on the arms and legs. Coagulation studies are as
follows: PT 24.4 seconds, APTT 52 seconds, platelets 46 ×
10⁹/l. Which of the following is most likely?
- (A) Warfarin therapy
- (B) Vitamin K deficiency
- (C) Von Willebrand's disease
- (D) Liver cirrhosis
- (E) Haemophilia A

95 A patient is tachypnoeic. Bloods results are as follows: Na
133 mmol/l, K 4.2 mmol/l, Cl 110 mmol/l, HCO₃ 12 mmol/l.
Which of the following is the most likely cause?
- (A) Morphine
- (B) Acetazolamide
- (C) Renal failure
- (D) Lactic acidosis
- (E) Frusemide

96 An 82-year-old man is admitted with pneumonia.
Examination of the neck reveals cervical lymphadenopathy.
He has hepatosplenomegaly. Full blood count shows WCC
42.8 × 10⁹/l, lymphocytes 33.2 × 10⁹/l, haemoglobin 10.6
g/dl, platelets 196 × 10⁹/l. Which of the following
underlying diseases is likely?
- (A) Myeloma
- (B) CLL
- (C) CML
- (D) Lung cancer
- (E) Rheumatoid arthritis

97 Which of the following statements about psoriasis is
correct?
- (A) Psoriasis rarely occurs in alcoholic patients
- (B) Most patients develop arthropathy of the hands
- (C) Characteristic plaque-like lesions develop on the flexural
surfaces
- (D) Guttate psoriasis is the most common type
- (E) Epidermal cell hyperplasia may be seen on skin biopsy

98 Which of the following is an example of type 3 hypersensitivity?

- ❑ (A) Goodpasture's syndrome
- ❑ (B) Myasthenia gravis
- ❑ (C) Pernicious anaemia
- ❑ (D) Rheumatoid arthritis
- ❑ (E) Rheumatic fever

99 Which of the following statements about the JVP is correct?

- ❑ (A) Cannon waves are a feature of TR
- ❑ (B) Large A waves are present in AF
- ❑ (C) Large V waves are present in tricuspid stenosis
- ❑ (D) Nodal rhythm causes cannon waves
- ❑ (E) Cardiac tamponade causes the JVP to fall on inspiration

100 Regarding immunodeficiency, which of the following statements is correct?

- ❑ (A) In common variable immunodeficiency the IgA is usually elevated
- ❑ (B) Patients with ataxia telangiectasia have a reduced incidence of malignancy
- ❑ (C) In Wiskott–Aldrich syndrome there are normal numbers of lymphocytes
- ❑ (D) Leukocyte adhesion deficiency typically presents with abscesses
- ❑ (E) Chronic granulomatous disease is characterised by low neutrophils

ANSWERS

1 **(E)** Alendronate can cause severe oesophagitis. Low-dose aspirin alone does not cause oesophagitis, but can cause gastritis or duodenitis. Nifedipine and isosorbide mononitrate can be used to treat diffuse oesophageal spasm. See page 133 for oesophagitis.

2 **(D)** This patient has achalasia (See page 134). Increased lower oesophageal sphincter pressure is typical, +/– abnormal peristalsis and dilatation above. Treatment for this includes oesophageal dilatation, botulinum toxin and surgery (Heller's myotomy).

3 **(A)** Whipple's disease typically causes malaise, arthropathy, malabsorption, and leads to villous atrophy. Other conditions cause diarrhoea but not arthropathy. See page 143 for Whipple's disease.

4 **(D)** Budd–Chiari causes exudative ascites, whereas the others typically cause transudative ascites. Serum albumin ascites gradient = serum albumin – ascitic fluid albumin. This is accurate for those with a low serum albumin in determining whether fluid is an exudate or a transudate. With a transudate gradient >11, exudate < 11.

5 **(E)** Hyperemesis can cause abnormal liver function tests and occurs in the first trimester. All others mentioned occur in the third trimester. See page 170 for liver disease in pregnancy.

6 **(B)** Probably azathioprine-induced pancreatitis. Small bowel obstruction would need to be considered in a patient with Crohn's, as strictures can develop. Gastroenteritis would not cause such severe abdominal pain. Toxic megacolon does not typically present with vomiting and abdominal pain, but presents with a severe flare-up of colitis and causes diarrhoea and abdominal pain, with evidence of a systemic inflammatory response.

7 **(C)** Low ferritin and folate suggests proximal small bowel disease, so duodenal biopsy should be the first investigation. 5% of patients with coeliac disease are endomysial antibody negative. Other tests could be considered later.

8 **(B)** MRCP – patient is likely to have PSC or microlithiasis. ERCP should not be used as a first-line test in the diagnosis of biliary disorders, as MRCP is much safer. Liver biopsy can be used to diagnose PSC but is more invasive.

9 **(A)** This patient has an unconjugated hyperbilirubinaemia. As the haemoglobin is near the upper limit of the normal range and reticulocytes are normal, haemolysis is unlikely. Gilbert's syndrome

is most likely. Rotor syndrome and Dubin–Johnson syndrome are causes of conjugated hyperbilirubinaemia.

10 **(C)** See page 156 for table about HBV serology.

11 **(D)** Blood pressure has a narrow pulse pressure, so aortic stenosis is most likely, which causes an ejection systolic murmur that radiates to the neck. AS presents with collapses. See page 13 for heart sounds.

12 **(D)** Sotalol and amiodarone can be used in the treatment of those with paroxysmal AF. As the patient is young and long-term side effects are fewer with sotalol, this should be used. Warfarin should not be given in view of the history of heavy alcohol intake. Digoxin does not prevent paroxysms of AF. The patient should be advised to reduce his alcohol intake, as this is the likely underlying cause.

13 **(A)** This patient has evidence of right ventricular hypertrophy. As she presents with a collapse and reduced exercise capacity multiple pulmonary emboli are the most likely cause.

14 **(C)** This patient is likely to have tricuspid endocarditis, and in IV drug users the most likely organism is *S. aureus*. See page 36 endocarditis

15 **(A)** Atenolol may be used in porphyria but the others can exacerbate it. See page 59 for drugs and porphyria.

16 **(B)** Adenosine will terminate most AVRIs or will slow the rate to show the underlying rhythm. If the patient has AF then digoxin or verapamil must not be used, as they can cause an extreme tachycardia.

17 **(D)** Ostium secundum ASD. Ostium primum ASD causes left axis deviation on the ECG. PDA cause a continuous murmur through systole and diastole. VSD causes a loud pansystolic murmur and would be unlikely to present at this age. Fallot's would not present at this age, or would have signs of correction.

18 **(B)** Hypertension and hypokalaemic alkalosis suggest Conn's syndrome, which can be diagnosed by serum renin and aldosterone. In the absence of protein or blood in the urine renal disease is unlikely.

19 **(A)** Erythromycin is an enzyme inhibitor so is most likely to be the cause of raised INR. Penicillins and doxycycline can cause an increase in the INR owing to the reduction in bacterial killing and reduction in vitamin K production from the gut. See page 51 for enzyme inducers and inhibitors.

20 **(E)** Tamoxifen increases the risk of thromboembolism. Patients with oestrogen receptor-positive disease should be offered treatment with tamoxifen or anastazole. Anastrazole has fewer menopausal symptoms than tamoxifen and is more effective at preventing recurrence; however, there is no difference in mortality. Tamoxifen should be continued for 5 years only, as it increases the risk of endometrial cancer. Hypercalcaemia may occur with tamoxifen. See pages 67, 71.

21 **(A)** Metformin is the first-line treatment for overweight type 2 diabetics who are not adequately controlled with diet.

22 **(B)** This patient has taken a salicylate OD. U waves suggest hypokalaemia. And there is a metabolic acidosis. Blood glucose is low. Theophylline causes hyperglycaemia but can cause all the other abnormalities. Amitriptyline reduces respiratory effort. See page 75 for salicylate OD.

23 **(B)** Patient is most likely to have sarcoidosis and CXR will show bilateral hilar lymphadenopathy. Skin biopsy will not be diagnostic of underlying cause. See page 412

24 **(D)** Psammoma bodies are a histological feature of papillary carcinoma of the thyroid. Hoarse voice suggests laryngeal nerve involvement. Anaplastic cancers can invade the larynx. Calcitonin is raised in medullary carcinoma of the thyroid. For thyroid cancer see page 105.

25 **(B)** See page 107 for diagnostic algorithm for Cushing's syndrome.

26 **(B)** Radioiodine is contraindicated in pregnancy. Propranolol is not recommended. Carbimazole leads to slow improvement in symptoms but can cause fetal hypothyroidism.

27 **(A)** Mucous membranes are often involved. High-dose steroids are effective. IgG antibodies are seen against the epidermis. Blisters are widespread and usually burst. See page 98 for pemphigus.

28 **(B)** Nearly all patients with MEN2 are thought to develop medullary carcinoma of the thyroid (MCT) and so should have prophylactic thyroidectomy to prevent this. Phaeochromocytoma is associated with MCT. Calcitonin is raised in MCT. Pituitary tumours, eg prolactinomas, are seen in MEN1. See page 110 for MEN and page 107 for thyroid cancers.

29 **(B)** This patient has Addison's disease (page 108), which can be diagnosed with a short synacthen test. Pigmentation, hypoglycaemia, hypotension, hyponatraemia and hyperkalaemia are features. Crisis can be precipitated in pregnancy or due to

intercurrent infection. Acute intermittent porphyria presents with abdominal pain, vomiting, confusion, hypertension and tachycardia.

30 **(B)** High C peptide and insulin are seen in insulinoma. Proinsulin is cleaved to produce insulin and C peptide, therefore endogenous insulin secretion raises the serum levels of C peptide also. Overdose of insulin will have high insulin but low C peptide, as insulin is exogenous. Phaeochromocytoma (raised urinary catecholamines) leads to hyperglycaemia. Raised cortisol and insulin antibodies would cause hyperglycaemia, not hypoglycaemia.

31 **(C)** Seizures, respiratory depression and arrhythmias and acidosis are features of TCA overdose. Arrhythmias should be treated with bicarbonate to correct the acidosis. See page 76 for TCA OD.

32 **(A)** This patient has neurofibromatosis type 2 (page 176); peripheral schwannomas are associated. Lisch nodules are seen in NF1. Ash leaf macules, subungal fibromas and adenoma sebum are seen in tuberous sclerosis.

33 **(A)** This patient has Turner's syndrome (page 180) and webbed neck is a feature. Rocker-bottom feet are seen in Edward's syndrome. Clinodactyly is seen in Down's syndrome.

34 **(B)** HIV is a retrovirus that has affinity for CD4 T-helper cells. Rotavirus is a reovirus. HIV is an RNA virus with reverse transcriptase and leads to depletion of CD4 cells. HIV1 is most common in the UK. HIV2 is common in West Africa. (See page 1)

35 **(C)** This patient has nephrotic syndrome, so 24-hour urine collection is required to quantify urine protein.

36 **(C)** This patient has hyponatraemia with a low serum and high urine osmolality suggestive of SIADH. Initial treatment is fluid restriction. (See page 280)

37 **(B)** This patient has Henoch–Schönlein purpura (page 445) and mesangial IgA deposition is typical, although crescents can be present.

38 **(C)** These features are typical of rhabdomyolysis. Very elevated serum CK with acute renal impairment is diagnostic. Urine dipstick will be positive for blood, but this is not specific. Urine myoglobin may be positive, but not in all cases. See page 295 for Rhabdomyolysis.

39 **(A)** Calcium gluconate should be given immediately to stabilise the cardiac membranes and reduce the risk of arrhythmia. Insulin and dextrose +/– salbutamol nebulisers should rapidly follow this to

lower the potassium. Calcium resonium is useful to slowly continue to lower the potassium when it is reduced below dangerous levels.

40 **(B)** Numerous eosinophils in the urine usually suggest interstitial nephritis secondary to a drug reaction.

41 **(A)** This is a picture of sepsis with ATN.

42 **(C)** This patient has diabetes insipidus because the serum osmolality is raised at the start of the test, indicating dehydration, and despite water deprivation the urine does not concentrate. The urine will concentrate after DDAVP, indicating there was a deficiency of ADH, so the diagnosis is cranial diabetes insipidus. See page 283 for water deprivation test.

43 **(C)** This is an anaphylactic reaction (type 1). Serum IgE is usually elevated. Serum IgE binds to mast cells, leading to release of histamine and other vasoactive substances. Antihistamines have some benefit by antagonising histamine, which is involved in the pathogenesis. Intramuscular not intravenous adrenaline is the treatment of choice.

44 **(A)** This patient has evidence of haemolysis and thrombophilia, which is typical of PNH. The others do not cause haemolysis but do cause thrombophilia. (See page 230)

45 **(E)** This patient has PCP (See page 5). The history is suggestive and chest X-ray findings would be consistent. Induced sputum for *Pneumocystis* is the first-line test. If this proved negative then bronchoscopy with BAL would be indicated.

46 **(D)** Propranolol is a good prophylactic treatment for migraine in those who have regular attacks. See page 328 for migraine.

47 **(D)** This patient has had a spinal stroke, which typically occurs from anterior spinal artery occlusion. Typical features are weakness with loss of pain and temperature (spinothalamic) but preserved vibration and joint position sense (posterior columns). See page 347.

48 **(A)** This patient has internuclear ophthalmoplegia (see page 353) caused by a lesion in the left medial longitudinal fasciculus. See page 353.

49 **(C)** Stevens–Johnson syndrome is a side effect of COX 2 inhibitors. COX 2 inhibitors increase the risk of cardiovascular death, so should not be used in patients with heart disease. COX 2 inhibitors have a reduced incidence of peptic ulceration, but it can still occur. COX 2s should be stopped in patients with active ulceration. COX 2 inhibitors have a similar incidence of renal failure as non-selective NSAIDs. Aspirin with COX 2s negates any

protective effect, so there is no benefit of using a COX 2 over a non-selective NSAID.

50 **(B)** Cauda equina syndrome (see page 348) presents with these signs and symptoms.

51 **(A)** MND does not cause sensory loss. Others cause sensory loss also.

52 **(A)** This patient has encephalitis. Patients present with seizures and reduced conscious level. HSV is the most common cause. HSV PCR on CSF is most likely to provide the diagnosis. Lymphocytic CSF can be seen in TB meningitis, but typically the glucose would be very low and the protein would be higher than 0.8 g/l. See page 333.

53 **(B)** The CSF biochemistry and microscopy are compatible with bacterial meningitis. Gram-negative diplococci in CSF suggests meningococcus. See page 367 for CSF results and page 332 for meningitis.

54 **(B)** This patient has lateral medullary syndrome caused by occlusion of the right posterior inferior cerebellar artery. See page 327 for features.

55 **(A)** Myotonic dystrophy causes small pupils and ptosis. Myasthenia cause ptosis but not small pupils. Third-nerve palsy and tropicamide cause large pupils. Pilocarpine causes small pupils but not ptosis. See page 350 for pupils.

56 **(A)** Retinal artery occlusion (page 375) causes a pale fundus, sometimes with a cherry red spot. An afferent pupillary defect is typical.

57 **(C)** Severe headache on one side and vomiting with evidence of a red eye suggests acute glaucoma. Urgent ophthalmology referral is required for ocular pressure measurement. (See page 379)

58 **(D)** Hypophosphataemia is common with alcohol withdrawal. Seizures and pyrexia and hallucinations are common. Antiepileptics are not indicated for withdrawal seizures, but patients should be treated with chlordiazepoxide or diazepam. Alcohol withdrawal, see page 388.

59 **(D)** Sulfasalazine is composed of 5ASA and sulfapyridine. which are cleaved by bacterial enzymes in the bowel. 5-ASA is not absorbed, but sulfapyridine is. 5-ASA is active in IBD, whereas sulfapyridine is active in rheumatoid disorders. Reversible azoospermia is a side effect. Patients with aspirin allergy will react to sulfasalazine. Black males are at risk of haemolysis owing to

G6PD deficiency, which is X linked. Acetylator status is important in the metabolism.

60 **(A)** *Staphylococcus aureus* is the most common organism in septic arthritis, especially with IV drug users. All the others do occur but are less common. *Haemophilus influenzae* is most common in <2-year-olds. See page 428 for organisms in septic arthritis.

61 **(E)** This patient has Reiter's syndrome (page 437). *Salmonella* is a cause.

62 **(D)** Hypomagnesaemia can be caused by ciclosporin and presents with tetany and causes prolonged QT interval on the ECG.

63 **(A)** This patient has limited systemic sclerosis (CREST), so anticentromere antibody is most likely to be present. See page 450 for autoantibodies and page 445 for systemic sclerosis.

64 **(B)** These features are typical of Kawasaki's disease. See page 453 Parvovirus B_{19} causes erythema infectiosum ('slapped cheek') and arthralgia. Scarlet fever (*Streptococcus pyogenes*) causes strawberry tongue and a diffuse macular rash. Scalded skin syndrome causes diffuse erythema with bullous desquamation over the body.

65 **(C)** Cryoglobulinaemia is associated with hepatitis C. These features are typical. See page 457 for cryoglobulinaemia.

66 **(B)** This patient has Guillain–Barré syndrome (see page 344). CSF protein is raised, but not WCC. Nerve conduction studies often show demyelination. Regular vital capacity should be measured, not peak flows. MRI spine is useful to rule out other causes, but is not the investigation of choice.

67 **(C)** This is Wegener's granulomatosis (page 454). Upper respiratory tract symptoms, pulmonary haemorrhage and renal failure are typical. cANCA (anti-PR3) is positive in 95% of cases.

68 **(E)** This young patient has evidence of severe chronic liver disease with some neurological symptoms. This is suggestive of Wilson's disease. Low alkaline phosphatase is typical. Low caeruloplasmin with Kayser–Fleisher rings is very suggestive. Diagnosis is made with high copper quantification on liver biopsy. (See page 272)

69 **(B)** This patient has acute intermittent porphyria. The abdominal pain is often very severe, requiring large doses of opiates. All the others can precipitate porphyria. The oral contraceptive is a common trigger for attacks. (See page 276)

70 **(A)** Familial hypercholesterolaemia is the most likely, as the

cholesterol is elevated but triglycerides are normal. All the others cause raised triglycerides. See page 265 for lipid disorders.

71 **(C)** *Clostridium difficile* is most likely. The white cell count is very raised, which is seen in *C. difficile* infections. MRSA enteritis is also a possible diagnosis but is less common than *C. difficile*. An increase in the WCC would not be seen in antibiotic-associated diarrhoea or overflow diarrhoea.

72 **(A)** Haemophilia A is most likely here. Factor V111:C levels are low and there is a prolonged APTT with normal bleeding time (prolonged in Von Willebrand's disease). This is suggestive of haemophilia A. PT would be prolonged in vitamin K deficiency or cirrhosis. Haemophilia B is Factor IX deficiency. (See page 208)

73 **(E)** This patient has a metabolic acidosis with high serum osmolality. The calculated osmolality is 2[130 + 4.0] + 6.0 + 6.0 = 280. The osmolar gap (measured serum osmolality – calculated serum osmolality) is 20, which suggests there is another osmotically active substance in the blood. The anion gap is 24 (high). Ethylene glycol is therefore the most likely cause. Patients typically present 'drunk', but there is no smell of alcohol. Ataxia, vomiting and convulsions follow. Salicylate overdose causes a high anion gap metabolic acidosis but does not alter osmolar gap. Amitriptyline causes metabolic acidosis but does not alter the osmolar gap, and other features are usually present, such as dilated pupils, dry mouth, urinary retention, arrythmias and seizures. Paraquat poisoning presents with burning of the mouth, vomiting, abdominal pain, and in severe cases pulmonary oedema, shock and convulsions. Digoxin causes confusion, vomiting, yellow vision, arrythmias, and in severe cases lactic acidosis. See page 74 for poisoning. See page 273 for acid–base balance and osmolar gap.

74 **(C)** This patient has Friedreich's ataxia. This is a trinucleotide repeat disorder, so the children of parents with the condition will have more severe disease. See pages 182, 349. The frataxin gene is responsible, which is autosomal recessive.

75 **(B)** This is hereditary angio-oedema. The oral contraceptive is a common trigger for symptoms. Typical presentation is with facial oedema, laryngeal oedema and abdominal pain (GI tract oedema). See page 229.

76 **(C)** Trimethoprim inhibits dihydrofolate reductase. Ciprofloxacin inhibits DNA gyrase. Penicillin inhibits transpeptidase. Isoniazid

inhibits cell wall synthesis. Erythromycin inhibits bacterial protein synthesis. See page 242 for antibiotics

77 **(E)** *E. coli* is the most common cause of UTI. All the others can cause UTI, but less frequently.

78 **(C)** Raised calcium with low phosphate is seen in hyperparathyroidism. Excessive vitamin D will not cause low phosphate. Renal failure causes hyperphosphataemia. Bone metastases do not cause low phosphate.

79 **(E)** This patient has falciparum malaria. The patient has a febrile illness with hepatosplenomegaly, anaemia and jaundice 14 days after leaving a malarial region. The confusion may suggest cerebral malaria, which has a high mortality and will rapidly progress to coma. See page 257 for malaria and other travel illnesses.

80 **(C)** Amoebic liver abscesses are more commonly seen in the right lobe. Daughter cysts are seen in hydatid liver cysts. Metronidazole and diloxanide (will eradicate luminal organisms) is the treatment of choice. Most patients present with RUQ pain and fever. US, CT, serology or aspiration of the cyst are the diagnostic tests of choice. See page 161 for amoebic liver abscess.

81 **(C)** Chancre is seen in primary syphilis, where VDRL and FTA will be positive. Gummas are seen in tertiary syphilis. The incubation period is 2–4 weeks. Generalised lymphadenopathy is a feature of secondary syphilis. See page 254 for syphilis.

82 **(B)** This is an exudate. Hypothyroidism causes a transudate. See page 423 for causes of pleural effusions.

83 **(D)** Paraquat poisoning, methotrexate and amiodarone can cause pulmonary fibrosis. Azathioprine is used to treat some cases of idiopathic pulmonary fibrosis. Carbamazepine may rarely cause pneumonitis.

84 **(A)** There is an association between Goopasture's syndrome and HLA DR2. Crescentic not focal segmental glomerulonephritis is typical of Goodpasture's. The anti-GBM antigen is type 4 collagen. Pulmonary haemorrhage is typical. Pulmonary haemorrhage is more common in smokers.

85 **(C)** This patient has the features *Mycoplasma* pneumonia (page 419), with SOB, headache, joint pain and erythema multiforme. Cold agglutinins may be present.

86 **(B)** Target cells are seen in thalassaemia. Helmet cells are seen in microangiopathic haemolytic anaemia. Howell–Jolly bodies are seen post splenectomy. Pencil cells are seen in iron deficiency. Burr

cells are seen in uraemia. Teardrop cells are seen in myelofibrosis. See page 200.

87 **(E)** Cavitating lung tumours are likely to be squamous cell. PTHrP is seen in squamous cell cancers. Voltage gated calcium channel antibodies suggest Eaton–Lambert syndrome, which is seen in small cell carcinoma. SIADH is common in small cell carcinoma. Hypertrophic pulmonary osteoarthropathy is seen in squamous cell carcinoma. See page 417 for lung cancer.

88 **(D)** This patient has symptoms of bronchiectasis (see page 404). High-resolution CT chest is the investigation of choice to make a diagnosis.

89 **(E)** This patient has a restrictive lung defect, so asbestosis is most likely. See page 396 for PFTs

90 **(A)** Skin necrosis can occur in patients with protein C deficiency who are started on warfarin. Protein C is dependent on vitamin K. Most patients with anticardiolipin antibody do not have SLE. Thrombocytopenia, thrombosis and recurrent miscarriage suggest antiphospholipid antibody syndrome. Factor V Leiden mutation is the most common inherited thrombophilic state.

91 **(D)** This patient has an exudative pleural effusion with a history suggestive of malignancy; thoracoscopy and biopsy is the best diagnostic investigation to be done here.

92 **(E)** Erythromycin does not cause haemolysis in G6PD deficiency (ciprofloxacin and nitrofurantoin do). Hereditary spherocytosis is AD. Methyldopa causes an immune-mediated haemolysis. Malaria causes haemolysis when parasites are released. Pyruvate kinase deficiency is a cause of haemolysis.

93 **(D)** Hodgkin's disease. Patients present with lymphadenopathy and B symptoms. Pain in lymph nodes after alcohol is suggestive of Hodgkin's disease. The others all cause lymphadenopathy and fever. (See page 205)

94 **(D)** This patient is most likely to have liver cirrhosis, as there is evidence of deranged clotting and reduced platelets, which are seen in cirrhosis. The others do not cause low platelet levels.

95 **(B)** This is metabolic acidosis with a normal ion gap. [133 + 4.2] – [110 + 12] = 15.2. Acetazolamide is a cause of this. Morphine causes a respiratory acidosis. Renal failure and lactic acidosis cause high ion gap metabolic acidosis. Frusemide causes hypochloraemic hypokalaemic metabolic alkalosis. See page 273 for acid–base balance.

96 **(B)** This patient has CLL. Bloods show lymphocytosis with mild anaemia. Lymphadenopathy and hepatosplenomegaly are typical examination findings. The pneumonia is precipitated by poor immune function as a consequence of the CLL. (See page 203)

97 **(E)** Epidermal hyperplasia is seen in psoriasis. Psoriasis commonly occurs in alcoholics. 10% develop arthropathy. The plaque-like lesions are on extensor surfaces. See page 81 and page 438 for dermatology and rheumatology.

98 **(D)** RA is an example of type 3 hypersensitivity. The others are type 2. See page 221.

99 **(D)** Large V waves (systolic) are typical of TR. A waves are absent in AF. Large A waves are seen in TS. In cardiac tamponade pericarditis the JVP may rise on inspiration (Kussmaul's sign). Cannon waves occur when there is RA contraction with a closed tricuspid valve. See page 12 for JVP.

100 **(C)** Common variable immunodeficiency leads to a reduction in all immunoglobulins. Patients with ataxia telangiectasia have an increased incidence of malignancy. In leukocyte adhesion deficiency pus cannot be formed effectively as leukocytes cannot leave the circulation. In Wiskott–Aldrich syndrome there are normal numbers of lymphocytes but signalling between lymphocytes is defective. In chronic granulomatous disease neutrophils are present in normal numbers but lack NADP oxidase, and so are unable to produce highly reactive oxygen species to kill micro-organisms. See page 226.

Index